Cooperative Veterinary Care

Cooperative Veterinary Care

Second Edition

Monique Feyrecilde

WILEY Blackwell

Published by John Wiley & Sons, Inc., Hoboken, New Jersey.
Published simultaneously in Canada.

For general information on our other products and services or for technical support, please contact our Customer Care Department within the United States at (800) 762-2974, outside the United States at (317) 572-3993 or fax (317) 572-4002.

Wiley also publishes its books in a variety of electronic formats. Some content that appears in print may not be available in electronic formats. For more information about Wiley products, visit our web site at www.wiley.com.

Library of Congress Cataloging-in-Publication Data is applied for:

Paperback ISBN: 9781394163595

Cover Design: Wiley
Cover Image: @Monique Feyrecilde

Set in 9.5/12.5pt STIXTwoText by Straive, Chennai, India

SKY10068810_030524

Contents

Preface

Thank you for taking the time and energy to care about the emotional and behavioral lives of pets. Veterinary care and husbandry, home medical care, and grooming are a necessary and important part of the life of every animal. By making space for the emotional welfare of the animal while focusing on providing high-quality veterinary care and husbandry, we can achieve *Cooperative Veterinary Care*.

Cooperative Care can be a series of complex behaviors, but it is limited neither to fancy trained behaviors nor to entirely voluntary and choice-based interactions. Cooperative Care is based in the understanding of how animals learn, how we can create the best possible experiences for them, and how our interactions in the present will inform the pet's decision-making process in the future.

I know some of the information in this book will be outdated even before the publishing process is complete! In a way, I find that very encouraging because it highlights the ever-growing community interest in *Cooperative Veterinary Care*. Innovation, exploration, and creativity abound. I welcome the contributions of my colleagues, clients, and the pet professional community as a whole in working to better the lives of our animal companions.

My hope is to bring to you a unique blend of my high-level clinical experience and a sophisticated understanding of learning and training to help my readers achieve their goals and have fun at the same time.

Happy training,
Monique Feyrecilde

Acknowledgments

I would like to thank my team at Mercer Island Veterinary Clinic for their ongoing support and desire to treat every patient and client with compassion. With your teamwork, my passion became our mission. Every patient, every day benefits from these methods and our desire to treat patients with gentleness and respect.

Thank you to Dr. Micah Brodsky for believing in me, for nurturing my ambitions, and for your friendship. Thank you to my wonderful friends for supporting me and this project, and my loyal clients for trusting and allowing me to care for their beloved family members. Thank you, my colleagues and mentors, for elevating the art of veterinary medicine to include the science of learning and behavior.

Thank you to Sophia Yin for all your support and encouragement. You are missed and remembered with great love and respect.

Thank you the entire team at Fear Free Pets for embracing change for the better and helping spread the word about Cooperative Veterinary Care.

Most importantly, thank you to my loving and patient husband, Salamandir, without whose support this project would not have been possible. My deepest debt of gratitude is to the animals, who are my most eloquent teachers and among my most treasured companions.

Monique Feyrecilde

About the Companion Website

This book is accompanied by a companion website:

www.wiley.com/go/feyrecilde/cooperative

There, you will find valuable material designed to enhance your learning, including:

- Videos showing procedures described in the book
- Puppy class syllabus
- Puppy Level One homework
- Patient Evaluation and Training Plan Worksheets
- Marketing and Client Education Materials
- Details of Stimulus Control
- Images

The videos are clearly signposted throughout the book. Look out for 👁.

1

Introduction to Patient Centered Veterinary Care

1.1   First, Do No Harm

1.1.1   Veterinary Technician's Oath

I solemnly dedicate myself to aiding animals and society by providing excellent care and services for animals, **by alleviating animal suffering**, and promoting public health. I accept my obligations to practice my profession conscientiously and with sensitivity, adhering to the profession's Code of Ethics, and furthering my knowledge and competence through a commitment to lifelong learning.

1.1.2   Veterinarian's Oath

I solemnly swear to use my scientific knowledge and skills for the benefit of society through the protection of animal health and **welfare, the prevention and relief of animal suffering**, the conservation of animal resources, the promotion of public health, and the advancement of medical knowledge.

First, do no harm. While these four words do not appear in the oaths, this short sentence certainly describes our mission as health care professionals. Our oath to prevent, relieve, and alleviate animal suffering and the oath's implication of doing no harm apply to both physical and mental or emotional suffering and illnesses of the body. Stress and fear are subjectively harmful and unpleasant on their own, but their physiologic effects of increased heart rate, respiratory rate, blood pressure, temperature, blood glucose levels, cortisol levels, and so many more clearly hold the potential for harm as well.

Recognition and treatment of stress and fear in veterinary patients is not a new concept, and the progress over recent years within our industry is admirable. Dr. Sophia Yin was a pioneer in this field, and the concepts highlighted in her work are still timely and relevant today. She brought the idea of low-stress veterinary care to the mainstream. Fear Free℠ has continued this work, providing visibility as well as educational content and certifications. A variety of organizations now offer education and even titling and award programs for pet owners in Cooperative Care. We owe thanks to these people and so many more who have come before us and walked beside us, supporting and contributing to this text which will continue the work of improving veterinary care for patients, clients, and the entire veterinary team. This guide will help the veterinary team take low-stress, compassionate, patient-centered handling to the next level. Creating a care model

Cooperative Veterinary Care, Second Edition. Monique Feyrecilde.
© 2024 John Wiley & Sons, Inc. Published 2024 by John Wiley & Sons, Inc.
Companion website: www.wiley.com/go/feyrecilde/cooperative

prioritizing patient welfare, developing training programs for fearful patients, and embracing the techniques used by progressive zoos and aquariums in their husbandry training programs will all be taught in this guide.

We deserve to take great care of ourselves as well. Veterinary professionals are at high risk for burnout, compassion fatigue, depression, and suicide [1]. Turnover in the veterinary profession is common, with technicians in particular citing burnout. Experiencing stress and potential emotional harm when we are trying to make patients healthy can take a serious toll on veterinary professionals. By using methods that allow patients to relax and cooperate for care, we can make it easier to fulfil our vocation of relieving and preventing animal suffering while keeping our own emotional and mental wellness.

1.2 Stress, Fear, and the Veterinary Clinic

Stress is how the body reacts to a challenge, or stressor. The stress response allows the body to be prepared and respond when necessary. Not every stress response is linked to fear, but in the veterinary setting that is often the case. The fear response is a mechanism that prompts an animal to flee, fight, hide, or react in another helpful way to defend its own safety and well-being. **Fear** and **anxiety** can be provoked by either real or *perceived* threats, or stressors. These stressors and potential threats are abundant in the veterinary setting. How an individual animal responds to specific events or stressors is unique to each pet, and can change over time with learning history – for better, or for worse.

While the stress of veterinary visits can provoke avoidance, hiding, and defensive aggression, stress and fear can also induce the state of learned helplessness [2]. **Learned helplessness** is a state where an animal (or person) learns that avoidance, escape attempts, or other responses to something unpleasant or threatening are ineffective, and eventually gives up attempts to escape [2]. In pets, this often looks like the pet is "a statue," "frozen," or "stoic." Learned helplessness can mask important findings on physical examination like changes in range of motion, pain in the abdomen, or other findings that rely on patient responses. Conversely, animals who are defensively **aggressive** because of fear may react by vocalizing, snapping, or moving away during examination. This response may be difficult to discern from a pain response, making diagnosis and treatment more challenging. Fear and stress impact blood test results, vital signs, cause changes in gastrointestinal and urinary signs, and more. Minimizing fear improves the validity of diagnostic processes. Every animal in our care deserves our empathy and respect. Each time the pet visits our office and has a negative experience, the fear will potentially worsen. This learned fear of the veterinary hospital is much easier to prevent than it is to reverse.

Preventing fear in the veterinary office isn't just about stopping the problems associated with fear; it is also about reaping the great benefits of working with patients who are less anxious. Patients who are comfortable and less anxious will allow more complete physical examination; allow better positioning for tests; have more accurate parameters, such as blood pressure, heart rate, temperature, and respirations; have more accurate lab results; and enjoy visits much more. Wouldn't it be wonderful to see patients who are happy to see you? We think so, too!

1.3 Freedom, Wants, and Needs

Dr. Temple Grandin is a world-renown expert in animal behavior and animal welfare. In her book *Animals Make Us Human*, she discusses what are called "The Five Freedoms" in animal care,

Table 1.1   The Five Freedoms.

Freedom from hunger and thirst
Freedom from discomfort
Freedom from pain, injury, or disease
Freedom to express normal behavior
Freedom from fear and distress

originally developed by Dr. Roger Brambell in 1965 (Table 1.1) [3]. When we cause fear and anxiety in our patients while we are trying to care for them, we are infringing on their freedom from environmental discomfort, freedom from anxiety and distress, and freedom to express normal behaviors. One of the first steps in restoring these freedoms is identifying the difference between wants and needs in the veterinary office.

Animal welfare is a crucial factor in animal care, and The Five Freedoms were developed by Roger Brambell and popularized by Temple Grandin.

To protect freedom from anxiety for our patients, we recommend setting up guidelines for assessing animals during procedures. We will discuss assessment tools throughout the book including a three-level system and the Fear Free Fear Anxiety and Stress (FAS) Scale. Patients should be observed and evaluated throughout treatment and handling to determine if it is appropriate to continue, or if a procedure should be paused. One guideline for when to stop a procedure involving restraint is to use the 2-2-3 rule. If it requires more than two arms to gently stabilize the patient, if a dog struggles for more than two seconds, or if a cat struggles for more than three seconds, pause the procedure, assess the patient and the situation, and then make a plan for how to best continue. Further guidelines and more detail will be presented in later chapters.

Determining when to perform a procedure relies on identifying the difference between wants and needs. **Needs** are urgent, life-saving treatments. **Wants** *are everything else*. While we may not want to pause or postpone some procedures, pause, retry, or postpone is always an option for wants. By keeping our priorities clear about wants versus needs, we can avoid causing unnecessary harm, and do our very best to keep the stress and fear levels as low as possible for our patients. Keeping fear levels low helps to protect our patients from emotional harm.

1.4   Iatrogenic Behavioral Injury

Iatrogenic means an illness or injury *caused* by medical treatment. Iatrogenic behavioral injury (IBI) is a term to describe mental, emotional, and/or psychological harm caused to patients while we are trying to provide veterinary care. Preventing IBI is one of our responsibilities as veterinary professionals. There are many modalities we can use to prevent IBI, including: recognizing the risks of IBI; using the human pediatric model for many treatments [4, 5]; embracing early and frequent medical intervention for fear, anxiety, and stress; and using **low-restraint** and **no-restraint veterinary care.**

The pediatric health care model has changed considerably over the past 20 years. A new emphasis has been placed on the importance of reducing stress for children and parents during medical care. Some techniques used in the pediatric model include explaining procedures to children using words and pictures prior to treatment, bringing comfort items such as a blanket or favorite toy from home, playing music clinically established to have a calming effect, allowing children to sit in a parent's lap and be held or hugged, using distraction techniques, practicing good caregiver continuity, and helping children to cope with pain levels [5]. Medication is given when needed for anxiety or fear, and ongoing research is investigating effective calming methods for children in medical settings. While we can't mirror all of these techniques in veterinary medicine due to the communication barrier between people and pets, we can certainly make use of the concepts to improve patient care.

Veterinary medicine will benefit from the experiences of pediatricians by implementing similar stress-relieving strategies. By explaining a treatment to a child, the doctor or nurse is telling the child what to expect and providing an opportunity for predictability and trust. The veterinary equivalent of this method is "explaining" procedures to pets by using touching and training techniques that help the pet understand what is expected, what to anticipate, and how to **cooperate**. We can allow pets to remain with their owners for many procedures and coach owners on how to remain safe and helpful during visits. Receptionists can instruct owners to bring a mat or bed, favorite treats or toys, and a hungry patient to each visit. Animal handling staff can become proficient in **distraction techniques** and training methods to reduce animal stress and promote cooperation. We can use medicines and supplements to mitigate fear and stress. For animals who need repeated treatments, we can help them cope by establishing a consent protocol for treatment, instructing the animals how to cooperate, and even sometimes teaching them to look forward to treatments.

It is the author's opinion that three components will promote the biggest improvement in patient welfare in the veterinary setting: veterinary professionals having a clear understanding of how animals learn, owner presence during examination and treatments (and observation from afar if hazard regulations prohibit presence), and the use of medication and sedation early and often. Working with animals with the owner present allows owners to see precisely what happens between person and pet, and opens the conversation when training and/or medical relief of fear, stress, and anxiety are needed. Allowing pets to remain with their owners does not mean expecting owners to assume the role of a veterinary professional. Owner presence can be done safely and has numerous potential benefits. When the owner is present, veterinary professionals are less likely to resort to "brutacaine" (strong physical restraint rather than appropriate medications) and excessive physical force to accomplish medical care. Furthermore, it helps clients bond with the practice and trust that we have their pet's best interests, both physical and emotional, at heart. Clients can learn how to participate in treatments when appropriate, and how to successfully performed prescribed treatments such as giving pills, ear medicine, eye medicine, injections, grooming and nail care, and much more at home.

1.5 Focusing on Welfare Rather than Animal Restraint

We will never be able to explain to our animal patients the important protection a vaccine provides, why an antibiotic is needed, what x-rays are for, or any of the other treatments we perform. In veterinary medicine, we have a history of being procedure focused. We tend to make a treatment plan and execute it, with the goal being skilled physical restraint for rapid completion of the procedure. Historically, the education provided was limited to how to perform a procedure without staff injury. Imagine you are sick and need to give a blood sample. You are on vacation and become ill, you must go to the hospital. You do not speak the language of the health care provider. You have never given blood before. The provider points to a chair with padded armrests. You sit and the provider reaches for your arm, pulls it out, and uses straps to secure your arm to the armrest.

Figure 1.1   Relaxed dog accepting food in the exam room.

When you are slow to comply or try to pull your arm away the provider says something to you in a language you don't understand. They place a tourniquet and poke your arm two or three times before getting a blood sample. This is an example of **procedure-centered treatment**. What might you feel during this encounter? Would your heart race and respiratory rate increase? Do you notice the pain of the needle more? Perhaps you experience fear, confusion, or the desire to escape the straps. How do you feel about the provider, the chair, the environment in general? This happens with veterinary patients regularly. They do not have the ability to understand what we are trying to do, nor why. Physical restraint is often unfamiliar to pets, and only paired with uncomfortable moments or potentially painful procedures. Look at the body language of the dog in Figures 1.1 and 1.2. Restraint alone causes a significant change in this dog's body language. Notice the ears pulled back, leaning away, and stiffness the animal shows in response to the restraint without any medical procedures being performed. By focusing more on **patient-centered treatment**, and less on the procedure, we can enhance care and well-being.

Working with animals comes with a risk of injury to the veterinary team and to the animals. We can decrease that risk and increase safety for both the team and our patients by skilfully applying methods which rely more on understanding the patient than on applying strong physical control or restraint. Skilful and effective restraint is an important part of what veterinary technicians should know for procedures which are *immediate needs* to save the life of a patient. For all other handling, a deep understanding of the alternatives to strong restraint will keep veterinary team members and animals safe. This author has almost 30 years of experience working full-time in veterinary medicine, and has sustained only three animal bites, with only one of those occurring during an actual interaction between the author and the animal. In the other two cases, the bite occurred without the author approaching the animal. The reason I have included this information is to highlight the fact these methods can indeed be applied safely. But they must be part of a larger vision of animal and human safety to be successful.

Animals use **body language** and body position to communicate with us. Animals can tell us if they are comfortable, **conflicted**, fearful, and anxious, all without any vocalizations or

Figure 1.2 The same dog shown in Figure 1.1 when restraint is applied. Note the change in body language.

aggression. Violence is a biologically costly strategy: it comes with risk of harm for the aggressor. Most animals will exhaust nonviolent means of communication before resorting to defensive aggression [2]. The exception is when animals have been scolded or ignored for nonviolent means of communication. When an animal feels its safety is threatened, the first response most animals use is the flight response: running away from the threat. When we remove the animal's opportunity to leave a threatening situation, we limit their available responses to **freeze** or **fight**. In the veterinary setting, we can become accustomed to ignoring nonviolent communication. When we ignore these important signs, we put ourselves at risk for injury, and the animals at risk for IBI as well.

When we move very close to an animal for manual restraint, we lose the ability to objectively observe the animal's responses and body language. We also send a series of potentially stressful messages to that animal. Research shows that using force when training dogs, such as attempting an **alpha roll** where the dog is forcibly placed on its side or back, can lead to aggression [6]. Placing an animal into **lateral recumbency** or **dorsal recumbency** can similarly provoke aggression. These dogs are not "bad" or "mean"; they are simply responding in a way that is normal for some dogs. When we are working with an animal in sternal recumbency or standing, and we "hug" them to provide restraint, what message does the hug actually send? The word *hug* may hold a positive connotation for humans, but for dogs, hugging is not a natural form of communication. Even for humans, only some people like hugs, and very few like hugs from strangers. If one dog grasps another around the middle, this is usually displacement, ritualistic conflict behavior, or sexually motivated [7]. It is easy to understand why a hug from a stranger at the veterinary clinic may not seem friendly, and may provoke avoidance or aggression.

There is no such thing as an unprovoked bite in the veterinary hospital. The simple act of bringing an animal into this environment is provocation in itself. It is easy to miss subtle signals in the hospital environment. When we are too close to the animal, we may not see all the signs. Restraint can mask warning signs as well. If the animal is leashed or held, the ability to flee is removed, which

Figure 1.3 Chloe, a young puppy, displays avoidance behaviors when asked to target the technician trainer's hand.

masks attempts at communication. Removing the option of flight is provocation. Animals who try to get away are warning us about possible future aggression. Animals who freeze, move away, turn to the side, yawn, look away, purse their lips, flatten their ears, vocalize, advance–retreat, snap, and more are all asking us to stop what we are doing. Chloe, the dog in Figure 1.3, is asking the trainer to move away and communicating she is uncomfortable with what she is being asked to do. If we ignore these requests, we run the risk of provoking the animal into self-defense.

Excessive restraint carries physical risks for the veterinary team, including bites and scratches, sprains and strains, and more. There are emotional risks to the veterinary team as well. When our mission, our vocation, is to relieve animal suffering, and we are constantly causing fear and distress in animals while we are trying to heal their bodies, it can take a significant emotional toll. Turnover in the veterinary profession is high [8]. Many technicians and veterinarians leave the profession after a short time, while others experience depression and compassion fatigue. Suicide rates among veterinary professionals are staggering [1]. Reducing patient stress may help protect us from these types of emotional harm.

In **Video 1.1,** the beagle Chloe is expressing anxiety by approaching and retreating. She will come to take food and will make contact with the technician, but immediately backs away between interactions. This backing-away behavior shows the internal conflict this dog is experiencing. She is very anxious, but has not yet escalated to threat displays or defensive aggression. The shepherd mix Max shows a similar pattern of approach–retreat and is conflicted, but he is also vocalizing and lunging, so some would describe him as more aggressive. Both of these patients are doing their best to communicate their discomfort and anxiety by leaving the situation. If we ignore these non-violent signals, and muzzle and heavily restrain these dogs, we are teaching them that nonviolent communication is ineffective. The dogs will learn the veterinary clinic is a place where subtle signals are ignored, and there is a real risk these dogs will escalate to biting in the future. We don't have to use heavy restraint as our primary tool for these patients. We can work with them and even train them to cooperate in their own health care.

Table 1.2 Steps for planning treatment.

Pause, assess, prioritize, proceed: steps for planning treatment
(1) Before treatment or if a treatment is paused: assess patient and plan
(2) Assess whether the planned treatment is a want or a need
(3) Prioritize needs first, then wants
(4) Prioritize wants in order of medical importance
(5) Evaluate the animal's stress level, and the anticipated response to the procedure
(6) Assess if medical therapy for fear, stress, anxiety, pain, etc. is indicated
(7) Make a training or handling plan to help the animal cooperate with as little fear and stress as possible
(8) Proceed with treatment in a fashion that considers the emotional welfare of the animal

If a patient is showing signs of stress or fear, remember to pause, assess the patient and the plan, prioritize, and proceed while observing the patient closely.

When working with little or no restraint, we will find some animals are unable to allow treatment. They may move away, they may never let us approach them, or they may become defensively aggressive. When an animal can't tolerate treatment, the veterinary team needs to have a plan of action. Table 1.2 provides a quick reference.

(1) Pause treatment, and assess the patient and the plan.

(2) Assess whether the planned treatment is a want or a need. If the treatment is truly a need, it is life-saving treatment. There are very few situations like this in veterinary practice. A few examples include Gastric Dilation and Volvulus (**GDV**) in distress, emergency **dystocia**, animals in severe **shock**, serious traumatic injury with significant active bleeding or respiratory compromise, or the animal is at immediate risk for severe self-harm.

(3) Prioritize needs first, then wants.

(4) Prioritize wants in order of medical importance.

(5) Evaluate the animal's stress level, and the anticipated response to the procedure.

(6) Assess if medical therapy for fear, stress, anxiety, pain, etc. is indicated.

(7) Make a **training plan** or handling plan to help the animal cooperate with as little fear and stress as possible.

(8) Proceed with treatment in a fashion that considers the emotional welfare of the animal.

Change is never easy, but it is also often extremely rewarding. This guide will give you the knowledge you need to understand how animals **perceive** their environments, how they communicate, and how they learn. You will learn how to assess a patient, how to tell when to stop a treatment, the steps for making a training plan appropriate for each patient, and assessment of the patient's response to training. Some training plans discussed may take only a few seconds, while others require several visits and compliance from the owner at home. We will also give you the tools you need to help introduce and promote change in clinic culture toward compassionate **cooperative care**. Methods for working with the veterinary team and for approaching topics of concern with clients will be discussed. The animals can be our very best teachers if we allow them, and the rewards associated with a move toward patient-centered practice for both pets and people are worth the effort.

References

1 Skipper, G. and Williams, J. (2012). Failure to acknowledge high suicide risk among veterinarians. *Journal of Veterinary Medical Education* 39 (1): 79–82.

2 Overall, K. (2013). *Clinical Behavioral Medicine for Small Animals*, 2e. St. Louis, MO: Mosby.

3 Grandin, T. and Johnson, C. (2009). *Animals Make Us Human: Creating the Best Life for Animals*. Boston: Houghton Mifflin Harcourt.

4 Kain, Z., Mayes, L.C., Caldwell, A.A. et al. (2006). Preoperative anxiety, postoperative pain, and behavioral recovery in young children undergoing surgery. *Pediatrics* 118 (2): 651–658.

5 Visintainer, M. and Wolfer, J. (1975). Psychological preparation for surgical pediatric patients: the effect on children's and parents' stress responses and adjustment. *Pediatrics* 56 (2): 187–202.

6 Herron, M., Shofer, F., and Reisner, I. (2009). Survey of the use and outcome of confrontational and non-confrontational training methods in client-owned dogs showing undesired behaviors. *Applied Animal Behaviour Science* 117 (1–2): 47–54.

7 Handelman, B. (2009). *Canine Behavior: A Photo Illustrated Handbook*. Spokane, WA: Direct Book Service.

8 Welborn, L., Brunt, J., Coffey, M. et al. (2013). 2013 U.S. Veterinary Workforce Study: Modeling capacity utilization. In: *Report for the American Veterinary Medical Association*. State University of New York: The Center for Health Workforce Studies.

2

Perception and Communication

2.1 Sensation and Perception

Sensation is the way we gather information about the environment around us. Think of sensations as the raw data collected by our sensory organs before the data is translated into meaningful information in the brain. When the sensory data travels to the brain via the nervous system, the brain processes this data into how we think, feel, and react to our environment: our perceptions [1]. One example is hearing. Sound waves enter the ear canal. The waves cause movement within the eardrum and middle ear, and eventually reach the **cochlea**. The waves then encounter the auditory nerve, which transmits the sound signal to the brain. The brain translates this raw sensory data into meaningful information, such as music or speech.

Pets, like people, have a variety of sensory organs. Their senses include vision, hearing, smell, touch, and taste. Animals can also sense **pheromones** using a specialized organ called the **vomeronasal organ (VNO)**, which is part of the **olfactory** system (Figure 2.1). Humans have a VNO as well, but experts disagree about whether humans communicate using pheromones in the same way animals have been confirmed to do. We will discuss sensation and perception in dogs and cats, to help us understand why animals may react in certain ways and make the decisions they do about their environment, particularly the veterinary environment. Dogs and cats have evolved specialized sensation and perception mechanisms.

Sensation and perception are how animals learn about the environment and develop feelings, opinions, and skills. Understanding how animals interact with the sensory environment, and especially noting individual variation, can significantly improve interactions between veterinary professionals and patients. Trying to understand the environment and experience from the animal's perspective is relevant to our work. Providing spaces, interactions, and experiences tailored to what pets most likely perceive will decrease stress and enhance safety for everyone involved.

2.1.1 Vision

Vision contains many separate components, each of which contributes to the total experience of sight [2]. These components include color, acuity (sharpness), brightness (luminosity), **depth perception** or depth sensation, and motion sensitivity. How an animal sees their environment depends upon the anatomy and placement of the eye, and how the brain processes visual data. Humans have a visual field of about 190–240°, with 120° of binocular overlap in the center, where both eyes can access the same visual data, combining the images to assess depth of field [1]. Table 2.1 shows differences between human, dog, and cat vision.

Cooperative Veterinary Care, Second Edition. Monique Feyrecilde.
© 2024 John Wiley & Sons, Inc. Published 2024 by John Wiley & Sons, Inc.
Companion website: www.wiley.com/go/feyrecilde/cooperative

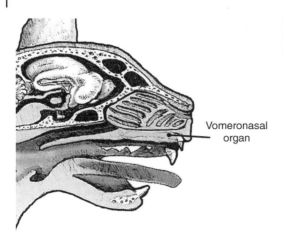

Figure 2.1 The vomeronasal organ location in the domestic cat. This organ is used to detect pheromones.

Vomeronasal organ

Table 2.1 Sensation: vision: a summary of human, canine, and feline visual sensations.

Species	Detail acuity	Color	Field of vision	Light receptors
Feline	20/100–20/200	90% fewer receptors than humans	200 – 295° total 130° binocular	High
Canine	20/80	Bichromatic blue-yellow emphasis	240° total 40 – 120° binocular	Moderate
Human	20/20	Trichromatic	190 – 240° total 120° binocular	Low

2.1.1.1 Canine Vision

How the eyes are placed in the head determines how much overlap there is between what each eye sees. Humans have forward-facing eyes and a 120° field of **binocular vision**, where what the left and right eyes see overlaps to allow depth perception and perspective. Dogs have a field of vision of about 250°, but only 40–120° of **binocular overlap**, depending upon breed and conformation of eye placement. For breeds with the eyes closer together (e.g. Pug), there is greater overlap, resulting in a broader binocular overlap and better depth perception but less peripheral vision. For breeds where the eyes are further apart (e.g. Greyhound), there is less binocular overlap but improved peripheral vision. In general, dogs have broader peripheral vision than humans [2].

Color is **bichromatic** for dogs. Many pet owners believe dogs see in black and white, but they actually do see in limited color. Based upon the distribution of cones in the dog's eye, they are thought to see the blue and yellow portions of the color spectrum best, with other colors lacking good differentiation [3]. When you see a dog's eyes shining at night, this effect is caused by light reflecting off of the **tapetum lucidum**. The tapetum lucidum and the number of **rods** dogs have, give them improved vision in low-light situations. This is an excellent adaptation for hunting, but not helpful for reading. Because of the ratio of rods to nerve fibers, dogs have decreased visual acuity for fine detail, and their vision is more focused on movement and contrast. Their vision is best in close-up situations. We would consider dogs to have 20/80 vision, while humans have 20/20 visual acuity.

In the veterinary setting, if we want to draw a dog's attention to an item like a mat, station, or target, choosing something blue or yellow in color, and placing it on a contrasting background, may help: for example, a yellow or white spoon or a blue plate to deliver treats. Conversely, items we do not wish to draw attention to should be low-contrast and in other colors. When moving ourselves or items around a dog, we can move smoothly and steadily, so as not to trigger a motion-activated overreaction. To draw extra attention to something like a piece of food or a toy, tossing the item so it has added movement, and choosing something of a contrasting color, can improve the dog's awareness of the item. For instance, tossing white cheese bits onto a dark-colored floor, or rolling a dark ball across a white floor, will make these clearer for dogs.

2.1.1.2 Cat Vision

Cats have a visual field of about 200–295°, with up to 130° of binocular overlap, depending upon the source cited [4]. Their peripheral vision field is similar to that of dogs. Like dogs, cats have less visual acuity for detail, and more focus on movement and contrast. They also have a diminished spectrum for color vision compared with humans. Based on the distribution and variety of cones present in the eye, cats are thought to see few colors. Having only about 10 percent of the color receptors that are present in the human eye, cats certainly see less differentiation in color than humans do, and based upon research findings, color seems to hold little importance for cats [3]. Like many other animals, cats have a tapetum lucidum that all primates lack, assisting with low-light vision. Even more than dogs, cats excel in low-light situations. Cats would be described as having 20/100 to 20/200 vision acuity if we attempted to classify it in human terms [4].

As when working with dogs, items that may be alarming to cats should be similar to the background in color, while targets, stations, feeding mats, and toys are best in high contrast. Toys and treats that move around and are high contrast will better draw a cat's attention as well, such as a white spoon or tongue depressor to give food against a darker mat or towel.

Figure 2.2 shows a simulation of the differences in color vision in a common clinic scenario: the exam room. Figure 2.3 demonstrates the comparison between visual fields in humans, dogs, and cats. Figure 2.4 shows a variety of dogs with different eye positions. Consider the impact these eye positions may have on the individual dog's overall field of view, and which areas have best depth perception.

2.1.2 Hearing

Hearing sensitivity or strength is generally defined in terms of what **frequencies** an animal can hear, and how broad the audible frequency range is. The frequencies heard depend upon the anatomy of the ear, which also changes over time. Humans can hear frequencies in the range of 20–20,000 kHz. Most human speech falls between 1000 and 5000 Hz. As humans age, our ability to hear higher frequencies diminishes. The fine hairs within the ear become stiffer, and the aqueous material in the cochlea thickens. This makes our hearing less acute and sensitive with age. Animals experience similar age-related changes. Like some humans, some animals may be born with changes in hearing or deafness, or may develop these problems prematurely [5]. Table 2.2 shows a hearing comparison between species.

2.1.2.1 Dog Hearing

Dogs hear a considerably larger frequency range than humans, at 67–45,000 Hz. The frequencies heard best by dogs are around 4000 Hz, which is well within the comfortable range of human hearing [5]. The ultrasonic scalers used in dentistry emit frequencies between 15 and 39,000 Hz. Think about how different your clinic may sound to a dog.

Figure 2.2 Color vision. Color vision based on anatomy of the eye. Top left: human view. Top right: what we believe dogs see. Bottom: what we think cats see.

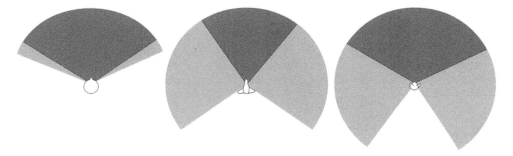

Figure 2.3 Field of vision. From left to right, human, dog, and cat field of vision. The darker shaded area is seen with both eyes (binocular overlap where depth perception is possible), while the lighter shaded areas are peripheral vision fields for each individual eye.

Figure 2.4 Comparison of canine eye set and head shape. Different head shapes and distances between the eyes, as well as where the eye is positioned on the head, will impact the dog's visual field.

Table 2.2 Sensation: hearing: a summary of human, canine, and feline auditory sensations.

Species	Frequencies (Hz)	Common sounds at this frequency
Feline	55–79,000	Piano's low a note: 55 Hz Bat echolocation: 50,000–100,000 Hz
Canine	67–45,000	Lowest cello note: 68 Hz Ultrasonic dental scaler: 18,000–45,000 Hz
Human	20–20,000	Lowest pipe organ note: 20 Hz Speech: 1000–5000 Hz

Figure 2.5 Equipment that may sound different or startling to animals in the veterinary clinic. Clippers, ultrasonic dental scalers, and x-ray machinery are a few examples.

2.1.2.2 Cat Hearing

Cats hear a considerably larger set of frequencies than even dogs, at 55–79,000 Hz [5]. While they may not be able to hear an elephant's long-range call at 21 Hz, they can hear everything happening inside our hospital. Cats can even hear the lower ranges of bat echolocation, which can span 50,000–100,000 Hz and is completely inaudible to humans.

Think about things in the hospital that may sound different to our patients (Figure 2.5).

2.1.3 Olfaction and Pheromones

Olfaction, or sense of smell, is our ability to sense and perceive odors in the environment. For humans, these smells are detected when molecules of volatile (floating) compounds reach a special area of nerve endings high inside the nose, which is about the size of a postage stamp and contains about 5 million olfactory receptors of 450 different types. Once the odor reaches the olfactory receptor, a chemical signal is sent to the nearby olfactory bulb in the brain. Humans can differentiate about 10,000 different odors, and some of the most noxious odors can be detected in very small quantities, such as one drop in a swimming pool of water! However, most odors are not so easily detected.

Pheromones are detected by the VNO. While humans have a VNO and also secrete pheromones, experts do not agree on whether pheromones are useful for intentional social signaling as an adaptation in humans. There is some evidence suggesting that stress-related pheromones trigger an enhanced startle reflex in humans, which may support subconscious pheromone communication.

2.1.3.1 Dog Olfaction and Pheromones

Dogs are the experts of olfaction. Their olfactory sensors cover a large part of the surface area of the nasal epithelium. Dogs have a staggering 220 million olfactory receptors in the nose, of about 900 different varieties [6]. Once the odor molecule reaches the receptors within the nose, signals are sent to a comparatively large olfactory bulb, and often the signal must traverse a tiny distance of only one neuron before perception can begin in the brain. Their nostrils can be used to direct and intensify certain odors, and sniffing is done intentionally to obtain olfactory information.

Pheromones are also used extensively by dogs [6]. Pheromones are secreted in association with estrus, pregnancy, lactation, fear, excitement, sexual maturity, health status, and more. When a dog is fearful, it may secrete pheromones associated with fear, and those pheromones can be detected by the next dog who is in that part of the hospital. Pheromone signals can trigger a fear response as the VNO is linked with the **limbic system**. The limbic system is a portion of the brain responsible for emotion, olfaction, long-term memory, and linking emotion with sensation. Synthetic pheromone products simulate the pheromone that mother dogs secrete when they are lactating, which is thought to calm the puppies. Using pheromone products in the hospital may help dogs to relax in this environment.

2.1.3.2 Cat Olfaction and Pheromones

Cats have considerably more olfactory receptors than humans: 150–200 million of at least 500 different varieties [6]. The have a similar percentage of their nasal epithelium containing odor receptors as dogs, and spend a similar amount of time investigating odor in their environments.

Cats also use pheromones extensively, to gather and give information about sexual and reproductive status, age, health, territory, and social cues. Pet owners are most familiar with the use of cheek and chin glands to secrete pheromones during rubbing or bunting, and glands on the paws used during clawing or scratching behaviors. Cats do secrete pheromones associated with emotional status as well, and these messages are left behind in your hospital by each cat who visits for the next feline inhabitant. Synthetic products to mirror pheromones in cats, such as Feliway® (facial pheromone) and Feliway Multicat® (mammary pheromone), can help cats relax in the veterinary setting [7]. When cats (and some other animals) are sensing pheromone information, they may display the *flehmen response*, a characteristic facial expression with the upper lip retracted and mouth slightly open.

2.1.3.3 Touch

The human body is covered in nerve endings that collect sensory information about touch. Receptors for pressure, contact, vibration, hair movement, heat, cold, pain, position in space, and more are all part of the sense of touch. When a touch receptor encounters a stimulus, a series of signals are sent to the brain for interpretation into a perception of the touch. How dense the nerve endings are in a certain area of the body, and how much of the brain is dedicated to interpreting that data, dictates how "sensitive" that area is to touch. For example, fingertips are very high resolution, packed with 2500 sensors per square centimeter, while the middle of the back may have as few as 500 [8]. As you would expect, the parts of the body used for manipulation, exploration, expression, and escape have the highest concentration of touch receptors in both people and animals.

Perception of touch is complex in humans and in animals. For example, if we touch someone who is ticklish under the arm with a feather, the person is likely to react strongly. Touching another subject who is not ticklish in the same way may elicit no response at all, or just a puzzled expression. These two people may have differences in sensation, perception, or both, which shape their responses. Animals are similar in their individuality.

2.1.3.4 Dog and Cat Touch

The distribution of touch receptors in dogs and cats seems to be similar to that of humans, with the lips, face, feet, and genitals all being quite sensitive. In addition, dogs and cats are special: their vibrissae, or whiskers, give them added sensitivity. These special sensory hairs are located around the face and front feet, and can trigger a strong response when touched or triggered [9].

When touching dogs and cats, many times the collar can be pulled tight, the paws grabbed, or the lips or face touched when an owner is applying punitive action or when the animal is being restrained or examined in the veterinary hospital. These sensitive areas require special consideration from the veterinary team, understanding how an animal may be startled or frightened by sudden touches. For both dogs and cats, starting touch in a less sensitive area and gliding to a more sensitive area can help the animal's nervous system acclimate to the type of touch required. Figures 2.6 and 2.7 show areas where the sense of touch is more intense shaded in darker colors, whereas regions with lesser density of nerve endings are lighter in color.

Figure 2.6 Sensitivity to touch in dogs. Darker shaded areas are often more sensitive for most patients, while lighter shaded areas are less sensitive.

Figure 2.7 Sensitivity to touch in cats. Darker shaded areas are often more sensitive for most patients, while lighter shaded areas are less sensitive.

2.1.4 Taste

Sense of taste is one area in which humans are the winners! While taste and olfaction are closely linked when it comes to determining if a flavor is pleasurable, humans distinguish at least five aspects of taste. Individual taste buds are responsible for detecting sweet, sour, salty, bitter, and savory. Humans have between 4000 and 9000 taste buds of different types located on the tongue, in the oral cavity, and in the nasal cavity. Each taste bud contains 10–50 individual receptors [8]. Taste information travels from these receptors to the brain via the facial nerves.

2.1.4.1 Dog and Cat Taste

Both dogs and cats have considerably fewer taste buds than humans, with dogs averaging 1700 and cats around 500. Their nerves also seem to process taste considerably differently than human nerves do. Because dogs and cats cannot talk, we must again rely on anatomic data and extrapolation to imagine what their sense of taste is probably like.

Studies of the facial nerve, nerve receptors, and brain activity when specific chemicals are offered suggest dogs and cats have the most receptors for sweet and savory. They also have many receptors for bitter, but these receptors are located far back on the tongue where plentiful ingestion or chewing is required. Dogs have more sweet receptors, while cats seem not to respond when the sweet chemical is given. Both cats and dogs have an inhibited response to salts when these chemicals are provided [10].

When providing foods in the hospital, providing sweet, fatty, and meat-flavored foods generally works best for most dogs and cats. Because olfaction is an important part of taste for pets as well as people, heating foods to increase odor can improve palatability and interest. Food is not the only thing we provide in the veterinary hospital that may trigger a taste response: medicines are important, too. Masking bitter medicines, or encasing them in a capsule so the animal does not encounter the bitter item, can be helpful.

2.1.4.2 Individual Variations: Nature and Nurture

Animals, like people, will have individual variations that may be **intrinsic** to the animal or learned through experience. It is important to note individual variations, whether they are natural or learned, to best serve every single patient. Some Basset hounds may resist nail trims, because their limb and foot conformation influences how that touch feels. Himalayans with a reduced visual field may startle more easily when approached from behind. Brachycephalic dogs and cats may resist traditional oral examination because it occludes the nares when the lips are lifted.

When a certain sensation predicts a specific experience, learned aversions can occur. When the odor of ear cleanser predicts a wrestling match followed by touching of a painful infected ear, the smell alone may become **aversive** even before any attempt to touch the animal. When the smell or taste of a specific cat food predicts nausea in a patient with renal failure, that smell or taste may become aversive in the future. When the sight of nail clippers predict touching of the foot and an accidentally painful experience if a quick is cut, nail clippers alone may cause the animal to anticipate a sensation of pain. (Refer to Chapter 3 for more information on classical conditioning.)

2.2 Stress and Fear

Many times when we think of stress or fear, we think of these as bad things. The negative emotions that come to mind when we remember being afraid or being stressed out can make us think stress or fear are always harmful. In reality, stress and fear exist to keep us out of harm's way. The stress response is a combination of instinct, **genetic predisposition**, and learning history. When we are faced with a threat, the sensory organs see, hear, smell, feel, and so on a certain stimulus or group of stimuli. The emotional part of the brain, the **amygdala**, sends a fear message to the hypothalamus, which is like the choreographer of the brain. The **hypothalamus** triggers the sympathetic nervous system to respond, and **adrenaline** is released. The adrenaline release leads to an increase in heart rate, blood pressure, and respiratory rate and capacity, and a release of a bolus of glucose for instantly available energy. In this newly heightened state, we are ready to fight or flee in response to a threat. This response happens extremely rapidly. In humans, the stress response can take less than 0.3 seconds! [11] If the perceived threat remains present after the initial stress response, **cortisol** levels are increased and the body remains ready to react in a state of heightened awareness and stress. If the perceived threat is lessened, the **parasympathetic nervous system** moves into action, calming everything down, and helping the body to relax [11].

This stress and fear response helps keep us safe, and it does the same for animals. Without the stress response, we would be unable to respond to immediate threats such as a knife being dropped while cooking, an oncoming car, or a fire alarm. Fear is an important default response, necessary for safety and survival. Especially in the wild, animals benefit from the fear response when it is appropriate. This adaptive trait is helpful, but can become a problem in certain situations.

Puppies and kittens who do not have the benefit of helpful genetic predispositions and positive **socialization** experiences during youth may never learn to be unafraid in new environments, meeting new people, being exposed to new sounds and surfaces, understanding different kinds of handling, and so much more. These stimuli may trigger the stress response even when the threat is not real. Stress and the fear response are coded in to be the default response when presented with "things" or "experiences" they did not learn were positive and harmless when they were young [6, 7]. Furthermore, some animals are genetically predisposed to be more fearful than others. Animals who are predisposed toward a strong fear response are at risk for increased unwanted behaviors at home, and increased handling and veterinary care problems as well [6]. These pets have an intensified feeling of fear in certain situations, which can be maladaptive and harmful to their emotional well-being over time. While careful and intentional socialization, training, and behavior modification can be of considerable help to such animals, we must remember that every pet is an individual and there is no simple single recipe for making novelty and handling experiences pleasant for every pet. Each pet must be observed and evaluated continuously for the best result.

When the fear response is triggered, most animals will try to flee (Figure 2.8). Fighting, as mentioned in Chapter 1, is biologically expensive, so most animals will not choose to fight as the first line of defense. If flight is not helpful in alleviating the perceived threat, the animal may feel no choice but to fight. There are a number of ways that the flight response may fail, particularly in the veterinary setting. Sometimes, the animal is in a confined space or wearing a leash. Other times, the animal may have learned that in the past, attempting to flee was not successful and only the fight response stops the threat from becoming worse. In any case, both flight and fight are methods of self-defense that exist to keep animals safe in the presence of a perceived threat.

Preventing fear in the veterinary office is paramount to providing patient-centered care using minimal restraint and intervention. One of the best services that hospitals can provide to prevent fear is positive socialization visits and classes for puppies and kittens, where puppies and kittens have the opportunity to visit the veterinary hospital and learn that the smells, sights, sounds, touches, tastes, and pheromones of the veterinary hospital are nonthreatening and actually predict good things like treats and favorite toys. Qualified team members can lead classes or offer happy

Figure 2.8 Flight response. This dog is fleeing from a fear-provoking stimulus (trainer).

visits, so puppies and kittens can practice skills like walking through the clinic, getting treats on the scale, going into the examination room, entering and exiting the cat carrier, and mock physical examinations. Team members can work together with pet owners to set up pleasant expectations about veterinary visits, handling, grooming, and general husbandry. These lessons can transfer in a meaningful way to the client's home relationship with the animal as well, helping to improve the bond between people and pets through good experiences surrounding necessary care for good health and comfort.

2.3 Body Language

Body language is the primary language our animal patients have to communicate with us. Becoming experts in body language can help us better understand our patients, recognize signs of stress and fear early, respond quickly to reduce fear in the veterinary setting, and prevent forming a learned response that can work against us in the future. The purpose of this guide is to help veterinary professionals understand the body language of relaxation as well as mild, moderate, and severe stress using a few key indicators. The guide provided will apply to a vast majority of patients, but individual variation can create animals who are more complicated to categorize. Learning history, differences in sensation or perception, physical illness or compromise, owner perception and communication, and what treatments are attempted will all affect how an individual responds in a given situation.

As we discuss body language, we need to remember that individual breed characteristics influence body language, and contextual cues are crucial to properly interpret body language cues. Some breeds are at a communication disadvantage because of structure. For example, Pugs, or Shar Pei have altered their expressions because of brachycephaly and excessive facial folds. A Pug with eyes that are bulging and showing the whites can be normal, but this would be a notable sign in any German shepherd dog. Basset hounds, Bloodhounds, and Scottish folds will have less ability to communicate using their ears because of ear size or shape. Breed differences in normal body posture also exist. Greyhounds holding the ears flat to the head can be normal, but a Corgi doing so is more likely to be fearful. A tail held low and loose between the hocks is normal for a Border collie or a Sheltie, but a low tucked tail for a Labrador or Golden retriever is likely a sign of fear.

Context and the total picture of the animal are very important for accurate interpretation of body language. For example, the author owns dogs of multiple breeds who fold their ears during walks. All of these dogs are eager to go for walks, and the rest of the body remains loose and relaxed during the walk. The ears alone are not enough information to interpret how the dog is feeling about going for a walk. The entire animal as well as the situation must be considered when making determinations about body language. No animal can be understood by observing a single body part.

Metacommunication is important, too. Metacommunication is the combination of signals, especially in sequence, to give context to what could be an ambiguous cue. For example, if a dog growls at another dog, growling alone is not complete information. If the dog first plays bowed before growling and moving in a staccato motion away, the growl is likely part of a play invitation sequence. Alternately, a dog who growls after moving away and slinking with a low tail and head is likely showing fear and distance-increasing behaviors [9]. A cat who crouches, wiggles the rump, and then claws or bites is probably engaging in a play or play-predation sequence. A cat who crouches, leans away, flattens the ears, and then claws or bites is showing fear and self-defense. A growl or bite alone is not useful information: metacommunication helps clarify signals [9].

In an attempt to make this guide easy to read, we will try to use consistent terminology throughout our discussions about evaluating an animal's emotional state, and choosing appropriate training levels for the state of the animal. There is no single consensus on exactly how to categorize body language and emotional states in animals. Common terms used include *appeasement*, *conflict*, *calming signals*, and *aggression*. Experts agree that conflict, appeasement, and calming signals are often prompted by the fear response [9]. This guide will use the following terms to describe and categorize fear and stress in veterinary patients:

- Relaxed or calm
- Mild stress (shows calming signals and/or appeasement behaviors)
- Moderate stress (shows conflict behaviors and/or avoidance)
- Severe stress (shows conflict behaviors, aggression, and/or learned helplessness).

We will describe in detail how to assess stress levels for each canine patient. Table 2.3 provides a summary that may serve as a quick reference guide.

2.3.1 Evaluation Tools

Several body language evaluation tools have been developed to assess a pet's emotional state based on observed body language signs. In this book, we will use the terms Relaxed, Mild stress, Moderate stress, and Severe stress. We will also refer to the Fear Free[sm] FAS Score.

Fear Free Pets provides education and professional certifications for veterinary professionals, trainers, shelter teams, groomers, pet sitters, boarding and daycare professionals, and more future programs are planned. Fear Free[sm] developed an evaluation tool called the **FAS Score**. FAS is the abbreviation for **F**ear, **A**nxiety, and **S**tress. The FAS Score is determined by observing the body language of the animal and categorizing it using a numeric value from 0 to 5. The benefit of this tool

Table 2.3 Canine body language: comparison of body language indications connected with different emotional states in dogs.

Emotional state	Proximity	Food acceptance	Body	Face	Tail
Relaxed	Approaches willingly Remains close Solicits attention	Readily accepts food Takes food gently	Front approach Side approach Soft muscles Hair lies flat	Normal pupils Soft eyes Relaxed ears Relaxed lips	Neutral Slightly elevated Wagging softly
Mild stress	Approaches willingly Remains close May lean away when touched	Readily accepts food May take food quickly or roughly during touching May or may not stop eating during procedures	Front approach Side approach Mild tension when touched Relaxed muscles when not touched	Normal pupils Pinched expression Forehead wrinkles Ears slightly pulled to the side or back Looks away when approached Closed mouth Lips relaxed	Neutral Slightly tucked Slightly raised Wagging with mild tension when touched Relaxed wag when owner touches
Moderate stress	May approach for treats Withdraws when food is not offered Leans or moves away when touched Prefers to stay near owner	May take treats Takes treats roughly Retreats after taking treats May refuse treats	Side approach if any Shaking off Panting Lips pulled back Dilated pupils Wide eyes Scratching Other displacement	Pupils dilated Eyes widened Whites of eyes may show Ears flat or pulled back	May wag with tension Tucked
Severe stress	Will not approach Hiding Attempts escape	Refuses most food Rarely accepts high-value food If accepts food, rapidly retreats	Exaggerated movement (fast or slow) Possible piloerection Freeze Vocalize Snap Bite Learned helplessness	Tight muscles Hard eye Dilated pupils Squinting Whites of eyes visible Looks away Stares	If wagging, stiff high wag Tucked tightly

and the corresponding numeric scoring is to standardize evaluation and descriptions of patients across multiple providers. The FAS Score can also be recorded in the patient's medical record, much as a pain score would also be recorded.

The FAS Spectrum illustrates and describes the body language signs observed for each FAS level. Spectrums are species-specific. Figure 2.9 shows the FAS Spectrum for dogs, and Figure 2.10 is the FAS Spectrum for cats. FAS 0–1 corresponds with relaxed. FAS 1–2 corresponds with mild stress. FAS 2–3 corresponds with moderate stress. FAS 4–5 corresponds with severe stress. Patients should always be evaluated continuously, and it's important to understand FAS Scores will fluctuate throughout an encounter with a patient. For example, a patient may be relaxed for pulse measurement with an FAS score of 0, and show severe stress with attempted nail care with an FAS score of 5. Emotional states and their corresponding scores are fluid and will sometimes change rapidly. Careful continuous observation improves safety for both the animal and the caregiver.

2.3.2 Dog Body Language

2.3.2.1 Relaxed or Calm, Dog (FAS 0–1)
2.3.2.1.1 *Overall Impression, Proximity, and Food Acceptance*
To read signs of stress through body language, we first must know what "calm and relaxed" looks like. When interpreting body language, first observe the whole body. Where is the animal in relation to you? Keeping the leash loose or opening carrier doors so the dog can move in the space gives the first clue in his comfort level. A relaxed dog will approach, and be willing to remain in close proximity to the team member without retreating rapidly or leaning backward. The relaxed dog will face the team member, and will approach forward or showing the side of the body. He may solicit attention. If he normally likes food treats or toys, he will accept them from the team member. Because the muscles are relaxed, the dog will take food gently or with some excitement, but will not bite hard. A dog with a relaxed body will sometimes lean against you, and will not feel stiff. He may get slightly more still when touched, but immediately soften again. The muscles should feel loose and soft under the skin rather than tense. The haircoat should be flat or in its normal position.

The relaxed dog will usually feel comfortable exploring the room. He is likely interested in investigating his surroundings without being hypervigilant. **Displacement behaviors** (Table 2.4) are absent, and the general impression should make the people in the room feel calm as well.

Training Tip: Normal Vital Signs

Interpreting respiratory rate, pulse, and temperature readings in stressed animals means knowing what normal is.

Canine	Feline
Temperature: 100 – 102.5 °F	Temperature: 100 – 102.5 °F
Pulse: Puppies 160–200	Pulse: Kittens 220–260
>6 wk 60–140	>6 wk 140–220
Smaller dogs higher	
than larger dogs	
Respirations: 10–35 bpm	Respirations: 20–30 bpm

THE SPECTRUM OF FEAR, ANXIETY & STRESS

RED: SEVERE SIGNS - FIGHT/AGGRESSION (FAS 5)
• Offensive aggression: lunging forward, ears forward, tail up, hair may be up on the shoulders, rump, and tail, showing only the front teeth, lip pucker - lips pulled forward, tongue tight and thin, pupils possibly dilated or constricted.

• Defensive aggression: hair may be up on the back and rump, dilated pupils, direct eye contact, showing all teeth including molars, body crouched and retreating, tail tucked, ears back.

RED: SEVERE SIGNS - FLIGHT/FREEZE/FRET (FAS 4)
• Flight: ears back, tail tucked, actively trying to escape - slinking away or running, mouth closed or excessive panting - tongue tight instead of loose out of mouth, showing whites of eyes, brow furrowed, pupils dilated.

• Freeze/Fret: tonic immobility, pupils dilated, increased respiratory rate, trembling, tense closed mouth, ears back, tail tucked, body hunched.

YELLOW: MODERATE SIGNS (FAS 3)
• Similar to FAS 2 but turning head away, may refuse treats for brief moments or take treats roughly, may be hesitant to interact but not completely avoiding interaction.

YELLOW: MODERATE SIGNS (FAS 2)
• Ears slightly back or to the side, tail down but not necessarily completely tucked, furrowed brow, slow movements or unable to settle, fidgeting, attention seeking to owner, panting with a tighter mouth, moderate pupil dilation.

GREEN: MILD/SUBTLE SIGNS (FAS 1)
• Lip licking, avoids eye contact, turns head away without moving away, lifts paw, partially dilated pupils, slight panting but commissures of lips are relaxed.

GREEN: ALERT/EXCITED/ANXIOUS? (FAS 0-1)
• Tail up higher, looking directly, mouth closed, eyes more intense, more pupil dilation, brow tense, hair may be just slightly up on the back and tail, may be expectant and excited or highly aroused.

GREEN: PERKED/INTERESTED/ANXIOUS? (FAS 0-1)
• Looking directly but not intensely, tail up slightly, mouth open slightly but loose lips, ears perked forward, slight pupil dilation.

GREEN: RELAXED (FAS 0)
A: Sleeping.
B: Neutral - ears in neutral position, not perked forward, brow soft, eyes soft, mouth closed but lips relaxed, body loose, tail carriage neutral, pupils normal dilation.
C: Friendly greeting - slow back and forth tail and butt wag, ears just slightly back, relaxed brow and eyes, may have mouth slightly open with relaxed lips and loose tongue.

FEAR FREE
HAPPY HOMES
Helping pets live happy, healthy, full lives

FEAR FREE
Taking the pet out of petrified

www.fearfreehappyhomes.com

Figure 2.9 The Fear Free[sm] Spectrum of Fear, Anxiety and Stress for dogs. Courtesy of Fear Free Pets.

THE SPECTRUM OF FEAR, ANXIETY & STRESS

RED: SEVERE SIGNS - FIGHT/AGGRESSION (FAS 5)

• Offensive aggression: pupils constricted or dilated, cat leaning forward, ears forward, moving forward, whiskers forward, tail is an inverted L (first inch of tail is horizontal with ground then the tail drops down), rump raised higher than front (on tip toes), staring, may be growling.

• Defensive aggression: ears back, pupils dialted, hunkered down, tail tight or tucked or tail thrashing, whiskers back, hissing, lips pulled back, staring, furrowed brow, could be swatting.

RED: SEVERE SIGNS - FLIGHT/FREEZE/FRET (FAS 4)

• Flight: actively trying to escape, pupils dilated, ears back, whiskers back, tail down and bottle brushed, fleeing, turning to look at stimulus.

• Freeze/Fret tonic immobility, dilated pupils, body flattened and tense, tail tucked, increased respiratory rate, ears back, staring, whiskers back.

YELLOW: MODERATE SIGNS (FAS 2-3)

• Ears further to the side, more pupil dilation but not completely dilated, increase in respiratory rate, brow furrowed, looking at stimulus instead of looking away, tail tight to body, possible tip of tail moving some, whiskers back. body crouched and leaning away.

GREEN: MILD/SUBTLE SIGNS (FAS 1)

• Avoids eye contact, turns head away without moving away, partially dilated pupils, head held just slightly down, slight brow furrowing, whiskers slightly back,ears partially to the side, body shifted slightly away, tail closer to body with possibly some slight flicking.

GREEN: PERKED/INTERESTED/ANXIOUS (FAS 0-1)

• Looking directly but not intensely, tail up and winding, mouth closed with loose lips, ears perked forward, whiskers forward, slight pupil dilation.

GREEN: RELAXED (FAS 0)

A: Sleeping.
B: Neutral - ears in neutral position, brow soft, eyes soft, mouth closed with relaxed lips, body loose, tail carriage U-shaped, pupils norm al dilation.
C: Friendly greeting - tail up and winding, may elevate rear end slightly by standing on toes, ears neutral, forward, or slightly back, might have squinty eyes, brow relaxed, might cheek mark or rub on person or object.

(A) (B) (C)

FEAR FREE
HAPPY
H❀MES

FEAR FREE

www.fearfreehappyhomes.com

Figure 2.10 The Fear Free[sm] Spectrum of Fear, Anxiety and Stress for cats. Courtesy of Fear Free Pets.

Table 2.4 Displacement behaviors: examples of behaviors that may communicate anxiety and discomfort when they occur in any context other than the appropriate one listed.

Possible displacement behavior	Appropriate context for this behavior
Shake off	Dog is wet
Yawn	Dog is tired and relaxed
Lick lips	Hungry, food is offered
Scratching	Itchy
Sniffing	Attractive odor present; dog is relaxed
Sneezing	Mechanical or chemical irritant
Grooming	Relaxed dog cleaning himself
Play signals	Relaxed dog inviting play at an appropriate time

Face The face of a relaxed or calm dog will have relaxed facial muscles. When the face is relaxed, the eye will be neutral. Neutral eyes are not bugged out and appear soft. The whites around the eyes should not show (unless they always do as a result of conformation). The pupils should be an appropriate size for the ambient light. The dog should be willing to look at the team member, or at least at their treats. Due to relaxed muscles, ears should be in a neutral position for the breed. Ears that are typically held upright should be in that position and not turned toward the sides or laying against the back of the head. Some dogs will flatten the ears when petted on the head, but remain relaxed. Floppy ears should seem forward and relaxed as shown in Figure 2.11.

A relaxed mouth is typically held softly closed or open a little. The lips seem soft and loose because the muscles of the face and neck are relaxed. The relaxed dog will not be panting unless he has been exercising or the temperature warrants panting to cool down.

(a) (b)

Figure 2.11 (a and b) Two relaxed canine patients.

Tail As we know from working with so many dogs, not every wagging tail is a happy tail. A relaxed dog has a loose wag with the muscles of the tail appearing relaxed. The tail should have some wave or flexibility, and sometimes will appear to "wag the dog" rather than the other way around. Some breeds will hold the tail loose and low when they are relaxed. Many dogs are missing a tail, and so this piece of information will be absent in those cases.

Relaxed Body: Video 2.1 Notice the body language of the puppy in this video. She is accepting food, seeking attention, and does not move away when touched. Her tail is relaxed and wagging softly, her muscles are relaxed and the overall impression is that her body is calm. The video is intentionally silent to encourage you to watch the body language signals the dog presents.

Excited, No Distress The excited dog who is not in distress, but is not calm, may be happy to see the team and eager to greet them. The dog may be pulling toward team members, jumping up, whining, barking with a high-pitched voice, and seeking attention. Often these dogs will convert to relaxed and calm body language when their social needs have been met. If the dogs do not become more calm and relaxed after the initial greeting, look for other signs that may indicate mild stress.

2.3.2.2 Mild Stress, Dog (FAS 1–2)

Dogs experiencing mild stress will generally show stress signals during interaction with the veterinary team and handling events, but will rapidly return to their baseline, more relaxed state when treatments are stopped. These changes can be quick and subtle.

Mildly stressed dogs will often show appeasement or displacement gestures. The body language of appeasement is meant to de-escalate stressful situations and communicate a signal of "no threat," or tolerance but discomfiture. Displacement behaviors seem completely out of context. For example, when the veterinary team member tries to touch the dog, he may return to his owner and offer a known action such as sit or lie down.

Body language such as raising a paw or placing a paw on the owner, leaning on the owner, licking of the chin or face of the veterinary professional, flicking the tongue, lip licking, turning away and sniffing, and yawning are all thought to be de-escalation responses to stress (conflict, appeasement). Several of these gestures, such as licking the face and leaning or pawing at the owner, can be misinterpreted as affection. In some cases, licking of the face can be a learned behavior to prompt a human to lean or look away. It is important to consider context: is the animal in a potentially stressful situation? Then the signal is probably a gesture of appeasement. For example, if a dog is turning and sniffing the ground when we attempt to touch him, he is probably stressed. If he turns and sniffs the ground where he found a piece of hot dog a few minutes ago, he could be investigating the environment. Context helps us understand behavior.

2.3.2.2.1 Overall Impression, Proximity, and Food Acceptance

A mildly fearful dog will approach willingly and usually look relaxed until you start to handle him. He may or may not explore the room. He will often allow petting, but may lean or walk away sometimes. He will usually approach facing you or with his side to you. He may lean away when petting is attempted, or stay near for petting with a single hand then retreat if a second hand is added. Once handling or procedures begin, stress markers may increase, but in most cases the dog will still accept food and remain nearby to receive it. Mildly fearful dogs will often remain interested in a distraction of delicious treats during handling or a procedure, but the dog will take the food more quickly or slightly more roughly during the procedure. The dog may also stop eating for brief periods during handling, then return to the treats between touches. When touched, the muscles

(a)   (b)

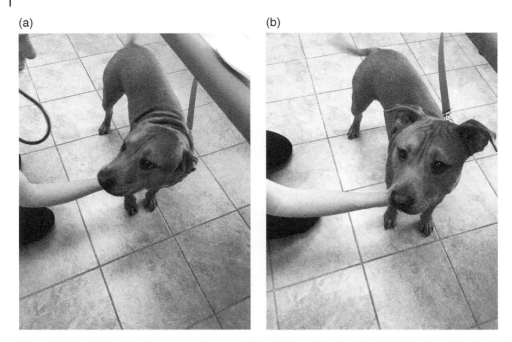

Figure 2.12 (a) The dog is nervous about touching. (b) Touching is paired with food, and the dog is visibly more relaxed.

have some tension, and the skin may crawl in an exaggerated **panniculus** response when touched lightly. The haircoat should be lying flat or in its normal position.

Face Mild stress will cause tension in the facial muscles. The eye may seem pinched, with a small forehead wrinkle. The ears may be pulled to the side or slightly back but not flat. If the ears are normally erect, they may point sideways or be laid back. The pupils may be normal size or slightly **dilated**, and the **sclera** (whites of the eyes) are unlikely to be showing. The mildly stressed dog will often look away from the veterinary team member, and frequently look at the owner.

Figure 2.12 shows a dog being touched by the veterinarian, and then being touched by the veterinarian while a treat is offered. The first picture shows taut facial muscles with the ears pulled slightly back. The dog is averting his gaze, avoiding eye contact. The second picture shows more relaxation in the facial muscles, and the ears are more relaxed. The dog will now make eye contact with the technician as well.

Tail The tail should be held in a neutral position for the breed. Tension through the muscles of the back and tail can cause the tail to be tucked tightly under the dog, or raised somewhat and wagged with mild tension. The tail will change based on what is being done. If the dog is being touched by a veterinary professional, it will probably drop or tuck slightly, and when the touching stops or the owner interacts with the dog, loose wagging or a neutral tail position is expected. Figure 2.13 shows two mildly stressed dogs.

 Canine Mild Stress: Video 2.2 Watch the dog in this video. He is interested in treats, interested in interacting, and chooses to approach Monique on his own. When handling is attempted, he shows a mild change in his body language: leaning away, walking away briefly, and turning to look

(a)

(b)

Figure 2.13 (a and b) Two mildly stressed dogs.

at the syringe, but after handling he immediately returns to his baseline behavior. The video is intentionally silent to encourage you to watch the body language signals the dog presents.

2.3.2.3 Moderate Stress, Dog (FAS 3)

Moderately stressed dogs may show any of the signals of a mildly stressed dog, plus additional displacement, conflict, and avoidance behaviors. Conflict behaviors are usually distance-increasing signals. The dog is asking for more space and for the threat to cease, but is not yet showing signs of overt aggression. When experiencing moderate stress, the dog may be of two minds, not sure how to respond. This indecisiveness is shown through body language: a mixture of signals will be observed. In general, moderately fearful dogs take longer to return to their baseline behavior after stressful experiences, and may not look relaxed while in the hospital at all.

2.3.2.3.1 *Overall Impression, Proximity, and Food Acceptance*

Moderately fearful dogs will often approach the veterinary team member for treats, but will repeatedly withdraw in between taking the food. These dogs may approach quickly (the "snake bite" for treats) or slowly, but they rarely choose to stay near the veterinary team member even when food is obviously available. A dog may stretch his neck way out to reach the food while keeping all his body weight away from the perceived threat so he can escape quickly. This can look like a middle ground between "fight" and "flight." Sometimes the dog is willing to try to approach, and then he may become overwhelmed and need to rapidly retreat. The dog will usually keep an eye on team members rather than turning to the side or away.

Very high-value food can sometimes have a masking effect on moderate stress. It is important to observe how a dog is taking food, and not just whether or not he is eating. To use a human example, we can discuss fear of spiders. If we take a large realistic toy spider and ask a friend who is fearful to touch it, she may refuse entirely, or touch it quickly. If we tape a $50 bill to the spider, she may approach more quickly and stay long enough to take the money, but will then back away again. When we ask our friend, "How do you feel about spiders now?" she will probably respond that spiders are just as scary as ever, but thanks for the $50. Just because she accepted the money, this did not diminish her overall fear.

Moderately stressed dogs may show displacement behaviors. Displaced behavior is out of context for what you would expect given the animal's emotional state. Examples include shaking off when the dog is not wet, yawning when the dog is not tired, panting when not hot, scratching when not itchy, or offering a play bow when not really wanting to play. Each of these signals could be signs of moderate stress.

Face   As stress increases, so will muscle tension. When the muscles of the face become more tense, the eyelids are raised, causing the eyes to widen. The dog will sometimes face away while looking at the threat, or face toward the threat while looking slightly to the side, causing the whites of the eyes to show. Pupils will often dilate, and the animal may be hypervigilant, frequently looking and listening in different directions and showing heightened awareness for what is going on both in the exam room and outside of it. Dogs may vocalize with a low distance-increasing bark.

The ears may be held to the side or back, showing the tension of the head and neck muscles. The lips can be pulled back in a grimace, tightly closed, or retracted, and the animal may be panting. Dogs who are stress panting generally have wrinkles at the corners of the mouth because the lips are very tense, and the mouth is halfway open with very little of the tongue protruding.

Tail   The tail on a moderately stressed patient may still wag, or it may be tucked or held low. If the tail is wagging, it looks more stiff and less fluid, because the muscles are tense. Figure 2.14 shows two moderately stressed dogs. In dogs with a low tail carriage such as a Border collie or greyhound, the tense tail may be pulled between the legs and up against the abdomen, with or without a wag or twitch of the tail tip.

Canine Moderate Stress: Video 2.3   Observe this puppy's body language. She seeks attention and seems interested in tactile interaction, but intermittently freezes and chooses to gaze off into the distance rather than glancing at Monique. After a moment of acclimating to the room, she comes to the mat, will interact but intermittently looks at Monique and away. She is accepting food, but she always looks ready to move away. Her tail tip is pointed toward the floor, but when relaxed she holds it parallel to the floor or with a slight upward curl so this tail carriage is an indicator of stress compared to her normal body language. She shows intermittent panting, her ears are held slightly to the side, and her brow intermittently furrows. This dog was scheduled for CVC appointments to

(a)

(b)

Figure 2.14 (a and b) Two moderately stressed dogs.

help intervene early and reduce her FAS level in the veterinary hospital. This video is intentionally silent to highlight the visible body language.

2.3.2.4 Severe Stress, Dog (FAS 4–5)

Dogs experiencing severe stress are in a state of significant emotional distress. These dogs may show defensive aggression and threatening postures, but this is uncommon. Usually dogs in severe stress due to fear will continue to use hiding and avoidance rather than overt aggression. Dogs in severe distress need relief from their stress prior to attempting any training and handling in most cases. A severe state of stress makes it difficult to relax enough to learn new skills and habits. When the emotion of severe fear is linked with the veterinary clinic, animals will find it difficult to cooperate and will often intensify in their reactions over time.

These dogs may show any of the signs described in earlier stress states, combined with those in the upcoming discussion. In addition to body language signals, severely fearful dogs may urinate, defecate, express anal glands, vomit, or even experience vasovagal fainting.

2.3.2.4.1 Overall Impression, Proximity, and Food Acceptance

A severely stressed dog will huddle in a corner, hide under a chair or table, or cling close to the owner. The body will be crouched into a ball or drawn in, and they may tuck a front paw under them. The dog will almost never approach the veterinary team member willingly, even when coaxed and offered food. In the rare instance when they do approach, they stay only long enough to grab food and then bolt away. Sometimes these dogs will take food from the owner, or will eat treats that you toss onto the floor, but most often they will not accept food at all.

Once a dog is severely stressed, you will notice everything about his body movements is exaggerated. The dog may move stiffly and slowly, or may frantically scramble at great speed. Some dogs will even enter a state called **learned helplessness**, where they no longer try to escape and seem like a statue. These dogs may appear cooperative, but are in a state of significant distress and suffering.

When approached, a severely fearful dog may become more stiffened or even freeze (FAS 4). *This form of freeze is a direct threat*, and when backed into a corner or restricted from escaping by a leash, the severely stressed dog may lunge, growl, snap, or bite (FAS 5).

Face When the muscles of the face are very tight, the eye can look hard. It may be very wide, showing the whites, or squinting. The pupils are usually dilated. The ears will be held tense and tight, usually flat, pulled back, or pulled far forward. Depending on the learning history of this individual, he may avoid eye contact or directly stare at the veterinary team. Often these dogs are hypervigilant, searching for escape routes. If the animal appears exceptionally stoic, he is likely in a state of learned helplessness and experiencing significant distress even if he appears cooperative.

When in severe distress and unable to escape, or having previously learned that escape is not helpful in minimizing the feeling of fear and threat, dogs may defend themselves. Staring directly at the threat, deep barking, growling, baring teeth, lunging, snapping, and biting are all signs of defensive aggression associated with severe stress. It is important to remember that dogs rarely "try to bite." If a dog snaps near someone without making contact, in most cases this is a threat that was intended to be an **inhibited bite** rather than a missed attempt at making contact.

In some cases, a dog may have been scolded in the past for trying to escape, or for growling or barking. Dogs with a learning history of scolding or punishment for these warning signs may appear to escalate to defensive aggression very quickly because the warning signs have been ineffective in the past or led to an unpleasant state of deeper distress for the dog.

Tail The tail on a severely stressed animal may wag in a staff-like shortened wag but will often be tucked up under the dog. Sometimes the tail is so tightly tucked that the tip touches the abdomen. Figure 2.15 shows two severely stressed dogs.

Canine Severe Stress: Video 2.4 shows the body language of severe stress. Notice that these dogs are described as experiencing severe stress, but are not showing any signs of defensive aggression. The dogs do not show aggression because the technician recognizes their distress and does not continue to press the handling scenario, which may prompt an escalation in their FAS level and create an unsafe situation for both human and dog. You may also notice the clips are quite short: this is because if we see signs of stress to this extent in our hospital, we immediately pause our handling and make an alternate plan. The body language labeled here as consistent with severe stress may appear more mild to some veterinary professionals, because so many patients present this way. We must remember dogs showing these signs are at enhanced risk for escalating to FAS 5 on this visit, and a significant risk of worsening fear and even permanent phobias about husbandry and veterinary care developing over time.

(a)

(b)

Figure 2.15 (a and b) Two severely stressed dogs.

The first puppy is showing inhibited movement. Puppies this age should be curious and willing to explore in new environments. She is stuck in one spot, scanning the environment. Her ears are folded, brow furrowed, and she licks her lips intermittently. She can't accept food. She does not move away, because she is essentially frozen in place. After about one minute of being allowed to just sit without being approached, she began to walk around the room. Observe her gait, it is stilted and cautious. She checks the exits and puts her feet up on the door to look for an escape route. We will show more video of this dog through the training process later in the book.

The next dog shows stress differently. She moves quickly, takes treats harder than usual, and pants heavily but intermittently. This dog is conflicted: she really wants the food but she is quite scared of the grinding tool the client has provided.

The third dog in this video shows another example of severe stress. She will come close but then move away. She is interested in contact but is panting with her lips pulled far back, notice the wrinkles at the commissure of her mouth. Her brow is furrowed, eyes dilated, and ears pulled as far back as she can pull them. She licks her lips, moves away, and shakes off frequently.

The last dog in the video shows fear of the blue platform. He will not approach: proximity is too intense. He will barely accept food, even though he really wants the treats.

Next is Coco, the Australian shepherd from a previous video, meeting a new team member. As soon as the stranger enters, the dog's eyes widen, she moves slowly, then she freezes. She vocalizes using an alarm bark.

2.3.3 Cat Body Language

Cats communicate through body language, olfaction and pheromones, and vocalizations. Olfactory communication is very important in cats. Each cat has his or her own smell, and cats in colonies have a communal scent, which is why it is important to methodically introduce a new cat into the household or re-introduce a cat that has been at your facility [12]. As with dogs, there is considerable individual variation among cats as well. Some cats are very social depending on their socialization history and genetics, while others are not social at all. Cats who are more social are often more comfortable in unfamiliar environments like the veterinary hospital, but these social cats also feel more confident showing how they feel, and when they are fearful this is often misunderstood as resistance or fractious behavior. As with dogs, signals from cats and the stress level of a cat can change rapidly. Watching for subtle changes and continuously monitoring the patient's state of mind by observing body language cues are the best ways to assess stress levels in cats.

As with dogs, we have divided the language of cats into four categories:

- Relaxed or calm
- Mild stress (mild conflict behaviors and/or avoidance)
- Moderate stress (conflict behaviors and/or avoidance)
- Severe stress (shows conflict behaviors, aggression, and/or learned helplessness).

We present a detailed evaluation guide here, as well as a quick reference summary in Table 2.5.

2.3.3.1 Relaxed or Calm, Cat (FAS 0)
2.3.3.1.1 Overall Impression, Proximity, and Food or Tactile Acceptance
A relaxed cat will come out of her carrier on her own at a moderate pace. She will not look rushed or panicked when exiting the carrier. The relaxed cat should slowly emerge while taking in the environment with her nose. She may approach and solicit attention by bumping the veterinary professional with cheek rubs or the top of her head. She will not retreat when you reach out to pet her, and will allow touching without retreating. When stroked, her muscles feel soft and relaxed to the touch. The relaxed or alert cat will often be sprawled out on the exam table or floor, lying on a hip with the legs relaxed and extended. She will also feel comfortable walking around the room with her topline or back level, parallel to the floor. She will rub on items in the environment, such as chairs or the corners of the exam table, and calmly investigate. Her haircoat should be lying flat and soft. She may try to initiate play by chasing or rolling. Relaxed cats will often accept food, and after several visits even begin to anticipate treats in the veterinary clinic. Many relaxed cats will eat food during handling procedures, or will just stop eating briefly for a few seconds during handling. Cats who prefer tactile rewards will accept cheek, chin, and/or head stroking before, during, and after handling and procedures.

Table 2.5 Feline body language: comparison of different signals associated with the emotional state of cats.

Emotional state	Proximity	Food or tactile acceptance	Body	Face	Tail
Relaxed	Exits carrier willingly Approaches team members Rubs Solicits attention Remains close	Will accept food May show interest in food but not eat Continues eating during handling May show interest in toys May show desire for tactile	Front approach Side approach Soft muscles Sprawls on floor or table Rolls Haircoat is flat	Normal slit pupils Soft eyes Relaxed ears Whiskers neutral	Relaxed Held soft and high Possible curled tip Away from body if lying down
Mild stress	Exits carrier willingly Approaches tentatively Slinky walk Retreats intermittently	May accept food May show interest but not eat Stops eating during handling May stop accepting tactile during handling	Side approach Mild muscle tension Sits or lies down with paws folded	Tense expression Shortened neck Squinting or slightly wide eyes Mild pupil dilation Whiskers neutral or pulled forward	Held low when walking Gently tucked around body when lying down
Moderate stress	Rarely exits carrier Retreats when approached Does not approach vet team Allows owner to approach and touch	Refuses food Refuses tactile	Looks away Hypervigilant Tense muscles Twitch or flinch when touched Mild piloerection	Moderate pupil dilation Widened eyes Ears to the side or back	Down Tucked Tip may twitch
Severe stress	Will not exit carrier Curls up small crouched in back of carrier Avoids approaches Avoids touch	Refuses food Refuses tactile	Tense muscles May crouch May arch back Piloerection Strike with paws Vocalization Bite Learned Helplessness	Dilated pupils Neck tense, short neck Wide eyes Flattened ears	Tucked tightly Stiff swishing Twitching Piloerection

(a)

(b)

Figure 2.16 (a and b) Two relaxed cats.

Face Relaxed cats will have relaxed facial muscles just like relaxed dogs. Cats lying on the table may roll onto one side, or rest their heads on the table. The eyes may be softly squinting or open, but do not appear wide. Pupils should be slit, and an appropriate size for the ambient light in the room. Ears should be held in the normal position of front facing and erect, or slightly to the side especially when touched. Whiskers will be held neutral to forward. Vocalization may occur in the form of friendly or inquisitive meowing or purring, but other vocalizations are uncommon in the relaxed cat.

Tail Relaxed cats have relaxed tails. If the cat is laying down, the tail will be laid on the surface in a line with a crook at the tip or a gentle C-curve. When standing, the tail will be held loosely down but not twitching. As a relaxed cat approaches and solicits attention, the tail will often be raised straight up, but feel soft to the touch, with or without a curled tip. Figure 2.16 shows two relaxed cats.

 Relaxed Body Language – Feline Video 2.5 shows a cat presented for examination. He exited the carrier on his own and began exploring the room. He rubs the walls and corners, solicits attention, and pauses to groom his paw. He does not accept food in this context but the remainder of his body language is relaxed for a cat in the veterinary clinic.

2.3.3.2 Mild Stress, Cat (FAS 1–2)

2.3.3.2.1 *Overall Impression, Proximity, and Food or Tactile Acceptance*

A cat experiencing mild stress may emerge from the carrier right away, or may take several minutes to walk into the room. She will move slowly or with caution, exploring and often looking for a place to hide. While she is walking around the room, the mildly stressed cat may look slinky, with the rear end held low in a crouched walk. The cat may tentatively solicit attention by bumping or rubbing. When stroked, her muscles feel slightly tense, and her skin may crawl slightly when she is petted. She may lean away without moving away. Her haircoat should be smooth and flat. The mildly stressed cat will often sit, or lie down on her belly with her paws folded. She will not sprawl on her side like the relaxed cat. The cat experiencing mild stress may accept high-value food, but will often pause eating during handling. She should return to her baseline easily when handling stops. Cats who prefer tactile may accept some cheek, chin, and/or head stroking before and after touching or handling, but during examination they may lean away rather than leaning into the touch.

(a)

(b)

Figure 2.17   (a and b) Two mildly stressed cats.

Face The mildly stressed cat will have tense muscles in her head and neck, causing a tense facial expression. Her eyes may be squinting or slightly widened, with mildly dilated pupils. Her ears may be soft and forward or slightly to the side. Whiskers are neutral to slightly held back toward the cheek. Some moderately stressed cats will purr.

Tail The mildly stressed cat will hold the tail low when she is walking, and will gently tuck it around her body when lying down, often with the tail tip flicking. Figure 2.17 shows two mildly stressed cats.

Feline Mild Stress: Video 2.6 shows mild stress in the cat. The first cat takes a moment to exit the carrier, and walks with his back arched and his tail down while scanning the environment. His FAS level decreases with a few minutes to adjust, and you see him much more relaxed in Video 2.5. The second cat is a kitten who is eating treats, but pauses eating and moves away with her tail held close to her body during the injection. She immediately returns to baseline eating when handling is stopped.

2.3.3.3   Moderate Stress, Cat (FAS 2–3)

2.3.3.3.1   *Overall Impression, Proximity, and Food or Tactile Acceptance*

The moderately stressed cat will rarely exit the carrier on her own. If she does, she will be tentative in her movement. She may initially move to come out, but then retreat to the back of the carrier again. When the carrier is disassembled and the top removed, often she will sit in the carrier bottom and look away from the veterinary professional. Sometimes, she will show a crouched body posture or nestling into her bed or the corner of the carrier, but still looking around periodically. She may also hide by pressing her head against or into a team member. Most moderately stressed cats will allow the owner to pet and touch them. She will not solicit petting or touching from the veterinary team, and will move away when handling is attempted. If she is moving around the room, she generally follows walls rather than crossing open spaces. When touched, she may flinch or twitch. She is often hypervigilant, noticing noises and movements and responding to them in an exaggerated way. Her coat may show mild piloerection. Most moderately stressed cats do not accept food.

Face   The facial muscles will be tense, so the eyes will appear wider. Her pupils will be mildly to moderately dilated, and she will alternate between looking away from the veterinary professionals and looking at them. She will hold her ears to the side or back, but they will not be completely flat. Whiskers will be in a neutral to flattened position; and if the cat is vocalizing, they may meow with what Kessler describes as a *plaintive meow* [13].

Tail   Her tail may be held down or tucked under her body, and if the cat is aroused it will twitch some. Figure 2.18 shows two moderately stressed cats.

Feline Moderate Stress: Video 2.7 shows two cats experiencing moderate stress. Notice the first cat is scanning the room looking for a retreat or hiding spot. Her ears are held slightly back, and she is moving away from Alicea with cautious motion. The second cat is relaxed and eating until Alicea tries to apply some eye medication. The cat switches to moderate stress markers, repeatedly trying to back away, licking her lips, and swishing her tail.

2.3.3.4   Severe Stress, Cat (FAS 4–5)

2.3.3.4.1   *Overall Impression, Proximity, and Food or Tactile Acceptance*

The severely stressed cat will generally try to escape, freeze, or show defensive aggression. She typically will not come out of her carrier by choice, so the carrier will need to be disassembled around her. When she is in the carrier, or if she is in the exam room outside of the carrier, she will make her body small and tuck her paws and tail close to the body. If moving around the room, the severely stressed cat will be crouched low to the ground, or possibly stand with the back arched and haircoat standing on end ("Halloween cat"). When the veterinary team attempts to touch the cat, she may rapidly try to escape, hiss, growl, yowl, or strike with a front paw.

When in severe distress and unable to escape, or having previously learned escape is not helpful in minimizing a perceived threat, cats may defend themselves. Staring directly at the threat; vocalizing, including meowing, hissing, yowling, and growling; showing the teeth with an open mouth; air biting; and biting are all signs of defensive aggression associated with severe stress. Like dogs, cats rarely "try" to bite. If a cat bites near someone or bites them softly, this is a warning associated with extreme stress.

In some cases, cats will also enter a state of learned helplessness or total immobility. Cats in learned helplessness look like they are trying to be invisible. A severely stressed cat in this state will seem like a statue, and will not respond in the expected way to a given stimulus. She will generally hide her head and look away, close her eyes, or stare off blankly into space. When touched, she

(a)

(b)

Figure 2.18 (a and b) Two moderately stressed cats.

will not react or will have a minimal or slow-motion reaction, and she generally does not notice things like vaccinations. Cats in learned helplessness are experiencing severe stress, even though they may look cooperative on the surface.

Face The head will often be lower than the body whether the cat is standing or crouching. The cat will usually either look completely away or directly at the perceived threat. She will open her eyes wide, with dilated pupils. The brow may be furrowed. The ears will be flattened to the side or fully back on the head. Due to the tenseness in the cat, the whiskers will be pulled back. She may hiss, show an open mouth with teeth exposed and a tense tongue, growl, or bite.

Tail The severely stressed cat will hold her tail close to the body and may tuck it under the abdomen, similar to a stressed dog. The tail may swish stiffly, twitch, or remain stiffly still. The cat may stand with an arched back and the proximal 1/3 of the tail held straight out

(a)   (b)

Figure 2.19 (a and b) Two severely stressed cats.

while the remainder points or curves toward the floor. Piloerection is common on the tail, making it look bigger, especially if the cat is arched. Figure 2.19 shows two severely stressed cats.

    Feline Severe Stress: Video 2.8 shows three examples of severe stress. The first cat's ears are held flat against her head. Her pupils are dilated, she licks her lips, and her front foot is ready for swatting in preparation for self-defense. The second cat's ears are held back but not completely flat. His pupils are dilated, his whiskers are forward, he hisses when the cage is opened, and he is ready to strike with a front paw. The third cat moves away from Alicea, demonstrating avoidance. She shows tail swishing once wrapped in a towel. During the injection, you can see the cat tense her muscles, back up, hiss, flatten her ears, and crouch.

2.4 Causes of Stress in the Veterinary Setting

2.4.1 Overview

This lengthy discussion of interpreting body language in our animal patients serves to help us identify their stress levels and stay safe, and improves their experiences in the veterinary hospital. Avoiding all stress in the veterinary setting is virtually impossible, but a great deal of stress can be mitigated through understanding, planning, and developing a great knowledge of learning and training. If we understand the causes of stress in our patients, and how the signs of stress can change over time, we can respond rapidly and with the necessary skills to decrease stress where possible, and treat it when needed.

2.4.2 Pain

Pain is a major source of stress in the veterinary hospital. Whether the pain is acute or chronic, even the most well-behaved patients can be stressed, including severe stress and defensive aggression, if they are in pain. Pain can be associated with injuries, infections, osteoarthritis, chronic illness, cancer treatments, gastrointestinal discomfort, pancreatitis, dermatologic disease, and glaucoma, just to name a few. Identifying pain in animals can be challenging at times. The physical signs of pain can have significant overlap with signs of emotional distress. Pain and emotional distress also worsen synergistically. Any animal suspected to be experiencing possible pain should be provided analgesia.

Patients who are aggressive because they are in pain due to an injury are learning that the veterinary hospital is a place where pain happens, and the people in the clinic cause painful experiences. Unpleasant experiences due to physical pain lead to lasting emotional responses even when the pain has been resolved, creating fear of the location and the providers. After a painful event, it is common to have patients who were once quite comfortable for veterinary care refuse to enter the building, or show extreme fear on subsequent visits.

We encourage liberal use of analgesics and sedatives for any patient who may be painful. A good pain management program can go a long way toward keeping team members and patients safer. If a patient is going to require repeated rechecks such as wound dressings, cast changes, **radiographs**, or lab work, it is a good idea to consider the use of **anxiolytic** medications along with the pain management protocol. Patients who struggle due to fear as well as pain are at a higher risk of physical injury in addition to the emotional consequences we have just discussed. If a procedure is anticipated to cause pain, such as removing a broken toenail, sedation or, anesthesia should be considered. Even a few brief seconds of pain create a lifelong memory for the animal. Whenever a patient is seen for an urgent care or surgical visit, it is a good idea once the animal has recovered to schedule some happy visits where no treatments are performed. This can help restore trust between the veterinary professionals and the patient, and improve emotional feelings about the environment.

2.4.3 Examination and Treatments

The stress of being touched, having to interact with strangers, and entering an unfamiliar environment can have a considerable impact on patients. It is common for animals to respond with fear or avoidance of simple procedures like coat care, ear cleansing, tooth brushing or nail care even from their most trusted humans and in a secure familiar environment. Many owners do not know how to provide this care for their pets in a way that is cooperative and fosters feelings of safety. Now the patient is in the veterinary hospital and needs many of these potentially scary types of handling, and they are being done by a stranger as well. Imagine that a patient, who is showing the signs of stress discussed earlier in this chapter, is in the hospital for an examination. The patient looks away, turns away, is panting even though she is not hot, and shows displacement behaviors like sniffing the ground when she is approached. Because the patient is not actively trying to escape, and is not behaving aggressively, veterinary professionals tend to soldier on, providing the physical examination. Imagine what might be going through this dog's mind: "I'm really uncomfortable and I keep telling you, but you are still touching me," or, "This is a really scary place! Please do not come any closer!" and yet we continue touching the animal. These animals are doing their best to communicate their mild and moderate fear to us, but we persist in our examination because we are not forced to stop by their behavior. Consider the learning history this animal is accumulating: nonviolent methods do nothing to prevent this discomfort and scary event. What is the motivation for the animal to continue using nonviolent communication with us in the future? Very little.

It is important to consider that the very things we are doing to try to help our patients, examinations and treatments, provoke a great deal of fear for some animals. Responding with respect to the signals an animal gives us about their discomfort is the first step in building trust and being able to provide more treatments with less stress over the lifetime of the animal.

2.4.4 Emotional Capital and Trigger Stacking

The ability to deal with stressors is finite. Every pet and person is working with a certain amount of "emotional capital" at any given time: we can show resilience and tolerance up to a point, but at some point the emotional capital is spent and we are unable to go further. Our emotional bank account is overdrawn and we must stop and escape.

We have all had that day. We get a speeding ticket on the way to work, the doctor is running 40 minutes behind on appointments, the phone is ringing off the hook, a dog in the kennels cannot stop barking, a coworker accidentally stole our lunch out of the fridge and ate it, and then we get a paper cut on our finger while unpacking boxes. That paper cut might cause quite an emotional outburst! Tears, swear words, or storming off might all happen, as a result of a tiny paper cut. But wait: is it really about the paper cut? No, it is about *trigger stacking*. The paper cut was the final withdrawal against our emotional bank account for the day. **Trigger stacking** is the process where many small stressors increase the emotional sensitivity of a learner (human or animal) over time, and when the learner goes over threshold for emotional resilience, even a small stressor can provoke a large, seemingly out-of-context response.

Trigger stacking happens in the veterinary hospital all the time. If a cat is brought into the hospital and experiences this tall stack of triggers, his emotional capital may be used up. Consider the following withdrawals from the cats emotional bank account:

- Capture by the client and being placed (possibly forced) into the carrier.
- Carrier slides around on the seat of the car while driving.
- A dog sniffs and barks at the cat in the lobby.
- The cat won't come out of the carrier so is pulled or forced out onto the slippery exam table.
- The owner's cell phone goes off during the history, causing a loud noise.
- A dog in the kennels is barking and can be heard from the examination room.
- The technician takes the cat's temperature and leaves the room.

After all this, when the veterinarian attempts to **auscult** the cat by sliding a hand under the chest to listen, the cat may lash out. The defensively aggressive display is probably not related exclusively to the auscultation, but rather is the culmination of all of the stressors erupting in an exaggerated response. Figure 2.20 illustrates an example of trigger stacking.

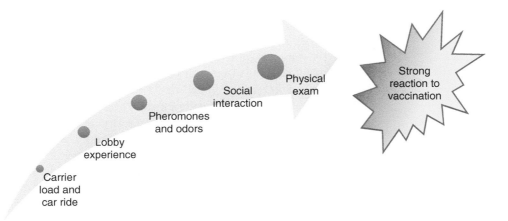

Figure 2.20 Trigger stacking occurs when stressors build one after another, until the patient has a strong response to what may otherwise be a mildly provoking stimulus.

An awareness of trigger stacking helps us keep patients calmer during visits. We can't eliminate all stressors from veterinary care, but by minimizing the environmental stressors we *can* control, we help preserve the pet's emotional resilience to cope with an examination and treatments. Furthermore, by using animal-friendly techniques during the examination and treatments, we can continue to expand the animal's emotional resilience. Awareness of animal body language will help us remain in touch with possible trigger stacking, and stay sensitive to an accumulation of stress that may harm the patient's ability to cooperate today and in the future.

Video 2.9 shows a humorous take on a veterinary visit from the cat's point of view. It is humor, but consider all the possible triggers this cat experiences, and how he might respond when it is time for his checkup and vaccinations. How many of the cats you work with experience some or all of these triggers during a visit?

2.4.5 Learning History

Multiple factors come together to build the learning history of the animal. Each visit, each experience, each event the animal is exposed to in the veterinary setting will contribute to the animal's overall body of knowledge. Every interaction we have with an animal is a training session, whether the training occurs by intent or by accident. We may be setting up the environment for success by making the clinic inviting: this is passive training. We may be taking a purposeful role to teach our patients we are nonthreatening and can be fun: this is active training. The veterinary setting is a perfect environment for accidentally using both kinds of training to teach our patients to dislike and fear us.

2.4.5.1 Normalizing Welfare for All

On social media, at continuing education conferences, and anywhere else a group of veterinary professionals gathers, people tend to start swapping war stories. Why do people do this? Are they proud of surviving a harrowing event? Does it show a level of bravery to return to work after being harmed by an animal? Is it a sign of willingness to put the safety of the animal above the safety of the human, allowing ourselves to be injured? Being injured while trying to fulfill our vocation of preventing and relieving the suffering of animals takes a serious emotional toll on veterinary professionals. It can help to know that we are not alone in having been injured in the past. Solidarity is healthy. However, human safety is supremely important in veterinary medicine. One way to be safe is what we have been taught in the past: how to apply strong restraint to prevent animals from hurting us. Applying that strong restraint can and does cause great emotional distress to many patients. Being the person who is asked every day to cause that emotional distress leads to emotional harm to the humans involved, not just the pets.

For each white ghost of a healed scratch drawn across a hand, every dented thumb-nail, every game of connect-the-dots of puncture wound scars, there is an animal who experienced that event as well. Every suture, every antibiotic pill, every ripped pair of scrubs or extra load of wash due to a patient releasing bladder or bowels is a sign of a pet who was terribly distressed while in our care. Our hope is we can begin to learn from our battle scars that there is a better way. Listening to our patients when they talk to us about stress and fear, developing new skills to use when we work together with the animals we love, pausing procedures much sooner, using medication and sedation to prevent and reverse fear early and often, and learning to set the stage for success for both people and pets will serve us all so much better.

By teaching animals that more good can come from the veterinary hospital than bad, we can help improve their opinions about the setting and the events that happen here. Ken Ramirez talks about

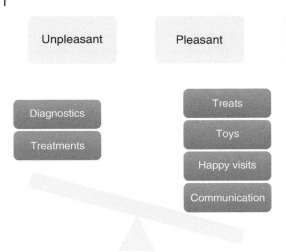

Figure 2.21 By providing more pleasant than unpleasant experiences in the environment, we can help tip the learner's emotional scales in favor of an overall pleasant emotional response.

the balance between pleasant and unpleasant in the learning environment. The goal is to make sure the pleasant side of the scale holds far more material than the unpleasant side (Figure 2.21) [14]. Veterinary care will never be entirely without holding still, being touched and manipulated, needles, clippers, pills, and more. Certainly, if we make an effort to balance the scales in our favor with treats, toys, play, desired touching, preventing pain and fear, and good communication, we can improve the overall experience of our patients and build a more favorable learning history over time.

2.4.6 Steps for Success

To successfully implement the strategies contained in this book, veterinary professionals will need to pay attention to our patients. We will need to assess and reassess pets as we work with them each day, each hour, each moment. We will try to set up the environment and our protocols to improve the patient experience, and we will write down our triumphs. Where? In the medical record! Dedicate a part of the medical record to the patient's likes, dislikes, emotional status, and handling history. These notes should be success based, not warnings. Avoid labels like "fractious," "bites," or "dangerous." Instead, select useful information to help the people who come after trying to handle the same patient. Table 2.6 shows some ideas for label replacements. Examples include: "will allow saphenous blood draw with peanut butter spoon," "allowed full exam after trazodone administered at home, remind owner to give trazodone," or "has muzzle from home, loves goldfish crackers." These messages still provide us with the information to approach an animal with caution (as we should with every animal), but serve the additional purpose of reminding us to approach the animal with compassion and a plan for success. Fear Free[sm] calls this the Emotional Medical Record. Maintaining an emotional record full of success notes is one important step toward maintaining an improved quality of veterinary experience for pets and people.

Table 2.6 Label replacements to use during conversation and in the medical record for patients.

Label or current language	Suggested replacement
Fractious, mean, stubborn, bad, spoiled	FAS score and context (e.g. FAS 5 for temperature)
Cautions	Success notes (and include a guide)
Needs muzzle	Is trained for a basket muzzle
Avoid <X>	Provide <Y>
Hates jugular blood draw	Standing saphenous with muzzle and spray cheese
Drugs required for visit	Calming medications prescribed
Sedate for everything	Medication prescribed for all treatments

References

1 Goldstein, E.B. and Brockmole, J. (2016). *Sensation and Perception*, 10e. Chicago: Wadsworth.

2 Miller, P. and Murphy, C. (1995). Vision in dogs. *Journal of the American Veterinary Medical Association* 207 (12): 1623–1634.

3 Jacob, G.H. (1983). Colour vision in animals. *Endeavour* 7: 137–140.

4 Peters, A. (2002). *The Cat Primary Visual Cortex*. Atlanta, GA: Elsevier.

5 Strain, G. (2011). *Deafness in Dogs and Cats*. London: CABI.

6 Overall, K. (2013). *Manual of Clinical Behavioral Medicine for Dogs and Cats*. St. Louis, MO: Mosby.

7 Martin, D. and Shaw, J. (2023). *Canine and Feline Behavior for Veterinary Technicians and Nurses*. Ames, IA: Wiley.

8 Noback, C.R., Ruggiero, D.A., Demarest, R.J. et al. (2005). *The Human Nervous System*. New York: Humana Press.

9 Landsberg, G., Hunthausen, W., and Ackerman, L. (2013). *Behavior Problems of the Dog and Cat*, 3e. Edinburgh: Saunders.

10 Serpell, J. (1995). *The Domestic Dog: Its Evolution, Behavior, and Interactions with People*. Cambridge: Cambridge University Press.

11 Gray, J. (1971). *The Psychology of Fear and Stress*. New York: McGraw-Hill.

12 Crowell-Davis, S.L., Curtis, T.M., and Knowles, R.J. (2004). Social organization in the cat: a modern understanding. *Journal of Feline Medicine and Surgery* 6 (1): 19–28. http://journals.sagepub.com/doi/abs/10.1016/j.jfms.2003.09.013.

13 Kessler, M. and Turner, D. (1997). Stress and adaptation of cats (*Felis silvestrus catus*) housed singly, in pairs, and in groups in boarding catteries. *Animal Welfare* 6: 243–254.

14 Ramirez, K. (2011). *Problem Solving: Full Course on Training*. Chicago: Shedd Aquarium Society.

3

Learning, Conditioning, and Training

Every interaction with our patients is a learning experience for them, which means it is a training opportunity for us. Understanding the science of how conditioning and learning happen allows us the best opportunity to assure great experiences for our patients. We are discussing the basics of learning theory in this book to help teams get started on the path to functional Cooperative Veterinary Care. There is an immensely deep and broad field of knowledge and concepts with respect to learning theory and behavior which are not addressed in this chapter.

Selecting appropriate methods begins with agreeing to "Do No Harm," and expanding protecting wellness to include emotional and psychological wellness, as already discussed. Understanding the how and agreeing on the why also let us select an appropriate what: what methods to use for our training. Dr. Susan Friedman provides a model for selecting methods that are most effective at achieving teaching, least intrusive to the learner, and lowest risk for the learner and the trainer.

Dr. Susan Friedman's "Hierarchy of Behavior-Change Procedures" (Figure 3.1) provides a roadmap for making the most ethical choices when training [1]. Along the road, the map shows a series of turns and speedbumps. Each turn represents a training method that can be employed. The first turns available have the least potential for harmful side effects, while later turns could have more concerning possible outcomes. Each speedbump indicates the need to slow down, and proceed with caution only after completely assessing the road ahead. To address a change in behavior, the first stops along the roadmap are to assure the animal's basic needs for wellness and nutrition are being met. Next come **antecedent arrangements**, **positive reinforcement**, **differential reinforcement of an alternate (DRA) or differential reinforcement of an incompatible (DRI) behavior**, **extinction** and **negative reinforcement**, and finally **positive punishment**. This is a lot of jargon packed into a few sentences. By the end of this chapter, you will be able to define each of these terms and many more, and apply them to common scenarios in a practical and scientifically sound way.

Terms in this chapter such as classical conditioning and operant conditioning are a framework we use to discuss, understand, and change the behaviors we see in learners. These processes are occurring all the time and simultaneously. We separate them linguistically for the purposes of discussion, but it is not possible to conduct them as isolated techniques or procedures. Rather, our understanding of the different types of learning lets us break down and better analyze a situation, and plan to better meet the complex needs of the individual learner at every level of learning.

Hierarchy of behavior-change procedures

Positive punishment

Extinction, negative reinforcement, and negative punishment

Differential reinforcement of alternative behaviors

Positive reinforcement

Antecedent arrangements

Health, nutrition, and physical setting

Figure 3.1 Roadmap of interventions. Dr. Susan Friedman's guideline for least aversive to most aversive procedures to change the behavior of animals.

3.1 Classical Conditioning

Classical conditioning, also known as Pavlovian or respondent conditioning, was defined by Ivan Pavlov while doing research on salivation and digestion in the early 1900s. Pavlov found that his dogs would begin salivating and producing digestive fluids at the sight of the experimenter or the sound of the bell long before any food was presented. While the experiment on digestion encountered a roadblock, Pavlov instead successfully defined a type of learning that was reflexive. He discovered that when a neutral stimulus is presented before an unconditioned stimulus, after repeated pairings the neutral stimulus will become a conditioned stimulus causing a conditioned response (Figure 3.2). These conditioned responses are reflexes, secretions, emotional responses, hormone responses, etc. The responses are not under the learners' control: responses happen *to* them, and they do not choose to respond [2]. For example, an owner opens the drawer and picks up the nail trimmers, catches the dog, and wrestles to cut the toenails, causing an emotional response of stress and fear. In the future, the dog may experience the emotional response of stress and fear by having a release of stress hormones, acceleration in heart rate and respirations, dilated

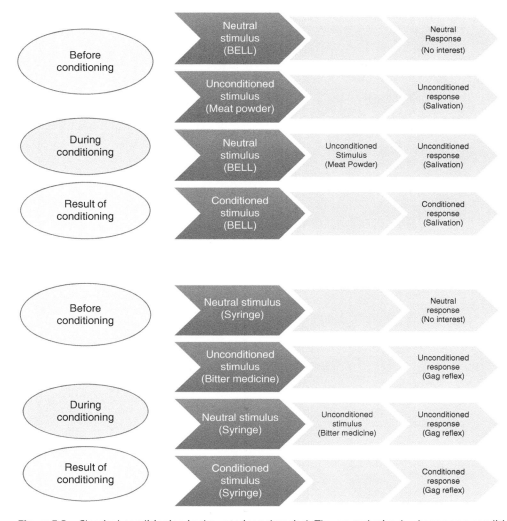

Figure 3.2 Classical conditioning in the veterinary hospital. The neutral stimulus becomes a conditioned stimulus through the conditioning process, resulting in a conditioned response. The first diagram shows Pavlov's familiar experiment on salivation in dogs. The second diagram uses the example of giving a cat bitter medicine.

pupils, and more, in response to the drawer being opened or the sight of nail clippers even if no nail trimming is attempted.

Classical conditioning is a powerful tool that can work for us or against us in veterinary medicine. Pavlov's dogs would hear a bell, and then salivate. Why? When Pavlov rang his previously neutral bell, it predicted meat powder. Meat powder causes salivation and the release of digestion compounds in the dog. When the bell was linked with meat powder for enough trials, the sound of the bell alone was enough to prompt the response of salivation, without the meat powder being present at all. The bell was no longer neutral: the dogs experienced a meat powder response to the *bell* instead of the meat powder.

Why is this relevant to training and to the veterinary environment? Associations are being made all the time by the animal's mind and body. Cats who perk their ears and purr in anticipation at the

(a)

(b)

Figure 3.3 (a) Classically conditioned gag response. (b) Classically counter conditioned pleasant response.

sound of the can opener or a dog who wiggles with excitement when his owner walks near where the leash hangs are good examples. If we think about associations and how they might form from the animal's perspective, we can work to encourage the responses we want and prevent potentially distressing or harmful responses when possible. We can also be more aware of situations where an existing problematic response exists, or where we see one emerging, and intervene in a helpful way. Classical conditioning is an extremely useful tool for preventing the development of fearful responses to veterinary handling or procedures (Figure 3.3).

Video 3.1: Feline Classically Conditioned Response. Video 3.1 shows a feline patient who has previously been given extremely bitter medication from a syringe. The cat responded by gagging and salivating. Now, when this patient sees a syringe – even an empty one or one with water or food in it – the cat gags and salivates. Previously the syringe was meaningless or neutral. It was associated with a noxious flavor which caused drooling and gagging. The syringe alone is no longer meaningless or neutral: it prompts the same response the bitter medicine did even when the medicine is absent. The cat does not choose or control this response.

3.2 Operant Conditioning

Operant conditioning, also known as instrumental conditioning, is based on E.L. Thorndyke's Law of Effect (1898) and B.F. Skinner's three-term contingency [3]. Unlike classical conditioning, which deals in unconscious responses, operant conditioning focuses on observable behaviors where the animal performs behaviors and these behaviors are followed by **consequences**. Trial-and-error learning is one way to describe operant conditioning. The learner performs behaviors, and depending upon the consequences, the learner will make future decisions about certain behaviors based upon how those trials and errors were perceived by the learner. Figure 3.4 breaks down the quadrants of operant conditioning as they generally apply to discussing animal training. The following includes basic descriptions of the quadrants and definitions, and a simplified real-life example to introduce each concept.

For the purpose of this discussion, we will look at two primary categories of consequences for any behavior: **reinforcement** or **punishment**. Reinforcement is anything that increases the future frequency, intensity, or duration of the behavior. Punishment is anything that decreases the future frequency, intensity, or duration of the behavior [3–5]. Consequences as perceived by the learner drive future behavior, whether the consequence is reinforcement or punishment. The trainer will be able to tell whether consequences were reinforcing or punishing by observing the frequency, intensity, and duration of the behavior throughout the training period. *Technically, we do not know in the moment if we are providing a reinforcing consequence. The animal's behavior over time is the only way to determine if a consequence was truly reinforcing or punishing.* There are

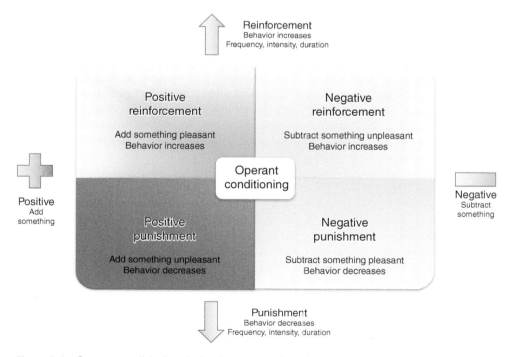

Figure 3.4 Operant conditioning. A visual representation of the quadrants of operant conditioning: positive reinforcement, negative reinforcement, positive punishment, negative punishment. Positive reinforcement is shown in green because it has the smallest probability of unpleasant side effects for the learner. Negative reinforcement and negative punishment are yellow because they present a medium risk. Positive punishment is shown in red because it presents the highest risk of unwanted side effects and potential welfare concerns for the learner.

two types each of reinforcement and punishment: positive and negative. With respect to operant conditioning, *positive* means adding something to the situation, and *negative* means removing something from the situation. These combinations result in positive reinforcement, negative reinforcement, negative punishment, and positive punishment.

3.2.1 Reinforcement

Acquiring and maintaining behaviors is best done from a welfare perspective by prioritizing reinforcement. For reinforcement to be effective, the learner must have a good "return on investment" for the behavior performed. The learner needs to be able to effectively understand the relationship between the behavior and its consequence. Rewards must be delivered promptly after the behavior, ideally within 1–1.5 seconds, for a reinforcement effect to be observed. Delaying the reward >2 seconds after a behavior is observed results in delayed acquisition or maintenance of behaviors. The reinforcement effect is weakened.

3.2.2 Positive Reinforcement

Remember: in operant conditioning, positive and negative do not mean good and bad. Instead, think of them as the math of learning: addition and subtraction. Positive means adding something to a situation, and reinforcement means the behavior strengthens over time. So positive reinforcement is the process through which a behavior gets stronger because of what was added to the situation [3–5]. Positive reinforcement training has been found to be extremely effective, and it is understandably popular with trainers around the world for all species [5]. This method helps the learner ascertain exactly what the desired behavior is, and allows the trainer and the learner to have a relationship based on predictability, pleasant interactions, and trust.

The process of positive reinforcement training relies on the learner performing different behaviors, and the trainer delivering consequences. When the consequence is positive reinforcement, the trainer delivers something they think the animal desires and enjoys. The animal performs a desired behavior, and the trainer immediately delivers a probable reinforcer such as a treat, a toy, praise, attention, or touch. How will the trainer tell if what she delivers is truly reinforcing? Observe the animal's response to the consequence. Are there signs of pleasure? Anticipation? Attempts to acquire the item again? Does the behavior which preceded the delivery increase? If these signs are seen, the interaction was likely reinforcing.

3.2.2.1 Example: Acquiring a Body Weight

A puppy is wandering in the proximity of the scale, which is covered with a comfortable nonslip mat. The puppy explores the area, and when he steps on the scale, the trainer delivers several tiny treats by dropping them right under the puppy's nose. The puppy eats the treats and wanders away. The next time the puppy wanders near the scale, she moves onto it more quickly, and more treats are delivered right under the puppy's nose.

Over time, if the puppy approaches the scale with more frequency, intensity, or duration, a positive reinforcement event has likely occurred.

3.2.2.2 Example: Teaching a Kitten to Target

The trainer extends an outstretched finger toward the kitten. When the kitten sniffs the finger, the trainer then immediately offers a lick of a delicious liquid treat. The trainer presents an outstretched finger a few inches away. The kitten reaches out and sniffs the trainer's finger, and another treat is delivered.

3.2.3 Negative Reinforcement

Negative reinforcement is the removal of something to increase the likelihood the behavior will happen again [3–5]. Remember: negative means subtract. Negative reinforcement can present ethical dilemmas, because we are sometimes removing something the animal will work to avoid. This means we have potentially applied something aversive, or put the animal in a situation where aversion is occurring. In general, when we work with animals, we want to choose the least invasive, minimally aversive, and maximally comfortable method for each individual animal. Negative reinforcement should be used with great care for this reason: it potentially compromises welfare and can cause harm.

3.2.3.1 Example: Fastening a Safety Belt

When the driver gets into the vehicle and starts the car, a harsh beeping noise occurs. As the driver fastens his seatbelt, the annoying beep stops. In the future, the driver rapidly fastens his seatbelt (increase in belt-buckling behavior) and the beep is subtracted, so negative reinforcement has occurred for the behavior of seat belt fastening. This example is relatively benign because the learner is able to comprehend the entire interaction in advance, choose to perform the desired behavior, and avoid the beeping entirely. Further, the aversive stimulus is a nonthreatening beep. Or is it? Some people might perceive the beeping as extremely aversive. Others may ignore the beeping completely. Individual preference and experience informs all learning events.

3.2.3.2 Example: Teaching an Animal to Stand Still When Restrained

The trainer can apply pressure around the animal's body while it is struggling. As soon as the struggling ceases, pressure is removed. The trainer removed something (pressure), and the animal stands quietly more in the future (increase in behavior), so negative reinforcement occurred for the behavior of standing still. The problem with this technique is that the trainer held the animal while he struggled. Struggling is likely a sign of stress or fear in this animal, and this method could damage the trust between the trainer and the learner because the feeling of fear or stress is unpleasant. Negative reinforcement requires the learner to want to avoid something and have it removed. *We must question the appropriateness of causing intentional avoidance, and be aware of possible fallout from doing so.*

Struggling or resistance to handling should follow the 2-2-3 rule. If more than two gentle arms are required to stabilize the patient, if a cat struggles for more than two seconds, or a dog struggles for more than three seconds, pause the procedure and make a new plan. A different technique is required, and negative reinforcement is contraindicated.

3.2.4 Punishment

Punishment by its very definition is effective in changing behavior: if the behavior does not decrease, punishment is not occurring. However, punishment, particularly intentionally using procedures with a goal of punishment carries disadvantages. Punishment can cause stress and conflict, which both reduce learning efficiency [5]. Punishment also inhibits behaviors, which can mask normal behavior and mask changes in behavior. Punishment procedures do not show the learner what the desired behavior is, but only aim to decrease or stop behaviors. Punishment-based training methods have also been correlated with increased fear and aggression in the learner including owner-directed aggression [6]. Fear may be of the trainer, equipment used, the environment, or a combination of these. Aggression may be displayed toward the trainer or redirected onto other people, animals, or objects. Increased fear and aggression can put patients, clients, and team members at risk. The fallout from punishment is not worth the risk, particularly with respect to Cooperative Veterinary Care training.

3.2.4.1 Negative Punishment

Negative punishment describes removing or subtracting a stimulus to weaken a behavior over time [3–5]. In general, negative punishment removes something the learner wants, so through trial and error the learner realizes his behavior does not achieve any pleasing result. By removing something a learner wants, we can communicate with a learner that a behavior is ineffective at obtaining rewards. However, this method does not teach the learner what the desired behavior is, and can result in confusion, frustration, and diminished trust between the learner and the trainer. Because the technique involves punishment, it deals entirely in reducing behaviors, but does not increase desired behaviors. While cessation of some behaviors is necessary, this method should be used with caution, as with all forms of punishment.

3.2.4.1.1 Example: Teaching a Puppy to Stop Jumping Up

Most puppies jump because they are seeking attention. If the puppy jumps and the trainer steps away, looking away and removing all attention, the puppy may learn that the behavior of jumping up results in removal of attention. If the behavior of jumping up gets weaker with time, this form of training is negative (remove attention) punishment (decreased jumping).

While this punishment is not directly or intentionally aversive to the puppy, it also does not teach him a preferred greeting such as sitting. The puppy may chase or continue to jump on the trainer as they move away, or may disengage and choose not to approach. As an alternative to punishment, using positive reinforcement by teaching the puppy to sit when a person approaches achieves the same result as forbidding jumping, with the added benefit of the puppy performing the correct behavior. It also avoids frustration and confusion and builds trust and understanding. The fastest route to right behavior is to define and then teach the desired behavior (**Video 3.2**).

3.2.4.2 Positive Punishment

Punishment, like reinforcement, can be positive and negative. Positive punishment is the addition of something to decrease the likelihood the behavior will happen again [3–5]. Positive punishment should be reserved for the last resort if it is used at all in training, and it is not appropriate for veterinary and husbandry training. The use of punishment, and particularly positive punishment, can be challenging. Difficulties include the fact that the trainer needs to be able to directly link the punishment with the behavior in the learner's mind. It is common for the learner to associate the aversive stimulus with the trainer, the environment, or an object rather than the behavior the learner was performing. In addition, the aversive stimulus must be sufficiently unpleasant that the behavior stops, and must occur as a consequence every single time the behavior occurs. Applying intentional and strong aversives is unethical and compromises animal welfare [3].

3.2.4.2.1 Example: Stopping Drivers from Speeding

Many drivers exceed the speed limit on a regular basis. If you are this driver, you engage in the undesirable behavior of speeding nearly every day. Occasionally you will get pulled over by a police officer, and given a warning or a ticket. Say this happens once every year or less. No one likes getting a speeding ticket, so why do people still speed even after having to pay a ticket? Because the speeding ticket does not meet the criteria for punishment. If it did, the speeding behavior would decrease!

Instead, the driver is being intermittently reinforced for the behavior of scanning for police officers and slowing down when they are visible. For speeding tickets to be effective, they would need to be delivered immediately every time the driver exceeds the speed limit, and the dollar amount would need to be high enough that it was truly aversive.

3.2.4.2.2   *Example: Stopping Drivers from Running Red Lights*

Red light cameras are popping up in neighborhoods all over the United States. Drivers know that if they run the red light, they will be mailed a ticket every time they choose to do the behavior. Because the aversive stimulus of the ticket happens every single time the behavior occurs, the punishment should be effective in reducing the number of red lights a driver chooses to run. However, not every light has a camera. The true behavior being changed is a decrease in running red lights where the driver knows there is a camera, not the behavior of running any red light. Some drivers may even choose an alternate route to avoid the lights with the cameras. Incorporating a planned punishment procedure is complex and must meet all criteria to truly and permanently diminish behavior.

3.2.5   The Role of Marker-based Training

Marker-based training is a positive reinforcement strategy used by trainers to improve communication between the trainer and the learner [5]. Any gesture, sound, word, signal, or touch can act as a marker if it is introduced as a consistent promise of imminent primary reinforcement. The animal experiences repeated pairings of the marker immediately followed by a treat (or other primary reinforcer), and through classical conditioning the animal learns the marker predicts a treat. In many cases, the marker itself will cause a visible pleasure response in the animal once it is truly a conditioned reinforcer. However, a marker is also a promise. A marker will always be followed by a **primary reinforcer**. Primary reinforcers are something the learner finds intrinsically rewarding. The easiest and most practical one of these to use during cooperative veterinary care training is food treats. If the pairing of the marker with a primary reinforcer is stopped, the value and importance of the click will diminish over time. The marker used most commonly in the videos accompanying this book is a **clicker**. The clicker is a small plastic and metal device used to make a "click" sound (Figure 3.5). In some videos the trainer uses a hand to work the clicker, in others it's under the trainer's foot. The second most common marker seen in these materials is a verbal marker such as "Yes" or "Nice." Animals can be conditioned to respond to multiple markers. For example, "Treat" may mean food will be delivered to the animal's mouth, while "Find" might mean the food will be delivered to the floor. It is not required to teach multiple markers, but this concept will appear in some of the example videos.

The purpose of the marker is to indicate the precise instant the learner has performed the desired behavior. Precise communication speeds learning. Further, some behaviors are incompatible with accepting reinforcement. The use of a marker allows the trainer to indicate which behavior was desired and then subsequently deliver a reward. Marker based training for humans is called TAGteach™.

In this text, the terms click and mark will be used interchangeably. Both indicate a communication to the learner a treat is promised. The term treat and reward will also be used interchangeably because treats are an expedient primary reinforcer most of the time.

A word on reinforcement. Whether something is rewarding or pleasurable is always the perspective of the learner. Building value for rewards is sometimes necessary. Training plans can be put in place to increase the value of some rewards, such as food. It is uncommon for this to be the case.

(a)

(b)

Figure 3.5 (a and b) Clickers are a tool often used in marker-based training. A treat pouch is a convenient way to store food rewards during training.

Generally if an animal is refusing food, there is an underlying medical condition, past learning history decreasing the safety or value of accepting food, or their fear, anxiety, and stress (FAS) level is too high. In later chapters, food refusal will be discussed.

Using marker-based training allows the trainer to communicate clearly and precisely with the learner. Rewards need to occur within two seconds of the correct behavior for the learner to properly associate the reward and successful reinforcement to occur, with a shorter interval such as 0.5 seconds being most effective [4]. A marker needs to be sufficiently brief to note a precise behavior. Longer words or phrases such as "Good Job" are too long to use as a specific marker. The clicker allows a great degree of precision. After we "charge" the clicker (or marker word, light, etc., as appropriate for the learner), we can use the click to tell the animal precisely when the right behavior occurred, and use the click as a bridge meaning, "That's right! A treat is coming soon!" The bridge helps span the time gap between the behavior and delivery of the primary reinforcer. Often, we will be training behaviors where the animal cannot eat at the same time he is performing the behavior. For example, nose targeting is impossible to perform at the same time a treat is being delivered: when the animal opens its mouth to receive the treat, the nose target behavior will be interrupted. We need a way to communicate with the animal that the right behavior has occurred, and a reward is on the way. The click, or marker, is how we can communicate this information, and can even be used when the animal is far away from the trainer or the treats.

Some research suggests that a click or whistle speeds up training when contrasted against a verbal marker or no marker. Other research asserts that a verbal marker, a click, and direct delivery of a treat are equally effective if the trainer is very proficient [7].

3.2.5.1 Marker-based Training: Mechanics Matter

Our companion animals are very attuned to our body language. Sometimes this awareness is for better, and sometimes for worse. If the trainer moves around a lot or talks to the animal frequently during training, the animal can become confused while trying to figure out what all the movements and words mean. If the trainer stands still like a statue or a robot, many animals will find this suspicious and unnatural, and be reluctant to participate. When initiating a training session, the trainer should be standing in a relaxed neutral posture, with a pleasant facial expression.

(a)

(b)

Figure 3.6 (a and b) Cutting treats into tiny pieces helps make the food easy to eat quickly and controls caloric intake from training sessions.

Training Tip: Treat Type Matters!

Select tiny treats the animal thinks are delicious. The treats need to be easy to eat quickly (Figure 3.6).

Animals quickly make associations between stimuli or actions, especially the ones that predict food or another primary reinforcer. For example, many animals come running at the sound of the crinkle of a plastic food wrapper, because that sound predicts food. Animals will often give the trainer extra attention when she reaches into her treat pouch or pocket, because that action predicts food delivery. When starting out with marker-based training, it is important the animal learns the click or marker is what predicts food, not another movement or hand-in-pocket. Choosing a home base position while introducing the concept of marker-based training is a useful way to prevent misunderstandings. Keeping hands at home base is an easy way to remember to keep the marker as the most important piece of information. Examples of home base include hands behind the back resting in the small of the back, hands at the sides, or hands folded in front over the waistband. Trainers need to be careful not to rest hands on the treat bag or pocket while at home base. When clicking, keep the clicker hand still, then deliver a treat following the click. Once both the trainer and the animal understand how to communicate using the marker, additional hand and body positions can easily be added to training sessions with less confusion.

The initial mechanics should look like: observe desired behavior → click while at home base → reach for and deliver treat → return to home base. Figure 3.7 illustrates this progression.

3.2.5.2 Marker-based Training: Capturing

There are two common marking methods trainers use to get behavior from an animal: **capturing** and **shaping** [5]. When capturing, we mark a behavior the animal is already doing in order to

Figure 3.7 Mechanics of marking and delivering rewards when introducing marker-based training. Begin in a "home base" neutral training position (example top left). Cue or wait for the learner to offer the behavior. Click when the desired behavior occurs. Deliver a reward, then return to "home base" for the next repetition.

strengthen the behavior [5]. The completed behavior is something the animal already offers. For example, puppies are born with the ability to sit. Getting puppies to sit on cue is easy using capturing.

Video 3.3 shows introducing capturing the behavior of moving onto a mat for the first time to a puppy and to an adult dog. In both cases, the environment is arranged to make the behavior both probable and easy for the animal through *antecedent arrangement*. A comfortable non-slip mat is placed on the floor, a person is nearby with treats and a pleasant expression, and then waiting for the dog to move around or prompting the dog to move around by rolling a treat. When the dog moves onto the mat, Monique marks with a yes or a click, then feeds immediately.

Capturing can be used in the exam room for those patients who are *already* relaxed and holding still. For example, the dog chooses to hold still while a nail is clipped. Click and treat for the stillness and cooperation to capture it, then proceed to the next toenail. If we take the time to capture the stillness for each nail and give a treat afterward, we are rewarding the desired behavior of calm stillness. When an animal is holding still and allowing a treatment, it's natural to want to just proceed. The difficulty here is it does not teach the animal that stillness is rewarding and desirable. If we ignore desired behavior, it will eventually fade away because it does not serve a useful purpose from the animal's perspective. Capturing is a great way to maintain or increase desired behaviors the animal is already offering. Furthermore, if we proceed while the animal is calm, and only pull out treats when the animal is wiggling or less cooperative, we are risk ignoring the calm behavior and rewarding the wiggling behavior. Stillness → clip vs. wiggling → treat. Watch closely to recognize when animals are already doing something right! We have so many opportunities to reward existing desired behaviors as long as we watch for them.

3.2.5.3 Marker-based Training: Shaping

Shaping is different from capturing because we build a complex behavior that is novel: the learner does not already perform this behavior. Shaping means breaking down the goal behavior into many tiny pieces, steps, or **approximations**. Pure shaping allows the learner to experiment in the environment, and the trainer will click when a step toward the goal occurs. The trainer will not be prompting, luring, or cuing during shaping sessions [5]. One analogy is the "Hot and Cold" game many of us played as children. The person who is the guesser tries to find or do a "secret" thing. The guide tells the learner they are "getting warmer" or "hot" when they are on the right track, and that they are "cold" when they are wrong. Clicks during shaping are like telling the animal he is "getting warmer," In shaping, we ignore the "cold" part of the game, and only focus on successful approximations of the goal behavior. As animals learn the shaping game, they begin to understand that a few seconds without a click means they aren't on the right track and need to try something else. For shaping to be successful, the trainer needs to have keen observation, good timing, and maintain a high rate of reinforcement. Frequent rewards are important! Late clicks, missed opportunities for clicks, and accidental clicks can lengthen the training process. If the rate of reinforcement is too low, the animal may become disinterested, distracted, or even frustrated. Frustration is not comfortable for the animal and should be avoided for cooperative care training. The good news is errors made using marker-based positive reinforcement methods are unlikely to be harmful to the animal or to the relationship between trainer and animal, unlike errors made using punishment.

Shaping allows training of simple and complex behaviors, and it allows the learner to discover the desired behavior through communication with the trainer. When working with an animal on a shaping project, it is important to remember that the learning track is not always linear. While the Hot and Cold game analogy assumes the learner makes constant progress toward the goal behavior, sometimes shaping is more like putting together a puzzle with many pieces. If the goal behavior is the entire picture in the puzzle, each puzzle piece may be an approximation. The shaping process allows the animal to obtain all the puzzle pieces, and learn how the pieces come together to comprise the goal behavior. To become proficient at shaping, a trainer must learn how to maintain the learner's motivation level, and develop a good communication style with the learner. We must watch for communication about what the animal understands, and what the animal has not yet grasped. Shaping relies on a good balance between rate of reinforcement and adjusting criteria. If the **rate of reinforcement** is too low (too much time between treats) or the criteria for reinforcement are too high (task too difficult to receive a treat), the animal may choose not to participate because the task is unclear or too difficult. If the rate of reinforcement is very high, the criteria may remain the same too long, and the animal may begin to think that the goal behavior has already been achieved. The rate of reinforcement must be kept high enough to maintain the animal's interest, but not so high that there is no desire on the part of the animal to try new behaviors or improve through the approximations to attain a more complicated goal behavior. When both the trainer and the animal understand the shaping process, achieving goal behaviors can be amazingly quick.

The key to using any training method successfully is defining what the desired behavior is, and building that behavior by design. Rather than asking ourselves, "How do I stop the animal from moving his paw?" the question should be, "How do I teach the animal to keep his paw still?" Instead of, "How can I hold the animal down to restrain it safely?" we should ask, "How can I teach the animal to stand still and volunteer for this procedure?"

Video 3.4 shows a young dog named Quill engaging in a shaping session to learn to put on an Elizabethan collar. Quill is familiar with the idea of shaping and marker based training, but not with the cone collar. Notice the approximations begin with just a glance or a sniff, then progress through approaching the cone, approaching the opening of the cone, approaching at different angles, offering to place a nose into the large end of the cone, and gradually all the way to placing his head into the cone. Monique also makes sure to have a good plan for removing the cone by providing a treat lure to keep Quill's nose still while removing the cone. Shaping relies on a high rate of reinforcement, plenty of approximations toward the goal, and patience on the part of the trainer.

Video 3.5 shows using shaping to teach a cat to go to a mat. The behavior is broken down into a number of approximations, and each approximation is marked with a click and a treat follows. The rate of reinforcement is kept very high, and the treat size is kept small to allow numerous reinforcers to be given during each training session. Going to a mat is an extremely useful behavior for any animal, and will be discussed at length in later chapters.

3.3 Habituation, Sensitization, Desensitization, Counter Conditioning, and More

3.3.1 Habituation

Habituation is a type of non-associative learning, and is largely a passive process. It is an adaptation where we learn to filter out unimportant information in the environment and stop responding to it. The learner may notice the stimulus at first and respond, but will stop responding with repeated exposures [5]. During habituation, the animal learns the stimulus has no consequences (good or bad), so no response is necessary. In habituation, the stimulus is always presented at the same level, with repeated exposures over time. For example, when you need to turn on your heat in the winter, your dog probably notices the first few times the furnace roars to life. However, this response quickly fades and the dog stops noticing. People who live near the airport may notice the sound of planes flying overhead for a few weeks, but then stop noticing this sound. Similarly, someone who lives near the railroad track may stop noticing passing trains with repeated consistent exposures. Consistent repetition is a key of habituation. If someone who lives near the airport goes on vacation in the quiet wilderness for a few weeks, the sound of planes will be noticed again when they return home. If the stimulus is too intense, for example a car alarm, habituation may never occur. It is very unlikely for a learner to habituate to a very intense stimulus. It is not appropriate to rely on habituation for cooperative veterinary care training.

3.3.2 Sensitization

Sensitization is a learning process in which repeated administrations of a stimulus results in the progressive **amplification** of a response [5]. The animal develops a stronger and stronger response over time to the stimulus (Figure 3.8). It is crucial to continuously observe animals during treatment for escalations in the fear response, or visible signs of stress during treatment. Professionals should actively monitor for the risk of and avoid sensitization during cooperative veterinary care training.

	Identify trigger(s)
	Break down into exposure ladder
	Identify nonstressful starting point
	Controlled exposures
	Monitor for emotional response(s)
	Develop tolerance to trigger(s)

Figure 3.8 The steps of desensitization. Desensitization is generally used in combination with additional classical conditioning or classical counterconditioning to establish a pleasure response rather than a calm or non-response.

One example is sensitization to storms resulting in storm phobia. At first, a dog may only "notice" a violent storm and show a mild response. Then the dog may show a stronger response like shaking, panting, and pacing during heavy storms, and "notice" small storms. Next, the dog may have full panic during large storms, and shake, pace, and pant during small storms. Eventually the dog becomes sensitized and may experience full panic even with a small storm. Sensitization can also result in generalization of similar stimuli. For instance, the storm-phobic dog may start to worry about other noises such as fireworks, the smoke alarm, a door slamming, and so on. Another example would be animals who respond progressively more strongly to having their nails trimmed with each event. At first, the dog may be mildly reluctant or withdraw his paw. Next, he might avoid all touching of the legs or feet. Eventually he may even show defensive aggression when we attempt to touch the feet. This is an example of sensitization because there is a stronger and stronger response to the same stimulus as it is presented over time.

3.3.2.1 Flooding

Flooding is exposing the learner to a feared stimulus at a high level of intensity until they stop reacting [5]. This type of exposure requires preventing the animal's ability to move away from the stimulus until the visible fear response has completely subsided. Most animals display a severe fearful response during flooding, followed by exhaustion and stop responding. The animal will generally try to escape, show visible signs of significant distress, and may become aggressive while trying to avoid the feared stimulus. Some animals will enter a state of learned helplessness, where they are still fearful but cease trying to escape. Flooding has many unwanted potential side effects, intentionally causes a distressed fear response, and can be dangerous to the animal and people nearby. For these reasons, *flooding is not recommended*.

3.3.3 Desensitization, Classical Conditioning, Classical Counter Conditioning, and Operant Counter Conditioning

3.3.3.1 Desensitization

Desensitization (DS) is a process where a stimulus is systematically presented repeatedly in a controlled and gradual fashion [5]. Because of the gradual exposures, the individual learns that the stimulus is not meaningful, and therefore stops responding to it. Systematic desensitization

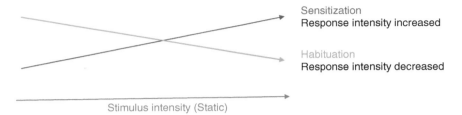

Sensitization
Response intensity increased

Habituation
Response intensity decreased

Stimulus intensity (Static)

Figure 3.9 Sensitization and habituation. When a stimulus remains the same, the learner's response may change over time.

requires that the stimulus be controlled in its intensity, and always kept a level where the learner does not show a response to the stimulus (Figure 3.9).

Controlling the intensity of the stimulus requires constructing a plan for graduated exposures, often called an exposure hierarchy or an exposure ladder. An exposure ladder may even contain subsets of exposures if the stimulus or end behavior is complex. Intensity of the stimulus can mean many different things. It may mean the duration the stimulus is presented, the environment in which the stimulus is presented, how loud a sound is, how soft or firm a touch is, which body part is touched based on nerve ending concentration and individual sensitivity, the distance between the learner and the stimulus, and how many factors are involved, such as equipment, odors, and more. In every case, there must be a zero-response starting point for desensitization to be effective. As an example, we can consider a possible exposure ladder and its subsets for nail trimming.

The components of the exposure ladder may look something like this:

- Touching of the target area of a toenail:
  - Touch shoulder, glide touch to elbow, carpus, paw, toe, and toenail.
- Introducing toenail clippers:
  - Touch shoulder, glide to elbow, carpus, paw, toe, and toenail while holding clippers.
- Trimming a nail:
  - While holding clippers, touch is tolerated up to and including toenail.
  - Trimmers approach nail, then approach and tap nail.
  - Trimmers approach nail, tap nail, encircle nail, and then trim a single nail.
- Trimming all nails:
  - Trimming a single nail is well-tolerated.
  - Trim two nails, then three, then four, then one entire paw.
  - Trim one paw, then begin a new paw.
  - Gradually work up to being able to trim all nails on all paws.

Desensitization takes time and patience, and the speed at which desensitization may proceed is dictated entirely by the learner. Some learners may be able to tolerate very rapid exposure procedures, while others require a slower approach. Desensitization will only be successful if the learner is carefully observed for signs of stress or response, and the stimulus intensity is carefully controlled. Sudden exposure to a high level of the stimulus can lead to a significant setback, or even sensitization. For practical purposes in cooperative veterinary care training, desensitization procedures are combined with additional conditioning plans to promote animal welfare.

3.3.3.2 Classical Counter Conditioning

Remember classical conditioning (CC) from earlier in this chapter? Establishing a physiologic response linked with a stimulus through pairing? **Classical Counter Conditioning** is the

Figure 3.10 Classical counterconditioning. Counterconditioning replaces an unwanted existing emotional response with a new, desired emotional response by linking the trigger with something that prompts the desired emotional response repeatedly.

technique of changing an *existing* classically conditioned response (emotion, reflex, secretion, etc.), and replacing it with a *new* response to the same stimulus [5]. By pairing a previously feared stimulus with something we know causes the *desired* emotional response, we can change the fear response to a happier one. Common tools used during classical counterconditioning include high-value treats, toys, pleasurable forms of touching, and happy verbal praise (Figure 3.10). **Classical counter conditioning** is a cornerstone of treatment for fearful animals in the veterinary setting and is almost always paired with some form of desensitization. Together, they are called desensitization and classical counterconditioning, or DS/CCC.

Classical counter conditioning is the *replacement* of an emotional response; there is no requirement or contingency that the animal performs a specific or desired behavior [5]. The goal is simply to form a pleasurable association with something he previously feared. In the examination room, every touch can predict something wonderful like a favorite treat. When the touch predicts the treat for enough repetitions, the animal should begin to anticipate something pleasurable associated with touching. If the animal is nervous about touching, the touch should be broken down into smaller segments (desensitization), and progress should be made at the animal's comfortable pace. DS/CCC to veterinary procedures will be described in depth using numerous examples in later chapters.

3.3.3.3 Operant Counterconditioning

Operant counter conditioning (OCC) is teaching the animal to perform a desired behavior in the presence of a previously important stimulus [5]. Some trainers call this DRA or DRI behavior, while others call it OCC or response substitution. OCC differs from CCC because we are paying attention to the specific observable behaviors the animal perform rather than responses the animal does not consciously control. By teaching the desired behavior, we can make it simple for an animal to comply with treatments. Furthermore, the desired behavior will not be possible while the undesired behavior is performed (Figure 3.11). For example, a dog who usually jerks his paw back when we try to touch a nail can be taught to stand and offer a paw. Standing and offering a paw is incompatible with jerking the paw away. If a cat runs away at medication time, teaching her to come to

(a)

(b)

Figure 3.11 (a and b) Differential reinforcement of an incompatible behavior. This dog cannot both jump up and sit at the same time. Reinforcing the sit rather than the jump will teach him to sit instead of jumping during greetings.

a medication station is a desired behavior we can reinforce, which is incompatible with running away (see **Video 3.6**). Using a training plan, it is possible to teach animals the desired behavior to cooperate for treatments.

3.3.4 Putting It All Together

Recall we discussed the idea each of these terms is used to *describe* components of the learning and behaving process. While we discuss them discretely, in reality *they are all happening simultaneously*. It is helpful to think about the different kinds of procedures we can plan out when developing a training protocol, but we cannot isolate parts of the animal's brain and physiology when training: all types of learning happen all the time.

3.3.4.1 Example: Leashing for a Walk

Owner picks up leash

Owner places leash on dog

Dog goes for a walk

On the walk, the dog receives the opportunity to sniff, explore, exercise, and receive treats.

Let us break it down a bit more:

The first few times the owner picked up the leash, the dog likely did not know what it was so there may be little observable response.

The owner then begins noticing the dog will approach, wag its tail, have a bright expression, and shift back and forth on its front paws.

We can infer from this body language the dog is likely experiencing emotions of anticipating something desirable. The "feelings" are evidence of the classically conditioned responses.

The dog also approaches, wags, perks its ears, and prances. These behaviors are followed by the leash being placed and the dog beginning its walk. These behaviors are observable and are likely being maintained through positive reinforcement.

Video 3.7: Operant Counter Conditioning. This 12-week-old Cattle Dog puppy is presented for vaccinations. Because the visit was curbside to comply with local and safety regulations, I took a video so the client could see the visit. The puppy showed no desire to avoid proximity and had excellent food acceptance. Blue's starting behaviors are to move around very quickly all the time, and to turn and place her mouth near my hand if I tented her skin to practice a vaccination. The behavior I would prefer is for her to hold still on the table rather than moving around, and to look forward when I am working with her skin to vaccinate her. I strategically position a nonslip surface, the location of my treats, the location where I place each reward, and the direction, speed, and location of how I am stroking her to promote this behavior. This is a combination of luring, capturing, modeling, desensitization, classical counter conditioning, and distraction which all combine to result in OCC. Watch for a very high rate of reinforcement, which stops when she is moving around a lot or if her head turns, and immediately resumes when she is still and facing forward.

3.4 The ABCs of Behavior

3.4.1 Functional Assessment

Learning terminology and theory can feel overwhelming at times. Behavior modification and training have plenty of jargon as well as scientific terminology. There is a great deal of conceptual overlap, and different experts may even describe the same situation using differing terminology. To help make understanding and remembering terms to physically change behavior in dogs and cats much easier, use a simple system to assess the learner's behaviors. The **three-term contingency** is used in **functional assessment**. The smallest meaningful unit of behavior analysis, the three-term contingency is not only a very useful tool but also easy to learn and remember: as easy as ABC. A is for *antecedent*, B for *behavior*, and C for *consequence*. The ABCs are not meant as a complete in-depth analysis of all behaviors occurring and their reasons, but they are an excellent starting point for the exercise of considering how behaviors develop and may be molded for the purposes of cooperative veterinary care.

3.4.2 Antecedents

Antecedents occur before a behavior or behaviors. They can be distant antecedents or immediate antecedents [4, 5]. Some are complex, while others are quite simple. Environmental changes or circumstances can act as antecedents, such as a drop in barometric pressure being followed by the onset of a bout of storm phobia. Other antecedents are social interactions between animals, interactions with a person, intentional antecedents like cues for a behavior (e.g. sit), tactile information, olfactory cues, and certain sounds provided by a trainer or caregiver. An antecedent is anything that precedes the behavior and predicts it will occur.

3.4.3 Behavior

Behavior is anything the animal does: the organism's response following the antecedent [4, 5, 8]. Keep in mind that behavior cannot be changed by anyone but the organism or learner itself. We can set up antecedents and deliver consequences in an effort to encourage behavior to be more or less likely to occur, but we cannot forcibly create the behavior. The learner is entirely in control of behavior, because behavior is simply the action of the learner. Prompts, cues, environmental setups, and more can all work in our favor in improving the likelihood of a desired behavior strengthening over time.

To modify behaviors, we must be able to observe and measure them. This means the animal is actually doing a behavior. It is not possible to observe or train the lack of a behavior. If an animal has a problem behavior the trainer wishes to decrease over time, it is important to decide what the desired alternate behavior is, and arrange the antecedents and consequences to support the desired observable, measurable behavior. Attempting to train and measure only the cessation of behavior is difficult and does not teach the learner how to succeed, feel better, or access rewards.

3.4.4 Consequences

Consequences follow behaviors [4, 5]. Each of the quadrants in operant conditioning is a type of consequence. These consequences drive future decision making by the learner. Consequences can be environmental, intrinsic, and **extrinsic**. The consequence may be under the trainer's control, or something in the environment outside the trainer's control. Remember: the animal or learner is the one whose perception of the consequence is important.

If a dog performs a given behavior such as seeing the scale and then following treats onto the scale, then receives a favorite treat, it is likely the dog will choose to move onto the scale in the future. If a dog sees the scale, is pulled by the leash onto the scale, and then slips or scrambles while being weighed, it is likely the dog will choose not to move onto the scale in the future (Figure 3.12).

In the first example, the salient antecedents are the presence of the scale and treats. The behavior is moving onto the scale. The consequence is receiving a delicious treat. In the second example, the antecedent is the presence of the scale and pressure on the leash. The behavior is moving onto the scale. The consequence is slipping and scrambling. The same antecedent of the presence of the

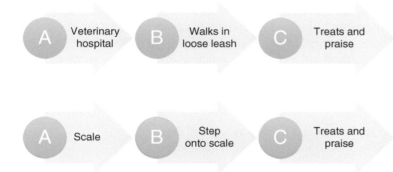

Baseline before training: Veterinary environment predicts avoidance, which are followed by unpleasant interactions.

Result after training: Veterinary environment predicts movement through lobby and placing paws on scale, which are followed by pleasant interactions.

Figure 3.12 ABCs. The antecedent, behavior, and consequence breakdown for entering the clinic and moving to the scale before and after training.

scale, and the behavior of moving onto the scale, resulted in two different consequences, which will drive two different behavioral choices in the future.

When we are considering the ABCs, first we observe the situation and make a map:

(1) Identify the **B**ehavior of interest.
(2) Identify the **C**onsequences which are likely maintaining the behavior.
(3) Identify the **A**ntecedents which predict the occurrence of the behavior.

Let us continue with the example of obtaining a body weight for a dog.

Observations: When the owner attempts to weigh a dog, it backs away from the scale.

(1) B = Backing away from the scale.
(2) C = Negative reinforcement – Removal of the proximity of the frightening scale: distance from a threat is increased.
(3) A = Collar pressure as owner pulls on leash, presence of scale.

A change in the antecedents may result in a change in behavior. *The goal is for the dog to move onto the scale to be weighed.* Which changes could we employ to encourage the behavior?

(1) B = Walking toward and then moving onto the scale.
(2) C = Treats delivered when dog is on scale.
(3) A = A non-slip mat is placed on the scale, a trail of treats is placed along the path to the scale and a small pile of treats are placed on the mat on the scale, the owner is coached by a team member to keep the leash loose.

In this example, a non-slip soft mat is placed on the scale. Treats are strategically trailed onto the scale. As the dog follows the trail of treats, he walks onto the scale and receives additional treats.

While this example is simple, it illustrates how changing the antecedents and the consequences can lead to a change in behavior.

Video 3.8: Body Language and Responses. Mushu is presented because he has intense fear of veterinary visits. Due to health department regulations, Mushu's owner may not accompany him into the examination room. He has a history of displaying aggression to his owner (growl, snap, bite) and veterinary team members at another hospital during attempts at handling. He also had a history of licking a distraction like cheese, allowing a touch but then snapping at the veterinary professional's hand during the touch. This clip shows part of his first introduction to the new clinical environment and to the author. Mushu loves treats and training at home, and knows how to offer a paw, offer a nose touch to hand, sit, and down based on training done by the client outside the veterinary environment.

Previous learning history in the veterinary environment:

B: Growl, bite, snap.
A: Veterinary team member approaches and touches any part of dog.
C: Veterinary team member rapidly withdraws their hand and moves away.

In the above contingency, negative reinforcement of the removal of a threat (hand approaching) will strengthen and maintain the growl, bite, snap behavior. However, failing to remove the hand is a major safety concern for the veterinary team member and welfare concern for the dog. A different plan is needed to allow Mushu to communicate both when he is uncomfortable with a touch and when he is ready to be touched.

Desired understanding when Mushu is uncomfortable:

B: Lean, look, or move away when uncomfortable with an approach.
A: Veterinary team member calmly shows a hand and approaches a small amount without touching.
C: Freedom from being touched, treat delivered away from veterinary professional.

Desired understanding when Mushu is ready to be touched:

B: Remain on platform with soft facial expression.
A: Veterinary team member calmly shows a hand and approaches as long as dog's body language looks comfortable.
C: Click at closest approximation of touch, treat delivered from veterinary professional's hand.

You will see more videos of Mushu and many other patients later in this book. By empowering Mushu to express his ability to move away from a threat, he did not have to use defensive aggression to stop the interaction. Over time, Mushu later learned to wear a muzzle, allow examination, blood collection, and vaccination without restraint.

3.4.4.1 Example: A Cat Avoids the Carrier

Current observations:

B: Cat moves away from carrier and hides.
A: Carrier is present and door is opened, owner approaches cat.
C: Hiding, feelings of improved welfare, increased distance from threat.

The behavior is entering the carrier. The consequence is being locked in the carrier, a car ride, a vet exam, some needle pokes, and another car ride. This consequence will likely result in a decrease in the behavior of entering the carrier, and an increase in the behavior of running away even at the sight of the carrier.

The current behavior of running away from the carrier and the emotional response of stress and fear can both be changed. The desired replacement behavior would be for the cat to enter the carrier on her own. The desired emotional response is pleasure when the cat sees the carrier. To break down the training picture, the antecedent would be the presence of the carrier. This antecedent is probably best accepted if the carrier is a normal part of everyday furniture, stored in one of the cat's living areas, near the cat's play area or climbing tree, or the like.

Desired scenario:

B: Cat moves into the carrier or allows owner to place cat into carrier.
A: Presence of carrier, owner, and treats.
C: Treats received inside carrier, feelings of safety.

Using desensitization and classical counter conditioning, the emotional response to the sight of the carrier can be improved over time. At first, the carrier may need to be covered or far away, then closer and closer, until the cat is happy near the carrier and willing to interact with it. Once the emotional response is improved, the behavior of following treats or a toy into the carrier, or even walking into the carrier as a trick, can be trained. The antecedent of the owner presenting the carrier would be followed by the behavior of the cat walking into the carrier. The consequence would then be receiving treats or a toy after entering the carrier, likely increasing the behavior of entering the carrier and decreasing the behavior of running away.

3.5 Fundamental Training Skills

When it's time to start training patients that need help, you'll need a training plan. It is imperative that we focus on positive reinforcement. While implementing your positive reinforcement training, keep in mind that capturing, shaping, desensitization, classical conditioning, counter conditioning, and response substitution will all be occurring at the same time. Focus on developing the desired behavior, and monitoring and assessing the patient's responses, emotions, and progression of learning.

3.5.1 Training Plans

Predictability and understanding are a good way to build trust and decrease fear, anxiety, and stress. By using a training plan, taking a systematic approach, observing the animal's responses during training, and going at a comfortable pace for the animal, we can provide veterinary care that is much less upsetting to our patients and often use little or no physical restraint. Before a trainer is ready to make a training plan, both the trainer and the animal need to have a good grasp of the fundamentals of training.

Making a Training Plan involves considering:

1. What rewards does the animal prefer?
2. A detailed description of the desired behavior including numerous hypothetical approximations?
3. What is the most feasible way to deliver the reward?
4. How can I arrange the environment to best support the animal to perform the behavior?
5. Does the animal have a pre-existing fear of any component of the environment or stimuli involved with the completed behavior?
6. Designing a detailed exposure hierarchy for any possibly FAS-provoking aspects of the completed behavior.
7. Will I need to lure, prompt, or otherwise arrange antecedents to promote the behavior in the beginning of training? If so, can I keep those lures or prompts in the long term or will they need to be changed?
8. A plan for fading or removing lures, prompts, or short-term antecedents if necessary.

The Training Plan will change after every session, and may even change mid-session. Observing the animal's emotional state and specific behaviors continuously, and adapting to what the animal needs in order to feel safe, remain engaged, and develop an understanding of how to access reinforcement is the key to good, patient-centered care and training.

3.5.2 Rewards and Reinforcement

Rewards matter. When starting a session with an animal, it's important to choose a reward that actually *reinforces* behavior. While you will not know if the reward you choose is truly reinforcing until you see the pattern of increased behavior emerge over time, you can often predict based on common preferences what an animal might find reinforcing for a given behavior. Developing a reinforcement hierarchy will be important when training new behavior with an animal. For instance, Monique's Border collie, Rye, prefers tugging in exciting environments, a tennis ball for moving behaviors, and food for stationary or lower energy behaviors. Invest some time to learn what the animal wants, then develop an order of preference. Consider how you can creatively use rewards that feel good to the learner. To continue with the example of Rye, he may love a tennis ball but the environment may not be appropriate for delivering it. Giving him a delicious treat by tossing or rolling it instead of handing it to his mouth might be a good way to use food for a moving behavior for this dog. Learning the effects of, and preferences for, different types of foods, treats, toys, touching, and other forms of potential reinforcement will speed up the training process, and give the trainer plenty of tools in the toolbox when challenges emerge. Table 3.1 shows examples of reinforcement hierarchies and how the skill and the environment may modify the learner's preferences.

3.5.2.1 Questions About Rewards
What if a pet likes treats, but will not eat them?

We should ask a few questions: is the animal hungry, or already satiated? Is the animal relaxed enough to accept food? Is the food a desirable treat for this animal? How can I make the environment calmer and less stressful to improve food acceptance? Is the behavior I am trying to train too difficult? It's important to persist in trying to help animals feel comfortable enough to take

Table 3.1 Example reinforcement hierarchies: Individual preference and the context of the situation will determine how patients are motivated.

Animal	Situation	High value	Medium value	Low value
Border collie (no prior fear of grooming)	Nail trim	Steak	Kibble	Tennis ball
Border collie	Recall away from squirrels	Tennis ball	Tug toy	Steak
Terrier	Going for a walk around squirrels	Cheese	Kibble	Tug toy
Terrier	Learning a new trick at home	Tug toy	Cheese	Kibble
Kitten	Learning a recall inside the house	Feather toy	Cream cheese	Cat treats
Kitten	Physical exam at the veterinary hospital	Cream cheese	Canned cat food	Feather toy
Cat	Learning to go into a carrier at home	Cream cheese	Kibble	Feather toy
Cat	Learning a medication station	Cream cheese	Facial stroking	Cat treats

treat. Experiment with a variety of different types of treats, reduce environmental stress as much as possible, and explore other reinforcement strategies until you determine what works best for each individual pet. Figure 3.13 is a quick reference for improving food acceptance.

3.5.2.2 If You Can Use Toys, Petting, and Praise, Then Why Use Food?

Not all rewards are equally reinforcing for certain behaviors. There are two types of reinforcers we will concentrate on for this guide: primary or unconditioned reinforcers, and secondary or conditioned reinforcers. Primary reinforcers are naturally reinforcing for the animal and do not require any training. Some examples of primary reinforcers include: food, water, reproductive opportunities, and shelter. Animals will naturally expend effort and work to access primary reinforcers (Figure 3.14). However, even primary reinforcers are not equally valuable to an animal. For example, hiking an extra 5 miles to have a bigger salad might not be so appealing, but doing so for some delicious ice cream may be more motivating for some people. Remember that what is reinforcing is up to the learner and not the trainer. The value of an item can also change as availability and access to the item change. For instance, if I am a millionaire, I will probably not be motivated to do an hour of work for $20. I can have money anytime I'd like it.

Novelty and "other people's cookies" can play a role. Clients should always come prepared with a favorite treat such as chicken, steak, canned food, or cream cheese from home. These are familiar items to the animal. In the hospital, we might offer something that seems lower value like cat treats, and the animal may prefer it simply because it is novel. The key to success is to be flexible and ready to change based on what the animal prefers during any given session.

Note: *When we use the word* reinforcer, *what we mean is something intended to provide reinforcement for a given behavior. If the behavior gets stronger over time, we will know reinforcement is successfully occurring.*

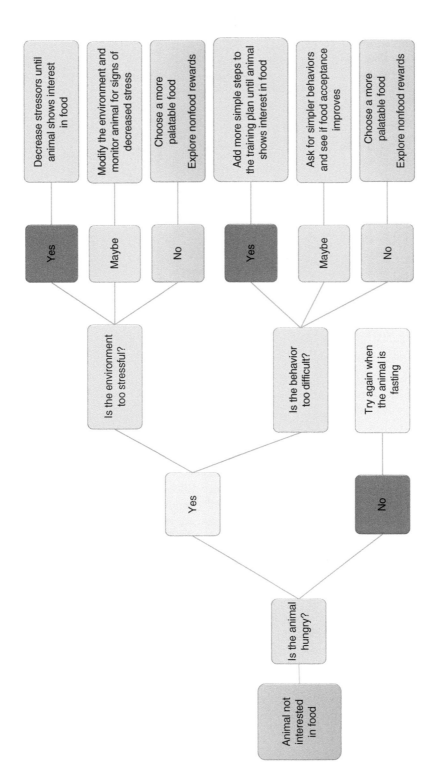

Figure 3.13 Flow chart to improve food acceptance. Animals will not accept food in the hospital for a variety of reasons. Use this chart to determine solutions to improve food acceptance.

(a)

(b)

(c)

Figure 3.14 (a–c) Primary reinforcers include food for most dogs and cats. Many cats also like this type of tactile interaction, and will work for tactile reinforcement.

3.5.2.3 What About Secondary Reinforcers?

Secondary reinforcers derive their value from being paired with primary reinforcers in a predictive relationship. For this reason, secondary reinforcers are also referred to as conditioned reinforcers [5, 8]. For example, the clicker is a secondary reinforcer. A click is heard; a delicious treat appears. The click predicts the treat often enough that the click becomes a conditioned reinforcer because it consistently predicts the appearance of a primary reinforcer. You will know the click has become a conditioned reinforcer when the animal responds to the click by anticipating a treat (orienting to the handler, raised ears, eager facial expression, tail wag, etc.) [5].

Money is a good example of a conditioned reinforcer for most people. We cannot eat money; it will not quench our thirst or give us shelter. However, money can predict the presence of a primary reinforcer because it can be exchanged for food, water, shelter, and much more. Think about how you feel when given a bigger paycheck or handed money for your birthday. Money is reinforcing because it leads to receiving the primary reinforcement of your choice, which triggers happy feelings. Money is only valuable if it retains its purchasing power, and in reality, the value of money is somewhat arbitrary and can change. If the money you received for your paycheck became

Table 3.2 Primary and secondary reinforcers: Primary reinforcers require no learning history, while secondary reinforcers have been classically conditioned to be reinforcing because they predict primary reinforcement.

Primary reinforcers	Secondary or conditioned reinforcers
Food	Money (humans!)
(and food acquisition sequences)	Click
Water	Verbal bridge
Reproductive opportunity	Known cue
Shelter	Location, odor, or object
Feelings of joy or welfare	Tugging, play, games
Rewarding without *any learning history*	*History of* predicting *primary reinforcers*

like every other piece of paper and you could no longer use it to buy anything, it would hold little value for you. This concept is important because it applies to the trainer's task of maintaining the value of secondary reinforcers. A click is a way for an animal to "purchase" a treat. It's important for the click to continue to allow the animal to buy treats; otherwise, the click will lose its value and the animal will be less motivated to try to earn clicks.

Other types of conditioned reinforcers used by trainers are praise from a familiar and preferred person, toys, and known cues. A cue such as "sit" can become a conditioned reinforcer when trained using positive reinforcement. The trainer gives the cue "sit," the pet sits, and a treat is given. The cue "sit" begins to predict a behavior that is linked to a primary reinforcer. Through classical conditioning, the cue "sit" and the behavior of sitting can cause a positive emotional change in the animal similar to what they experience when receiving the treat that generally follows. After the cue is well understood by the learner, it can reinforce and mark the previous behavior like a clicker would [8, 9]. Using behaviors as conditioned reinforcers is how we chain multiple behaviors together and give only one food treat at the end. Table 3.2 shows a comparison between some primary and secondary reinforcers for most animals.

3.5.3 Building Behaviors: A Good Foundation

A complex behavior like reading requires us to first learn the foundations of the alphabet, how to make words, what the words represent and mean, and how they connect together forming sentences and paragraphs. As we become more advanced readers, we learn that similar words or chains of words can have different meanings depending upon context. Just like learning to read, to become a proficient in teaching cooperative veterinary care, you'll need a good foundation made up of many component skills. Good trainers understand learning theory, and also correctly observe and accurately interpret communication from their animal learners. Constructing training plans, using marker-based training, using lure-reward training, and applying basic behavior modification techniques are all critical materials for building a well-rounded veterinary trainer.

Like the trainer, the animal needs a good foundation as well. For an animal to engage in veterinary training, useful foundation behaviors include paying attention or attending to the trainer, the ability to be still or stationary, responding to the clicker or other marker, responding to cues, stationing, and targeting. A good foundation for trainer and learner will help your team build complex behaviors. If you want to teach complex behaviors, you will need to train the foundation behaviors separately first.

3.5.4 Foundations for the Trainer

3.5.4.1 Methods

For veterinary training, we suggest three main methods of applying positive reinforcement to teach an animal a behavior: lure-reward training, shaping, and capturing. Shaping and capturing have already been described earlier. **Luring** is suitable for basic or simple behaviors and behaviors that are needed only once, while shaping is more appropriate for complex behaviors and serial behaviors. Shaping and capturing have been detailed earlier in this chapter, and we will discuss luring here.

Lure-reward training uses strategic movement of food lures to encourage an animal into a certain position or location [5]. A few examples of luring include encouraging a cat to follow a treat out of a carrier, or a dog to follow a treat while walking to the exam room. The position of the lure, what is being used to lure the animal, and the eventual training goals for the behavior all combine to determine the proper luring technique. Because the lure can easily become part of the cue for the behavior, it is important to limit the use of luring to select appropriate situations [5].

Correct luring will show the animal where to go or what position to assume, be physically comfortable for both the trainer and the animal, deliver a primary reinforcer once the animal is in position, and allow for the addition of a cue during the training process (Figure 3.15). Luring the animal means delivering treats at a rapid enough rate that the animal makes progress in the correct direction, while staying interested in the process. A good lure is like a pact or a promise. It acts as a magnet the pet *wants* to follow. When the animal gets to the point where the lure was offered, a small amount of food is given. One analogy is that luring is like following stepping stones across a stream. Each stepping stone is a stopping point along the path where reinforcement happens while you are on your way to the goal of getting across. If the animal is reluctant to make forward progress, assess the animal and the environment. Assuming the animal's overall stress level is low

Figure 3.15 Correct luring means the animal is willing to move freely toward the treats, and they are positioned so the animal will perform the desired behavior.

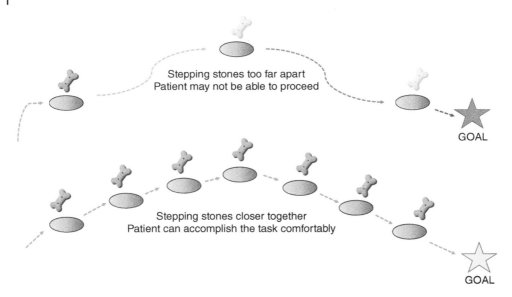

Figure 3.16 Stepping stones. When luring, shaping, or trying to achieve any goal behavior, the process must include enough incremental steps so the patient can achieve success. Assure each step feels comfortable and possible for the learner. Keep the stepping stones close enough together for the patient to successfully reach the goal behavior.

and the environment is sufficiently welcoming to allow training, animals who will not follow the lure are communicating they are confused or lack motivation. In these cases, we can refer back to the stepping stone analogy. Either the stepping stones are too far apart, they are trying to span a gap that is too wide (we are asking too much of the learner), or the reward found when the learner gets to the stepping stone is not sufficiently desirable (Figure 3.16).

Video 3.9 shows two methods of luring a puppy onto the scale. In the first example, the puppy is reluctant to move. The environment is not overly stressful, and the puppy is motivated by the tasty canned food, but the "stepping stones" are too far apart. Each time the puppy gets to the point where the lure was presented, the treat is pulled further away before he can eat anything. The puppy is reluctant to move because the rate of reinforcement is too low, and the distance he must move for a small bite of food is constantly changing. In the second example, the video shows the correct way to lure the puppy. The trainer makes the lure increments closer together, and assures the puppy is allowed to eat something at each stopping point.

3.5.5 Modeling

With **modeling**, the trainer uses a body prompt or light touch to demonstrate what we want the animal to do [9]. Modeling a paw lift or hug is a quick way to get started training a behavior, but the training plan needs to include a plan to fade the prompt over time. Because modeling is one of the few times we will start by touching the animal, it is important that we closely observe the animal's response to touching and assure there is no unwanted sensitization.

Whether using lure-reward or modeling, the best practice is to use the smallest amount of prompting necessary to elicit the behavior. Gradually, use smaller and smaller amounts of prompting until the animal is offering the behavior without the prompt. As with other methods, modeling uses a combination of positive reinforcement with desensitization and classical conditioning or counter conditioning to achieve the result of a happy patient performing the desired behavior at the end of the training process.

- Modeling can also be used to teach acceptance of touch, as in **Video 3.10**, Monique uses modeling by touching Barley's elbow to show him how to raise a front leg for cephalic access. Many dogs are sensitive to having their feet touched, but more tolerant of touching of the proximal limb. Over time, the prompt of raising the leg from the elbow can be faded to the cue of a light touch to the elbow will elicit the dog to raise the front limb for cephalic access.

Luring, Shaping, and Capturing: Teaching a Puppy to Go To a Mat

Luring
- Hold a delicious treat close to the puppy's nose
- Puppy is "magnetized" onto the treat
- Trainer slowly moves treat toward the mat
- Puppy receives a lick or nibble of the treat every few steps toward the mat
- Once the puppy has moved onto the mat, mark, and treat
- Tossing a treat onto the mat rather than using it as a "magnet" on the puppy's nose is also luring

Capturing
- Place the mat in an area ahead of time
- Puppy is allowed to freely explore the area
- Observe the puppy's movements
- When the puppy explores the area and coincidentally moves onto the mat, mark and treat

Shaping
- Trainer is ready with a mat down, treats, clicker, and puppy
- Puppy is free to explore the area
- Trainer carefully watches puppy's movements
- Any behavior which could lead to the goal of being on the mat leads to mark/treat
    - Glance at mat
    - Sniff mat
    - Turn toward mat
    - Look at mat
    - Coincidentally move toward mat
    - Intentionally move toward mat
    - Lean over mat
    - Step toward mat one or several steps
    - Place a paw on mat
    - Place multiple paws on mat
    - Place all paws on mat
    - Place all paws on mat and remain there

Modeling
- Put mat down, place puppy near mat
- Gently place a finger under the puppy's harness and guide it to step onto the mat
- Mark/treat on mat

3.5.6 Cues and Cueing

If we remember the ABCs of behavior – antecedent, behavior, and consequence – we know that behaviors follow antecedents, and consequences follow behaviors. A cue is also called an antecedent or **discriminatory stimulus** [3, 5, 8]. A cue is something that comes before the behavior; it is a clue to the animal that "if you perform this behavior, reinforcement may occur." Essentially, a cue is a signal to the animal that reinforcement is available for a certain behavior. Cues can be intentional or accidental, and can be environmental or handler-based. Cues that come from the trainer are generally signals, tactile information, words, sounds, or a combination of these. Animals are usually more sensitive to signals and body movements or postures, while people communicate primarily with words. In the training videos, you will note the technicians speak frequently, but this is largely for the benefit of observers.

For an animal to understand a cue, it needs to be consistent. The same signal, gesture, word, or combination should mean reinforcement is available for one consistent behavior. As the trainer, we need to be mindful of what we would like the cue for a behavior to be, and make sure we present the cue in the same fashion for every repetition so it is easy for the animal to understand what we mean. There are a few behaviors that require the animal to tolerate variety. For example, auscultation requires the stethoscope in several different areas, and not every veterinarian may perform auscultation in exactly the same way. The "cue" for auscultation in this case may be the presence of a stethoscope and a word rather than a precise body movement or signal.

Sometimes it is impractical to teach the final cue from the beginning of the training process. For example, say we want a dog to step onto the scale with the verbal cue "mat." In the early stages, the cue for this may look like me standing near the scale and pointing, which is a prompt most dogs would understand. To change the cue, we can use a process called a *cue transfer*. The cue transfer is simply giving the new cue, then giving the current cue, waiting for the behavior, and then reinforcing the behavior (Figure 3.17). For this example, we would say "mat," then we would stand in the prompt position and point. After a few repetitions, the animal will offer the behavior preemptively in response to the new cue, rather than waiting for the initial cue. Once this occurs, the new cue can be used exclusively.

Lastly, cues are related to stimulus control. Establishing stimulus control is an advanced training skill, and may be useful in some circumstances or unnecessary in others. **Stimulus control** means the behavior occurs on cue, only on cue, not in response to a different cue, and not when the cue is not being given (Table 3.3) [8, 9]. Often animals will offer behaviors that the trainer has reinforced in the past, even when the behavior has not been cued. Some behaviors are desirable when the trainer or owner wants the behavior, but problematic if the animal offers them at the wrong time

Figure 3.17 Cue transfer steps. A known behavior can be placed on a new cue by using the new cue to predict the old cue. After several repetitions (more repetitions for more complex behaviors), the learner should begin to offer the behavior in response to the new cue.

Table 3.3 The four factors of stimulus control.

• When the cue is given, the behavior occurs promptly	• When the cue is absent, the behavior does not occur
• When the cue is given, only the cued behavior occurs and no other	• When a different cue is given, the behavior does not occur

or in the wrong context. One example is if a trainer teaches a dog to "speak." Barking may be desirable when the cue is given, but if the dog offers barking off-cue to try to obtain reinforcement, or "push the cookie button," it can present problems in the wrong context. When you see stimulus control mentioned in this book, it is for practical reasons rather than academic training reasons. *Refer to the Appendix for details on achieving stimulus control.*

3.5.7 Foundations for the Learner

Like the trainer, the learner will need a few foundation behaviors to achieve the best results for veterinary training. These foundation behaviors are helpful for almost every veterinary patient, and it is helpful to teach them as early in the training process as is feasible and safe. Foundation behaviors can be used to prompt and build new behaviors and improve communication between the veterinary team and the patient in a variety of different situations. The foundation behaviors are nose targeting, paw targeting, stationing, response to cues, stillness, and attention to the handler.

3.5.7.1 Nose Target
Nose target refers to the behavior of teaching an animal to touch her nose to something. Sometimes the target is the trainer's hand, or a target stick, or a specified object like a training disc or paper marker (Figure 3.18). Nose targeting is useful because it allows the trainer to change where the animal is, direct the animal to orient a specific way, and show the animal how to move from point A to point B without using a food lure and without touching the patient.

Figure 3.18 A variety of objects used to train nose targeting.

Figure 3.19 This dog is targeting the trainer's hand with his nose.

3.5.7.1.1 *Teaching Nose Targeting: Canine*

First, assess the environment. Work in an area that is not too distracting, and where the learner feels comfortable. Remember: if stress levels are too high, it will be difficult for the dog to focus and learn something new. Assure the dog is motivated and likes the rewards you have, but keep your hands empty and away from your pockets. Hold a clicker in one hand; the opposite hand should be empty. Most dogs are naturally curious and have a terrific sense of smell. Open your empty hand and show your palm to the dog. The curious dog will generally sniff or lick your hand (Figure 3.19). Click the instant you feel contact with your hand to capture the nose target, and then reach into your treat bag for a reward. The click should occur while the dog is in contact with your hand, and the treat will follow afterward. Repeat this process for several repetitions, until the dog participates without hesitation.

Once the dog is happily targeting one hand, change hands and reinforce her for targeting the opposite hand as well. Next, assure the dog is touching the hand quickly when it is presented. Offer the hand target, and count in your head to five seconds. If, within five seconds, the dog has not touched, remove access to your hand target for five seconds, and then try again. The goal is for the dog to promptly touch either hand. Once the dog is promptly touching either hand, you may wish to introduce a verbal cue for this behavior in addition to the visual cue of the flat palm. Many trainers use the word "target" or "touch" for this behavior. At the same time the palm is presented, speak the verbal cue as well so the dog has a chance to learn both cues for this behavior.

Training Tip: Getting The Target

Some pets may be distracted, or have trouble noticing the hand target at first. Wait until the pet is looking at you, then present your hand. The movement of your hand will often entice the animal to investigate, leading to a nose touch.

Once the dog is willing to touch either hand, and do so promptly, begin offering the hand target in a variety of different positions: high, low, left, right, forward, and backward. Reinforce the behavior with a click/treat for every touch, while teaching the dog to reorient to find the hand target that has been offered.

Video 3.11 shows Monique introducing a patient to the clicker and hand target during her first visit to the hospital. The dog is naturally curious and sniffs Monique's hand. A click during the sniff after two repetitions turns into a nose touch. By the fourth click, the dog shows anticipation of food after the click. Off to a great start!

3.5.7.1.2 Teaching Nose Targeting: Feline

As with dogs, assure the environment has few distractions, and is a comfortable place for the cat to work. It is important to be sure the cat is hungry and interested in the treats you are offering. Like dogs, cats are curious, but they tend to explore by sniffing and cheek rubbing rather than licking like a dog would. Offer an empty hand toward the cat, with one finger outstretched. Click for any interest shown in your finger, and then treat after the click. If the cat does not immediately make contact with your finger, make this a shaping exercise. At first, any interest in your finger earns a click and treat. The next steps are moving toward your finger and making contact with your finger. Once the cat will target one finger, as with dogs, change hands and offer a finger on the opposite hand.

After the cat is touching a finger on either hand, you may wish to introduce a verbal cue. In addition, begin offering the target finger in different locations such as up, down, left, right, forward, and back. Some cats may prefer to target an object rather than the trainer's hand. A target stick is useful to teach nose targeting for these individuals (Figure 3.20). A pen, chopstick, or other small thin object may also be used.

Video 3.12 shows a client using her target stick to show her dog how to move onto the scale and then into an exam room. The dog has learned through a series of clicks and treats to touch her nose to the ball on the end of the target stick to earn a reward. She can now follow the target stick in motion as well.

3.5.7.1.3 Alternative Targets

Hands and fingers are just the beginning as far as nose targeting goes. Target sticks, large spoons, tongue depressors, and pens are all examples of alternative targeting items. In some cases, it is not

Figure 3.20 This cat is targeting the stick with her nose.

appropriate to allow the patient to approach the trainer's hands. In other cases, the patient may be small, and reaching out to offer your hand will cause the trainer to loom over the patient in a counterproductive way. In addition, target sticks can be easier to use when having a patient follow, as this keeps the hands free for a leash, a clicker, and treats. Target sticks can also be used through kennel run doors or cage bars for cases in which protected contact is desired between the animal and the trainer. This technique is used in zoos and aquaria around the world every day.

    Video 3.13 shows using a target stick to teach a cat how to move into a carrier. The target stick is a good choice for this behavior because it can reach into the carrier without blocking the opening like a hand and arm would.

3.5.7.1.4 Following a Target

For both dogs and cats, once the pet understands how to touch a target in a variety of orientations, the pet is ready to learn to follow. Following a target can be used to move onto the scale, from the floor to a mat or the exam table, from the exam room to the treatment room, and anywhere else you need the patient to move.

It is important for the animal to be able to easily meet criteria when introducing this exercise. Remember the stepping stone analogy for luring. The same principles apply to following a target. Only ask the animal to move a few inches or a few steps at first, and proceed at the rate the animal is prepared to move.

First, present the target, whether it is your hand, a target stick, a spoon, and so on. As the animal shows interest in the target, move it an inch or two so the animal moves forward to reach the target. When the animal moves toward the target and approaches it, click and treat. With subsequent repetitions, gradually move the target greater distances for the animal to follow prior to reinforcement.

Training Tip: Targeting, Not Treating!

Remember, targeting means the animal is *choosing* to touch a target with a specific body part. Never place food on the target. Placing food on the target teaches the animal to eat food, not to make the choice to move to the target and touch it.

3.5.7.2 Paw Targeting – Canine and Feline

Paw targeting is the behavior of placing a paw on a designated target, such as the trainer's hand, a target disc, a mat, a washcloth, a towel, a paper target such as a sticky note, and so on. Paw targeting using a small mobile target is useful in getting animals to move around in the exam room, onto the scale or examination table, and into and out of kennels or carriers, and even to present paws for nail care training and peripheral venous access training.

3.5.7.2.1 Teaching a Paw Target

Work in an area that has few distractions, and assure the patient is interested in the rewards you have to offer. Select something to use as your paw target, such as a FitPAWS® target disc, a small section of a yoga mat or rug, or a small fabric or paper target such as a sticky note (Figure 3.21).

When working in a small area, capturing is often effective at teaching a paw target. Place the target in the area where the dog or cat is likely to be moving around. When the pet incidentally steps on the target, click during the instant the paw is touching the target, then follow the click with a treat. After a few repetitions, the animal will begin intentionally touching the target with

Figure 3.21 A variety of objects used to train paw targeting.

a paw. At this point, you may wish to add verbal cues and/or signals as cues in addition to the presence of the target, to allow flexibility later in your ability to determine when the animal will perform this behavior.

Shaping can also be used to teach paw targeting through successive approximations. When shaping, the target will be presented and the animal will earn clicks and treats for progressively approaching the desired behavior. For example, at first simply looking at the target would earn a click, then moving one step toward it, then moving several steps toward it, then raising a paw near it, and finally touching the target with part of a paw and the entire paw. At this point, you may wish to add a word and signal to use as the cue for paw targeting. Once the animal is approaching the target closely or stepping on it, it can be helpful to give the treat by rolling it or tossing it a short distance away as a "reset" point to begin another repetition.

In both cases, once the animal is offering the paw target behavior promptly when the target is presented or the cue is given, begin moving the target small distances, so the animal learns to traverse the distance to complete the target behavior. As with the process of teaching following a nose target, keep the distances short at first, and make sure the animal can easily achieve the goal. Gradually, the animal can be asked to move greater distances, and even up onto a platform or table, and in or out of a kennel or room.

Whether the capturing or shaping method is used, realize that many patients have a dominant paw preference, much like most people have a dominant hand for writing. If there is a particular paw you would like the animal to use for this behavior, select it early and only reinforce for the selected paw. In advanced training situations, it may be helpful to have an animal offer more than one specific paw. Patients are capable of learning to differentiate between each paw as a distinct targeting behavior with training.

Training Tip: Paw Targeting

Paw targeting (Figure 3.22) is a foundation behavior for many more complex skills, including nail board training. Nail board training is an alternative to nail trimming. Refer to Chapter 7 for more information.

(a)

(c)

(b)

Figure 3.22   (a–c) Three different stations. These are just a few examples among many possibilities.

Video 3.14 shows teaching paw targeting with a dog. The paw target is placed on the ground in an area the dog is likely to investigate. The target is big enough the dog can easily touch it with a paw. Once the dog begins to show understanding by repeating the paw target behavior several times, the target size can be faded and the target can be moved to new locations to show the dog how to place their paw in a designated location.

Paw targeting is an example of a skill that may benefit from stimulus control, or at least partial stimulus control. Some owners may object if their pet is offering the paw target behavior in new places or new situations, such as pawing at the owner to seek attention or request food. As a technician, it might be difficult for me to clean an animal's ears if he is trying to give me his paw in my hand. Most animals will learn the proper context for this behavior, but if the animal is offering the behavior at inappropriate times, an effort to achieve stimulus control may be helpful. (See "Stimulus Control" in the Appendix.)

3.5.7.3   Other Body Targets

As with teaching a nose target or paw target, other body targets can be taught. For example, chin or "chin rest," collar, side of neck, side of body, shoulder, hip, each leg, rear, or tail, etc. These advanced skills are discussed later in this book.

3.5.7.4   Go to Mat or Go to Station

Using a mat or station is teaching the animal how to move to a location or surface and stand, sit, or lie down on the target. These behaviors are to move the animal move around the room, onto the exam table, onto the scale, to a medication or treatment station in the clinic or at home, in and out of the kennel, to their bed to relax out of the way at home, and much more. Mat or station can be trained using lure-reward training, consider using capturing and shaping to train this behavior for best understanding on the part of the patient and for the most durable behavior under mild stress such as during veterinary procedures.

3.5.7.4.1   Teaching a Station

Work in an area with few distractions, and assure the animal is interested in your rewards in that environment. Choose a surface that is large enough the animal can simultaneously place four paws on the station with a little extra room. Particularly if the animal has little history of training, using a very large station such as a yoga mat, beach towel, or unfolded blanket can be helpful. These can then be folded into smaller sizes as the animal becomes more proficient. Introduce the mat, bed, rug, or other target, and wait. At first, click for any interest in the station such as looking at it, sniffing it, moving toward it, or moving around it. Gradually increase the criteria to leaning over the station, stepping onto the mat with part of a paw, then a whole paw, then more than one paw, and eventually all four paws. Once the animal is moving to the station reliably, ask for a known behavior with a strong history of reinforcement such as a sit or a down on the mat.

Placement of reward is important when teaching stationing. Some animals do best when receiving the treat on the mat, while others benefit from the treat being tossed away from the mat to reset for another attempt. Often, both are used: one on the station for the behavior, and a second rolled or tossed away to "reset" for a new repetition. Following food that is tossed is another useful foundation behavior.

When shaping, we need to find the balance between rate of reinforcement, increasing and decreasing criteria, and getting understanding from the animal without confusion. Finding the balance can seem overwhelming at first! Take the time to experiment and practice. You will not do any harm by practicing, and you'll build your skills and your confidence.

The rate of reinforcement needs to remain high enough that the animal can sustain interest during the session, but low enough that the animal is willing to offer "improvements" on the behavior. If looking at the target earns 20 clicks and treats in a row, the animal will be less likely to try to move toward the station because the reinforced behavior is looking, not moving. However, if the criterion is too difficult, such as expecting the animal to place four paws on the mat immediately, the rate of reinforcement will be too low and the animal may lose interest, or try offering other known behaviors instead of exploring this new skill.

Video 3.15 shows Monique working with a dog on her first visit to the hospital. The goal is to use a shaping procedure to encourage the dog to walk onto the mat, then use known cues to encourage the dog to lie down on the mat. Lying down on the mat is a form of targeting where the animal's whole body is on the designated destination or target area. Notice the clicks at first are for a glance, then movement, then placing one paw, multiple paws, and all paws onto the blue mat. Between each repetition, a treat is tossed away for the dog to follow to set up for a new opportunity to try the behavior again.

3.5.7.5 The Station as an Introduction to the Concept of Opting In

Once an animal knows how to move onto the station, it is the area where most veterinary training and handling will occur. Some people call this the "Medication Station." For veterinary training, we are focusing on specific behaviors that are useful for veterinary care and animal husbandry. Throughout the training plans presented later, you will see stations used to give animals the option to move into or out of a handling or training session. Stations are not the only way an animal can tell us if they are ready or not ready, but they are a great starting point. Choose a station that makes sense for the animal and the trainer, as well as the owner if the behavior such as taking medication will need to be repeated at home. In the clinic, common choices for a station include a rug, mat, yoga mat, nonslip exam table cover, low platform, or exam table (Figure 3.23).

Stationing allows the animal to opt into a procedure and choose to engage in training, or send a clear signal to the trainer the animal is uncomfortable and not ready for what is being asked. By giving the animal some control in this situation, we can reduce stress and anxiety, decrease fear, increase comfort, and increase the animal's ability to cooperate.

To introduce the station as an opt in or opt out signal, work in an area with few distractions, and make sure the animal is interested in your rewards in this environment. Make sure the animal is comfortable moving onto and off of the station, and that you have a clear mental image of what "on" the station looks like: ideally all the animal's paws are on the station, at least to begin (some animals may roll into a hip down, or fold back into a sit or down and end up a little bit off the mat but still look relaxed and willing to work). The patient should be free and unrestrained whenever this is safe. The patient may be tethered to a secure anchor if necessary. The use of protected contact may also be necessary at first (for example a basket muzzle). For patients requiring a tether or basket muzzle for safety, consider referral to a veterinary behaviorist, Veterinary Technician Specialist (VTS) Behavior, or other experienced professional if you are new to cooperative veterinary care and just getting started in your training journey.

Figure 3.23 Nail boards are an alternative to conventional nail trimming.

Once the animal is at the station, begin interacting. Coming to the station signifies an opportunity for considerable reinforcement. Reinforce every one to two seconds at first simply for remaining at the station. If the animal chooses to leave the station, pause giving treats and wait to see if they return. If they return to the station or show interest in the handler within five seconds, resume. Invite the animal back onto the station. If the animal is reluctant to return to the station, assess the animal, yourself, and the environment for sources of increased fear or stress.

When the patient is comfortable remaining at the station for several seconds in a row, begin introducing nonthreatening touching while the animal is stationed. This should be touching you know the animal will allow, tolerate, and hopefully enjoy. For dogs, this generally means a low rub on the chest between the front legs, or a gentle stroke along the sides. For cats, this generally means a light touch along the cheek or chin, or a gentle stroke along the back. Help the animal learn the "touching game." Touch, click, treat. Touch, click, treat. Each touch predicts a click and a treat. Very rapidly, the animal will begin happily anticipating touching. After five touches, toss a treat away to reset for a new round. The reset gives the animal an opportunity to choose if they would like to continue by opting in again, or if they would like to take a break. This method uses a combination of operant conditioning, desensitization, and classical conditioning to encourage a positive emotional response as well as the behavior of remaining at the station for touching.

If when you reach toward the animal their body language changes to show signs of reluctance or concern, stop reaching toward them and toss a treat away to encourage them to leave the station. If the animal chooses to leave the station when you reach for them, reward them for moving off the station when they are uncomfortable. Using a station gives the pet a voice: I am Ready or I am Not Ready. We must respect and appreciate when the animal communicates with us this way. If the animal does not know how to tell us they are not ready or are uncomfortable, they may escalate up the FAS Ladder, showing signs of self-defensive behavior. This compromises both handler safety and animal welfare.

The "Touching Game" is the very first introduction of stationing for consent to interact. Later in this book we discuss and show stationing as consent for veterinary procedures. Those exercises have their foundation in Touching Game.

Video 3.16 shows a kitten's first exposure to the idea of stationing. In this example, a combination of luring, capturing, and shaping is used to encourage the kitten to station. As the technician consistently rewards him when he comes to the blanket, he begins to return to the blanket more frequently.

3.5.7.6 Adding Duration

Nose targeting, paw targeting, body targeting, and stationing are all wonderful foundation behaviors. However, there are few medical tests and treatments we can accomplish in one to two seconds. Over time, it will be necessary to teach an animal how to hold the target position or station for gradually longer periods of time, until the release or end-of-behavior cue is given. Because a click is a signal that the behavior has been completed, adding duration is often as simple as *briefly* delaying the click. Using the example of Go to Mat, ask the animal to move onto the station, then mentally count "One banana." Click and treat at the end of the held position, and then gradually begin adding time before each click.

Tasks that always increase in difficulty can be demotivating for some learners. When adding duration, gradually ask for longer behaviors, but intermittently sneak shorter durations in as well. For example, if we are training for a 10-second hold, we may reinforce after 2, 5, 1, 10, 3, 9, 15, 11, 4, and 7 seconds. This is an average of 7 seconds of holding over 10 reinforcement events, which is close to the goal of 10 seconds without wearing out the learner by continuously asking for more and more difficult repetitions.

3.5.7.7 Attention to the Handler

Working with an animal on foundation behaviors will naturally cause her to check in with the handler more often. By teaching the animal that attending the handler is also a way to earn clicks and treats, we are giving the animal a reliable way to earn rewards between exercises, and establishing a way to begin training again if for some reason the patient opts out or becomes distracted. To teach attention to the handler, simply be aware of the patient's attention and focus. Anytime the patient checks in with the veterinary team member by looking at or turning toward them, click and treat. The animal should begin checking in more and more frequently with the veterinary trainer as the reinforcement history for this behavior grows. (This is also a great life skill for pet owners and their pets out in the world!).

For example, if a dog has come to the station and we are practicing ear handling, and the dog leaves the station, this is an opportunity to reinforce attending the trainer. As soon as the dog turns toward or looks at the trainer, click and treat. Now the dog will have returned his attention to the trainer and is showing he is likely ready to return to work. Invite the animal to station again and see what happens: usually an animal who is attending the trainer is ready to try again.

 Video 3.17 shows rewarding a young dog for attending the handler and following her. Notice the trainer moves around, which gives the puppy an opportunity to repeatedly orient toward the handler, showing she is ready to work. The trainer waits for the puppy to reorient and pay attention after each treat, then reinforces for attention.

Refer to the "Puppy Class Syllabus" in the Appendix for more detailed information about attention training.

3.5.7.8 Stillness

For most veterinary and handling procedures, it is quite helpful if the animal will remain stationary. Stillness is a learned skill! Teaching animals that stillness is rewarding helps build the foundation for care behaviors. Teaching stillness is an extension of stationing and the Touching Game to start.

Once the animal will come to the station and is comfortable with the Touching Game, gradually increase the duration of each touch. When you can touch the animal for one to two seconds, it's time to add stillness as a criterion for the click and treat. Touch the animal using a mild to moderate pressure and nice slow hand movements. Monitor the animal, and click when they are both allowing touch and have a still, stationary body. Deliver the treat calmly to encourage the animal to remain calm rather than moving excitedly to get the treat unless you choose to toss the treat to reset for a new repetition. Over time, you can add duration to the touch, move your hand around so there is motion in the touch, tenting skin, and other small changes to the touch while also watching for stillness.

3.6 Conclusion

Every interaction we have with a patient is a training opportunity. Unlike punishment-based methods, positive reinforcement and marker-based training do not carry serious risks when training mistakes happen, and will not result in harm to the patient if errors occur. The concepts introduced in this chapter of classical conditioning, desensitization, classical, and operant counterconditioning, and operant conditioning will all combine to make more advanced training plans for patients in subsequent chapters. By understanding the science of learning and applying the science, we can provide patient-centered veterinary care. Mastering these skills empowers technicians to provide the very best-quality care available for patients and clients.

References

1 Friedman, S. (2010). What's wrong with this picture? Effectiveness is not enough. *Association of Pet Dog Trainers Journal* 41–45.

2 Kalat, J. (2010). *Introduction to Psychology*. Independence, MO: Cengage Learning.

3 Skinner, B.F. (1945). The operational analysis of psychological terms. *Psychological Review* 52 (4): 270–278. https://doi.org/10.1037/h0062535.

4 Skinner, B.F. (1966). *The Behavior of Organisms*. New York: Appleton-Century-Crofts (First published in 1938.).

5 Martin, D. and Shaw, J. (2023). *Canine and Feline Behavior for Veterinary Technicians and Nurses*. Ames, IA: Wiley.

6 Herron, M., Shofer, F., and Reisner, I. (2009). Survey of the use and outcome of confrontational and non-confrontational training methods in client-owned dogs showing undesired behaviors. *Applied Animal Behaviour Science* 117 (1–2): 47–54.

7 Gilchrist, R.J., Gunter, L.M., Anderson, S.F., and Wynne, C.D.L. (2021). The click is not the trick: the efficacy of clickers and other reinforcement methods in training naïve dogs to perform new tasks. *PeerJ* 9: e10881. https://doi.org/10.7717/peerj.10881.

8 Ramirez, K. (1999). *Animal Training: Successful Animal Management through Positive Reinforcement*. Chicago: Shedd Aquarium Society.

9 Pryor, K. (1999). *Don't Shoot the Dog: The New Art of Teaching and Training*. New York: Bantam.

4

Successful Visits: Environment and Protocols to Prevent Fear and Stress

Prevention is always the best medicine! Why treat what we can prevent? In general practice, we spend a great deal of time preventing common diseases and parasites, and setting up preventive nutrition protocols, educational protocols, and testing protocols for monitoring health. Preventive medicine can and should also encompass behavioral health, inside, and outside the veterinary hospital. Compliance is a sizeable issue in veterinary medicine, and clients who own fearful pets are less likely to present them for wellness or interventional care, because of perceived stress [1]. Setting up the environment and basic protocols to prevent fear and stress in the veterinary hospital will prevent problem behaviors for many patients.

Pets of all ages can benefit from prevention, not just puppies and kittens. Preventive behavioral care geared toward making veterinary medical treatment easier and safer for people and pets as well as toward keeping pets in their homes and protecting against relinquishment starts with making a plan. Remember, fearful behaviors tend to intensify with time and repetition, especially when no intervention is provided. Every pet has a certain amount of "emotional capital" they can spend during a veterinary visit. Preserving emotional capital so it can be used for examination and treatments will make veterinary visits easier for patients, clients, and, veterinary professionals. Every interaction, from our first meeting with a client and patient, is an opportunity for success. While some animals may need extra training and medical management even when we have done everything we can for prevention, many patients will respond well to these preventive protocols. For those animals who need intervention, Chapters 5 through 7 will outline interventional plans suitable for every patient.

4.1 Setting Up for Success: Before the Visit

4.1.1 At Home

Imagine every time you get into the car, you go to the dentist's office or to pay your taxes. You might learn to have an unpleasant opinion of car rides because they predict something unpleasant. It's easy for dogs and cats to learn to fear travel in the car, harnesses, and carriers if they always predict something unpleasant. Puppy and kitten owners as well as new clients should be advised to make wearing a harness and collar fun. Clients should take time to teach pets to enjoy short rides in the car by visiting enjoyable locations such as going for a pleasant walk or visiting a favorite location. Cat carriers should be kept in the main living area of the cat's quarters, incorporated with a normal resting place such as a cat tree, and paired with enjoyable items like catnip, cat treats, and special toys. Treating cat carriers with a synthetic pheromone product prior to travel may help cats relax.

Cooperative Veterinary Care, Second Edition. Monique Feyrecilde.
© 2024 John Wiley & Sons, Inc. Published 2024 by John Wiley & Sons, Inc.
Companion website: www.wiley.com/go/feyrecilde/cooperative

CALM or FEAR?

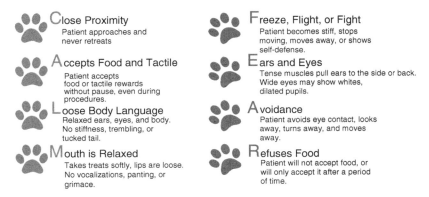

Close Proximity
Patient approaches and never retreats

Accepts Food and Tactile
Patient accepts food or tactile rewards without pause, even during procedures.

Loose Body Language
Relaxed ears, eyes, and body. No stiffness, trembling, or tucked tail.

Mouth is Relaxed
Takes treats softly, lips are loose. No vocalizations, panting, or grimace.

Freeze, Flight, or Fight
Patient becomes stiff, stops moving, moves away, or shows self-defense.

Ears and Eyes
Tense muscles pull ears to the side or back. Wide eyes may show whites, dilated pupils.

Avoidance
Patient avoids eye contact, looks away, turns away, and moves away.

Refuses Food
Patient will not accept food, or will only accept it after a period of time.

Figure 4.1 CALM or FEAR? Patient assessment is complex and fluid. Use these basics as a good starting point.

Help clients know what kind of cat carrier is best. A hard-sided carrier with quick-release clips on the sides and back is easiest to use at the veterinary hospital. These carriers are safe and secure, and quick and easy to disassemble for veterinary visits allowing the cat to sit in the familiar carrier bottom during most of the visit. Soft-sided carriers can be useful as well, especially for cats who already have a conditioned emotional response to a hard-sided carrier, or cats who require sedation on arrival for examination. Figure 4.1 shows a cat carrier that has clips which are easy to open for veterinary visits, and provides safety during travel. Cats and small dogs can also use the SleepyPod carrier, a crash-tested carrier in which the bottom of the carrier is a comfortable bed and the top of the carrier zips on and off for transportation.

If a dog is so fearful of car rides that the owner has difficulty loading him, or a cat is so concerned about a carrier she disappears as soon as she sees it, intervention rather than prevention is needed. Desensitization and classical counterconditioning will help, and sometimes in-home coaching is needed to help clients learn to load pets into the carrier or the car. Many pets will benefit from a prescription medication and supplements to help them relax and ease loading. In severe cases, consultation with a **veterinary behaviorist** may be indicated.

4.1.2 Making the Appointment

Our first opportunity to set up a successful appointment is when the client calls. A knowledgeable receptionist is crucial for successful patient visits, particularly for first-time clients and patients. Clients should be instructed to make sure their pets (both dogs and cats!) are hungry when they come to the clinic, and to bring some of the pet's favorite treats and a toy if the pet loves toys. Ideally, one pet should visit per appointment to reduce any social pressure in the exam room. One exception to the single-pet guideline would be bonded pets who are allies and are more anxious when they are separated but more relaxed when they visit together. Anxiety can be contagious between pets, and one nervous animal can spread the nervousness through the whole exam room. Also, multiple pet visits prolong the time each pet must spend in the hospital. Lastly, each veterinary team member can only devote his or her full attention to one pet at a time, including monitoring for and reducing fear and anxiety. If multiple pets must be scheduled, make a plan to keep the pets as comfortable as possible. Cats should each have their own carriers rather than being transported together.

Table 4.1 Checklist for scheduling appointments.

☐ Check medical record for notes
☐ Schedule special needs patients accordingly
☐ Remind client to give any necessary medications
☐ Remind client to bring a hungry pet
☐ Remind client to bring favorite treats and toy
☐ Calling from the parking area helps with traffic control
☐ Ask for any questions or concerns before the visit.

Dogs need to be leashed, and may even be seen one at a time rather than simultaneously if a safe nonstressful arrangement can be made for each dog to wait while the other is being treated. Fear Free[sm] has developed a Pre Visit Questionnaire which can easily be adapted to send via email with appointment reminders, and asks clients about what will work best for their pets well in advance of their arrival.

Ideally, a portion of the medical record should be dedicated to use as the Emotional Medical Record. The Emotional Record is a good place to record the patient's preferences (favorite treat, location, provider), concerns (triggers of escalation of fear, anxiety, and stress [FAS]), and special needs (no contact with other pets, pre-visit prescriptions, sedation for examination, etc.) If a dog needs extra space and is stressed by the presence of other dogs, there will be a note in the medical record indicating this need. The receptionist should schedule this dog's appointment at a quiet time when no other dogs will cross paths with the dog who needs space. Waiting in the lobby can expend a great deal of emotional capital for pets and people. Consider having clients check-in when they arrive by calling or texting, then wait to invite them inside until an exam room is ready. If the hospital has a separate entry through a side door, this can also help diminish stress by preventing social interactions between patients or between pets and other clients. Table 4.1 provides a checklist for scheduling appointments.

When transporting patients to the veterinary hospital, clients should be instructed to make sure the car is a comfortable temperature before placing the pet there. Any music playing should be considered calming for pets. The pet should be safely contained in a pet carrier or transport harness. Clients should take care with driving maneuvers. Fear Free Happy Homes provides a very nice client education video about how to make the trip to the veterinary hospital less stressful. A link is easily shared with clients via email.

4.2 During the Visit

4.2.1 Patient Assessment Tools

Assessing the patient is a key in determining what interactions will be most appropriate. The Fear Freesm FAS Spectrum was introduced in Chapter 2 to offer a numeric scoring system for a pet's emotional state. This chapter is all about prevention, and Chapters 5 through 7 will each be dedicated to progressively more fearful, anxious, or stressed patients. To determine the patient's stress level, we suggest the following evaluation criteria:

Dogs:

(1) Food acceptance
(2) Body language
(3) Proximity preference.

Cats:

(1) Food acceptance and/or toy acceptance, tactile interaction acceptance
(2) Body language
(3) Proximity preference and exploration versus hiding.

During each interaction, every team member should be familiar with these three criteria, and monitor them throughout the visit. As discussed in Chapter 2, changes in food acceptance, body language, and proximity preference are cues to the veterinary team about the animal's emotional state and comfort level. The goal of prevention is to set up an environment and set of protocols such that the animal's stress level remains low or absent as a baseline in the hospital whenever possible (Figure 4.1 provides a quick reference graphic for patient assessment).

Dr. Colleen Koch has developed a useful algorithm for making decisions about what treatments are appropriate at each stage of a visit, and taking into consideration wants versus needs (Figure 4.2). This algorithm provides helpful suggestions in a succinct manner. The concepts introduced in this algorithm will be revisited repeatedly. The vast majority of what we do in regular practice are wants. Needs are lifesaving measures for unstable patients. Temperature measurement, vaccination, conscious x-rays, oral examination, and lab work on healthy or chronically ill patients are all examples of wants. Wants can always be rescheduled, postponed, or abbreviated for patient well-being. A training plan and possibly medical intervention can be set up, and then the patient can be better prepared for treatments in the category of wants.

4.2.2 The Lobby: Setup and Equipment

Make sure there are plenty of tasty treats available in the reception area, in addition to any treats the owner may have brought along from home. In a perfect world, patients spend very little time in the reception lobby, but in case of waiting the lobby should be set up and marked with separate areas for dogs and cats. Figure 4.3 shows an example of a reception desk with a selection of treats above the scale, and a reception area divided into smaller waiting areas. These areas can be separated quite simply by using the positioning of chairs into two distinct seating areas, planters, displays, solid benches, half-walls, screens, and more. An elevated area to place cat carriers is helpful, rather than placing carriers on the floor or the owner's lap. Pheromone diffusers can be used, and if music is played it should be relaxing.

Social contact should be minimized in the waiting area. Social stressors such as interacting with other pets or with strangers can increase anxiety and decrease the patient's ability to cooperate for treatments. Dogs should be on a short leash (no retractable leashes) attached to a harness, martingale, or flat collar. Cats should be in a cat carrier or harness and leash. Prong collars, choke collars, and electronic collars are not appropriate for the veterinary environment. The client services team should monitor pets and people, to assure no inappropriate interactions occur, and kindly interrupt inappropriate interactions by redirecting and escorting the client to a different area or to an exam room. Table 4.2 shows a checklist to begin setting up the lobby.

4.2.3 The Entrance: Dogs

Our first interaction with the patient begins in the parking lot or the reception area. A properly trained team member should greet the patient and client. It is crucial for the client services and reception team to be trained in the evaluation tools of food acceptance, body language, and proximity preferences. It can be easy to accidentally overwhelm mildly nervous dogs with good intentions. The receptionist may choose to offer treats and a greeting if the dog is comfortable and happy

Algorithm for handling patients

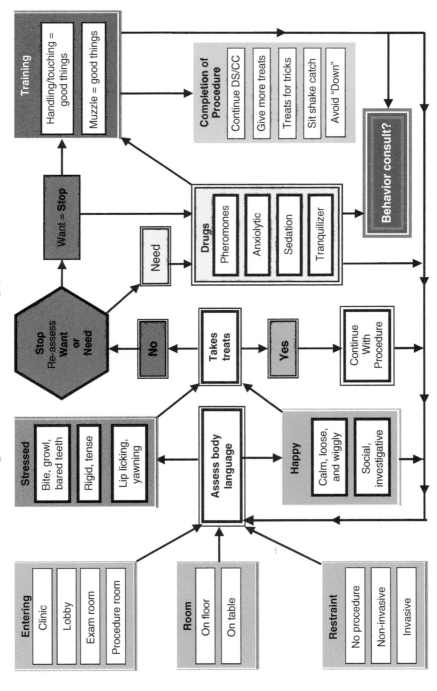

Figure 4.2   Patient-handling plans. This detailed algorithm outlines planning patient care based on patient assessment, medical therapies indicated, and tools available. Source: Courtesy of Colleen Koch DVM DACVB.

(a)

(b)

Figure 4.3 Reception area. (a) Divided waiting area at Mile High Animal Hospital. (b) Wide variety of treats in the reception area at Mercer Island Veterinary Clinic.

to receive them, and should discontinue any interaction that increases the dog's stress level. The receptionist should direct the owner to an examination room, or to appropriate waiting area until an examination room is ready.

4.2.4 The Scale

Have you ever wondered why dogs hate the scale? Unlike us, it has nothing to do with the number on the display. Consider the scale from a dog's perspective. A stranger or your owner pulls you to

Table 4.2 Reception and lobby checklist.

☐ Nonslip surfaces
☐ Variety of treats
☐ Pheromone product diffusers
☐ Calming music (if any)
☐ Separate areas by species, or visual dividers
☐ Elevated area for cat carriers
☐ Loaner leashes and carriers available
☐ Signs reminding about appropriate collars.

---

a wall or a corner, and pushes you onto a slippery, unstable surface. Every time this unpleasant experience happens, it is followed by the even more unpleasant experience of going into the exam room for temperature measurement, needle pokes, and a probing and prodding examination. If we consider it from the dog's point of view, it makes sense. When going onto the scale is an unpleasant experience that predicts an even more unpleasant one, classical conditioning will cause the dog to become frightened of the scale itself.

To correctly weigh a dog, we must abandon the pushing, pulling, and the owner scolding, "Sit. SIT. SIT!" We need to assure the scale is as inviting and comfortable as possible for the dog. The scale should have a nonslip surface and should be in an open area when possible. Many clinics, including the clinic of the author, have recessed scales so the top is flush with the floor, making the transition easier for dogs. Keep treats near the scale, and use a treat trail to encourage dogs to walk onto the scale. If the dog already has the foundation skill of following a target, hand targeting, or stationing on a mat, these skills can also be used to make weighing a breeze (Figure 4.4). If the dog is mildly anxious, having the owner make the treat trail is sometimes helpful. If a patient shows ongoing or escalating fear of the scale, consider postponing the weight until later in the veterinary visit. Carefully observe and coach the owner when necessary, as sometimes owners will escalate out of frustration or embarrassment when a dog is difficult to weigh, worsening the experience for the dog.

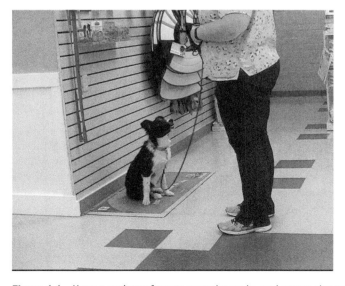

Figure 4.4 Keep a variety of treats near the scale, and assure the scale has a nonslip surface.

4.2.4.1 Video: Weighing a Large Dog

In Video 4.1, you will see a new technician working to get a large dog onto the scale. The greyhound is friendly, but confused about what he is supposed to do and reluctant to step onto the scale. Eventually, the technician lifts the dog by herself onto the scale, which presents a risk for injury as well. During the second attempt, the technician uses a treat trail to encourage this dog to move onto the scale. Notice how she positions her body to make the path onto the scale obvious without looming over the dog, and allows him to move at his own pace. The dog freely follows the treat trail on a loose leash, and has a positive experience on the scale. This takes less than half the time of physically manipulating him onto the scale, and causes none of the associated stress. After a few examples like this one, most pet owners can walk their own dogs onto the scale in a gentle and effective manner.

4.2.5 The Entrance: Cats

In contrast to dogs, who usually will wish to greet the reception team, most cats will be in a carrier, and many cats experience a higher level of stress at the veterinary hospital. The client services team should greet the client in a calm and friendly manner, and either invite the owner and cat directly into an exam room, or provide a quiet area in the lobby to wait until a room is ready. Many owners will try to lift the cat carrier by the handle, which allows the carrier to swing in an unsettling way. Encourage clients to lift the carrier from the bottom like carrying a gift. When inviting cat owners to the exam room, the client services representative may wish to carry the cat herself, or instruct the owner to carry the kennel from the bottom using both hands to avoid swinging movements that will make the cat feel unsteady.

4.2.6 The Exam Room

Moving into the examination room can be frightening for some animals, especially those who have had negative experiences in the past. To make the exam room as inviting as possible, follow these simple tips. First, when possible, have species-specific exam rooms. Particularly cats will benefit from having their own room. Interspecies social signaling is decreased, which can reduce stress levels for some patients. Always cleanse examination rooms thoroughly using a disinfectant to remove odors and pheromones. Select a disinfectant free from harsh fragrances and which does not cause "nose-blindness." Use synthetic pheromone diffusers or other preparations in each exam room. It is ok to use canine and feline synthetic pheromones in the same space: they are only perceived by the target species. Provide nonslip, comfortable surfaces for patients, including on the floor, on the exam table, and anywhere else the pet is expected to spend time. To avoid patients getting trapped or stuck in tight spaces, select closed-bottom furniture and position it to limit the risk of cornering pets. Store a variety of delicious treats of different flavors and textures in the exam rooms, and means to administer them such as dishes, paper plates, sturdy plastic spoons, tongue depressors, syringes, and pretzel rods. Keep a few likely favorite toys in the rooms as well, such as tennis balls, squeaky toys, and a cat fishing pole. Store the basic equipment you are likely to need during visits in the exam room, or gather all the equipment needed for a patient at the beginning of the visit to minimize the need to relocate the patient or repeatedly enter the exam room.

Figure 4.5 shows examples of a variety of nonslip surfaces in the exam room, and suggestions for a variety of treats, toys, and treat delivery options to keep in each room. Table 4.3 provides a checklist to begin setting up the exam room.

(a)

(b)

(c)

Figure 4.5 (a–c) Nonslip surfaces should be provided in the exam room, as well as a variety of treats and toys close at hand.

4.2.7 The Exam Room Experience: Dogs

Dogs should be encouraged to move around the room and explore. Larger patients should be allowed to stay on the floor or a low platform, while smaller patients might be more comfortable beside the client on a bench or elevated on the exam table. Select an area to work based on the dog's preferences. Food acceptance, body language, and proximity preferences will tell you where the dog feels most comfortable.

Table 4.3 Exam room preparation checklist.

☐ Nonslip surfaces on floor and table
☐ Wide variety of treats
☐ Toys, including food-dispensing toys
☐ Treat delivery tools (spoon, target, and pretzel rod)
☐ Pheromone products
☐ Calming music (if any)
☐ Separate areas by species, or visual dividers
☐ Syringes, needles, blood tubes, etc.
☐ Otoscope, ophthalmoscope, etc.
☐ Scissors and zip ties to open/close carriers if needed
☐ Body language posters
☐ Passive educational materials about care planning
☐ Signs reminding about appropriate collars.

When collecting a history, the technician should be multitasking. When safe, allow dogs freedom to explore, approach, or retreat. Use treats tossed around the room to promote exploration and comfort, and offer food to assess food acceptance. Make note of the dog's body language and proximity preferences to you, as well as which treats the dog prefers. When the history is completed, if the dog is comfortable being approached and touched, collect the vital signs as appropriate.

With any touching, begin in a less sensitive area before moving to a more sensitive one. For example, when palpating a femoral pulse, begin touching along the shoulder, then glide your hand down the back to the flank and then to the medial femoral area. During touch, assess, and reassess the dog's body language and food acceptance. Ideally, limit the number of times touch is started and stopped, and instead maintain at least some contact and glide between body areas. Fear Free[sm] refers to these methods as using the Touch Gradient.

Pair touching with something wonderful! In many cases, the owner can be helpful if instructed in proper techniques for giving food, where to place the food, how quickly to give the food, and to notify you if the dog stops eating. The same principles can be used to measure body temperature. Begin touch in a less sensitive area, and make sure the touch predicts wonderful treats. Minimally displace the tail laterally or elevating it if it is wagging, and then measure the temperature. If the dog is not comfortable with temperature measurement, save this procedure until the end of the visit, or omit it if the information is not truly necessary. In some cases, the risk to the patient and staff of measuring rectal temperature far outweighs the benefit of collecting this information. New products measuring axillary temperature, TempScan[tm] microchips, and ear thermometers can be good alternatives to rectal temperature measurements, particularly in healthy and higher FAS patients.

In Chapter 2, Figures 2.6 and 2.7 showed a gradient example of relative sensitivity in dogs and cats. The lightest shaded areas have the lowest concentration of nerve endings, while darker shaded areas contain a higher density of nerve endings. The darkest shaded areas will be the most sensitive to touch for most patients, while the lightest areas are the least sensitive. One exception is the cheek of the cat, which is rich with nerve endings, but a pleasurable area when touched for many cats.

Video 4.2 shows measuring the temperature of a puppy on her first visit. Not only is this the puppy's first visit, but also the clients are first-time dog owners. The owner has been instructed to keep treats near the puppy's nose, keep the treats stationary, and provide treats repeatedly until the procedure is complete. The technician begins touch along the puppy's back, then slides to the rump, and gently moves the tail prior to measuring the puppy's temperature. This puppy is learning many things in these brief seconds: how to enjoy being on the table, touching predicts wonderful things, temperature measurement is associated with wonderful things, and how to hold still for treats. The client is also learning: that the team cares about this puppy's experience, the technician loves puppies, the puppy can learn to like veterinary care, and how to properly deliver treats to encourage a dog to hold still.

Once the history and vital signs measurement have been completed, it is time to round the veterinarian. When providing the medical history, also provide information about the dog's emotional state, preferred working area, treat preference, and how he responded to touch. Good communication helps each team member save time, improves efficiency, and improves the patient experience.

Plan the physical examination like every other aspect of the visit: to build the most comfortable experience for the patient. To improve cooperation and decrease fear and anxiety in the exam room, start with the least invasive touches, such as checking the skin and coat, lymph node **palpation**, and auscultation. Gradually work up to more invasive touching, such as the abdominal palpation, ear examination, oral examination, or any painful areas. During each phase of the exam, teach the dog that touches predict wonderful treats, working to classically condition a positive emotional response to examinations. Monitor the dog continuously for changes in food acceptance, body language, and proximity preferences. If signs of stress and anxiety emerge, pause the exam and make a handling plan to improve the dog's experience during the exam and any future visits.

Video 4.3 shows a brief example of Monique working with Border collie puppy Kestrel to introduce a few components of her physical exam. Notice that each touch predicts a delicious treat.

During regular exam visits, many dogs need to give a blood sample or allow vaccination. Applying the same principles used during the exam will help dogs feel comfortable and cooperate. Vaccinations and venipuncture should be paired with wonderful treats for every patient, and the procedure should be done gradually. Desensitization and classical conditioning can be used preventively from the very first visit. For example, before giving a vaccination, touch a nonsensitive area, touch the injection area, pinch the skin tent lightly, pinch more firmly, simulate the injection with a capped needle, and finally inject. Each step of the process should predict a small wonderful treat. This injection process in a comfortable dog will take about 10 seconds, and will teach the dog that injections are nothing to fear. In many cases, the owner can assist with feeding treats during this process.

Video 4.4 shows a Poodle mix puppy receiving her first vaccination. Her owners have been instructed how to give small delicious treats throughout this process. She wiggles a small amount because she is following the treats, but does not even notice her vaccinations. This is a good example of a prevention protocol for vaccinations in young dogs.

Venipuncture requires more planning because the dog must hold still enough for the technician or veterinarian to access a vein, whereas subcutaneous injections like vaccines do not need to be nearly as precise. Many owners do not understand this important difference, so take time to explain precisely what the dog will need to do and what your job is before you begin. As with the vaccination process, allow the dog to become comfortable with light stabilization, then with holding off the vein, followed by alcohol application, touching and pinching the site, and then finally venipuncture. Each step in this process should predict wonderful treats, and many dogs will stand, sit, or lie still for venipuncture if the owner or a team member distracts them with food.

In **Video 4.5**, we see a senior dog named Lucy being vaccinated and giving a blood sample. She is standing on a nonslip mat, and a pet owner is feeding treats at nose level. A technician gently stabilizes the dog for the vaccination. She is supporting the dog without restraining her, but has one hand ready just in case the dog responds to the needle sensation. A second technician touches the injection area and gives the vaccine. This dog responds to the needle sensation by turning to look at the injection site, but rapidly returns to eating. A few seconds later, the team works together to collect a blood sample. The same technician is stabilizing the dog and occludes the vessel, while a second technician gently touches the area, pinches to assess the dog's response, and then collects a small blood sample. The dog eats treats during the entire procedure, and does not respond at all to the needle sensation this time. Her positive experience during the vaccination made the blood sample collection go more smoothly.

4.2.8 The Exam Room Experience: Cats

Cats should be allowed the opportunity to explore the exam room, or be allowed to hide if they prefer to do so. Hiding is a stress-reducing coping mechanism for cats, so let the patient show you what makes him most comfortable. Once the cat has been invited into the exam room, the owner should place the carrier on the floor, bench, or exam table and open the carrier door. Treat a towel with Feliway, and place it over the carrier, leaving part of the door opening uncovered so the cat can choose to come out. Ideally, the owner will bring this towel from home. Place a small amount of highly palatable food such as canned food, cream cheese, or a butter pat outside the kennel door to encourage the cat to explore.

Many cats will choose to exit the carrier and explore after a few minutes. Be patient, and discuss the history questions with the owner while you allow the cat to acclimate. This is a good multitasking opportunity. During the history, assess the cat's food acceptance, body language, and proximity preferences. While talking with the owner, use the time to offer treats and toys for cats who will explore. If the cat chooses to remain in the carrier, this is a sign of stress. Do not force the cat to exit the carrier, but rather plan a single handling event for these cats: vital signs, exam, sample collection, and weight.

For cats who choose to exit the carrier, many can be lured onto the scale with a small amount of the same palatable food offered to encourage them to come out. For those who choose to stay inside the carrier, gently disassembling the carrier around the cat and allowing him to stay inside where he is comfortable will help reduce anxiety. Refer to Chapter 2 for signs of moderate and severe stress in cats, as these indicate the need to pause and make a new plan.

Sometimes pet owners bring carriers with difficult bolts or broken clips, or held together with zip ties. Keep nail clippers and zip ties in each exam room to disassemble and quickly reassemble carriers in disrepair. Figure 4.6 shows a carrier with quick-release clips, which are the easiest type to disassemble during veterinary visits.

Video 4.6 shows a kitten during her first and second appointments in the clinic. The beginning of the video is the kitten coming out of her carrier for canned food at the start of her very first appointment. She is a little nervous but comes out to get the canned food. The second half of the video shows the same kitten three weeks later. Even though this cat received vaccines during her first visit, she came right out for food treats again at the second visit. Her first associations with the exam room are yummy food treats and gentle handling. Allowing the kitten to come out at her own pace and pairing the experience with something wonderful helped her make a positive emotional response. Working hard to help kittens feel comfortable is an investment in the future: cats who feel comfortable in the veterinary clinic.

Once the history and weight are completed, it is time for vital signs measurement for cats who come out of the carrier. Just like with dogs, begin touches in less sensitive areas before moving to more sensitive areas and use the Touch Gradient. For example, when palpating a femoral pulse, begin by touching along the shoulder, then glide your hand down the back to the flank, and then to the medial femoral area. Continue to monitor the cat's response to you. Is she still interested in food and facial petting? What about her body language: is it relaxed or more nervous? Is she trying to move away, or willing to stay nearby? Use these assessments and reassessments to guide your handling plan, and listen to the cat if she asks you to stop. As with dogs, pair touching with

(a)   (b)

Figure 4.6 (a–b) Using carriers with quick-release clips and alternate openings simplifies visits for cats.

something wonderful when possible. The owner can be instructed how to help give food or the cat's favorite tactile interaction. Teach the owner how to keep the cat interested. Some cats will even eat while you measure their temperature. Begin touching the cat in a less sensitive area, working down to the rump. Minimally displace the tail to the side, and then measure the temperature. If the cat is uncomfortable with temperature measurement, save this procedure until the end of the visit, and ask the veterinarian to assess whether temperature measurement is crucial information during this visit.

When the history and vital signs are complete, or the history and assessment show the cat should only be handled once, it is time to round the veterinarian. When providing the medical history and presentation, team members should remember to provide information about the cat's emotional state as well. Whether the cat is accepting food and play, how the cat responds to touch, and if the cat is choosing to hide should be communicated along with health information. Good communication makes it easier for the veterinarian to create an efficient handling plan prior to interacting with the patient.

A good physical examination is brief and pleasant, and does not require restraint. Work where the cat is comfortable. This may be the floor, the owner's lap, the exam table, the bottom of a carrier, or even hiding under a towel. The American Association of Feline Practitioners/International Society of Feline Medicine (AAFP/ISFM) Feline Handling Guidelines updated in 2022 are an excellent resource for detailed instructions regarding keeping cats as comfortable as possible within the veterinary environment [2].

Figure 4.7 shows several places a cat might like to be examined: on the table in a soft bed, in the bottom of the carrier, or on the owner's lap. Begin the exam with gentle touching in the least sensitive areas, and work to more sensitive spots. The oral examination and any painful areas, or areas noted in the record as stressful in the past, should be reserved for last. For cats who will accept food and toys, each portion of the exam should predict something pleasant happening, to encourage the cat to develop a positive emotional response. Many cats are more sensitive than dogs to the introduction of touch. Once contact is established, try to maintain at least one point of physical contact with the cat, using a gentle glide with the grain of the fur, or lightly swapping

(a)   (c)

(b)

Figure 4.7 (a–c) Choose a place where the cat is comfortable, such as in a soft bed or on the owner's lap. Source: Courtesy of Landon.

hands, to avoid startling the cat. Watch for signs of startle such as a flinch, the skin crawling, or moving away from newly established touch.

Vaccinations, venipuncture, and cystocentesis are often part of wellness visits for cats. In the chapters for Type One, Two, and Three training (Chapters 5–7), we will discuss providing these procedures for cats. Many kittens and some adult cats will allow these procedures using distraction techniques like those discussed for dogs.

4.2.9 The Trip Home: Cats

The visit to the veterinary hospital is not over when the cat owner receives the receipt and goes home, especially for multicat households. Social groups of cats develop a group odor as well as a group pheromone profile. This group odor is one way that cats identify one another as members of the accepted social group. When one cat visits the veterinary hospital and then returns home, sometimes other cats at home may act aggressively toward the returning cat. To prevent this, apply Feliway to the cat carrier before the client leaves the clinic, and advise the client to use something with the home scent to rub on the cat when she arrives home. Place the newly arrived cat in another room like a bedroom for a few hours while they acclimate to being home again, and gradually reintroduce the cats under supervision. Intercat aggression secondary to reintroduction can have lasting emotional effects for both cats, so prevention is important. A single fight can lead to long-term problems with intercat aggression [3].

4.3 Happy Visits and Other Preventative Planning

4.3.1 Happy Visits

Happy visits are a great way to prevent fear of the veterinary hospital. Happy visits are free of charge for the client, and have a great value for the patient, client, and veterinary team. Any patient is welcome to come for happy visits to form or maintain positive emotional responses about the veterinary clinic. In a happy visit, the patient should visit the hospital, and have a pleasant interaction with a team member such as receiving treats and a quick play session. Depending upon the layout of the hospital and current caseload, having the dog hop on the scale or walk into an exam room for a few treats are also great experiences during happy visits.

The purpose of happy visits is to show the puppy or dog (rarely, cats) they can visit the veterinary office, have a great experience, and then go home. These visits help tip the scales in favor of good experiences at the hospital rather than worrisome ones. Animals with a history of negative experiences at the vet, including recent surgery or treatment for injuries, and those who display moderate stress signals will often benefit from happy visits. Some veterinary clinics even instituted a Happy Visit Punch Card. When the client comes for five happy visits, they receive a discount off their next veterinary care appointment. Positive reinforcement works on clients as well as patients! However, if an animal is showing moderate or severe stress before approaching the clinic or in the lobby, happy visits may *not* be a good starting point, and repeated exposures without more planning could do more harm than good, running the risk of sensitization or even flooding events for these patients. Dogs with moderate or severe stress should be signed up for medical intervention and training visits rather than passive happy visits.

Happy visits help add value to your practice in the eyes of the client as well as the patient. Public perception is that the veterinary office is a frightening place, and that animals fearing the veterinary clinic is normal. Happy visits are one way to show clients that pets can learn to like the veterinary hospital, and how important pet well-being is to the veterinary team. When clients see the veterinary team's deep and genuine love and compassion for patients, it will help bond clients to the practice. For animals showing moderate or severe stress during attempted happy visits, this is an opportunity to open a dialog about scheduling training appointments prior to the next veterinary care appointment. Figure 4.8 shows a puppy interacting with a team member during a happy visit.

4.3.2 Puppy and Kitten Visits

Puppies and kittens present a wonderful opportunity for the veterinary team: the opportunity to make a great first impression. The great opportunity to make a good first impression is also a

Figure 4.8 Happy visits help build positive associations with the veterinary hospital.

big responsibility. Puppies and kittens are in a critical developmental stage during their juvenile wellness visits. The developmental stages include **sensitive periods**, where young animals easily become fearful of novel things. It makes sense, if we consider the wild counterparts of our canine and feline pets. Novel things can be dangerous, and learning to be cautious of them is a functional fear response, as we discussed in earlier chapters. If puppies and kittens learn the veterinary clinic is a place where frightening things happen when they are young, fear of the veterinary clinic can last a lifetime. To help puppies and kittens learn the veterinary hospital is nothing to fear, and a source of pleasant experiences, make a plan for puppies and kittens with behavioral wellness at the core.

To make sure each puppy and kitten gets the care he or she deserves, and each client receives the proper information, schedule extra time for new puppies and kittens. During the initial visits, the technician should take time during the history to assess what treats, toys, and other forms of possible reinforcement the puppy or kitten prefers, and note these in the record. If the patient is wary or fearful during greetings or vital signs, this should also be noted. Worry in puppies and kittens is a sign the animal may be at risk for developing worsening fear, both in the veterinary clinic and at home. Each time the patient is handled by a technician or the veterinarian, the handling should predict the animal's preferred treats, toys, or other rewards to assist in building a positive classically conditioned emotional response to veterinary care. If a puppy or kitten is too stressed to eat or engage in play in the veterinary clinic, it may be necessary to intervene with the more advanced training techniques discussed in subsequent chapters.

Unwanted behaviors are a common cause of animal relinquishment. Preventing unwanted behaviors at home protects pets and preserves the **human–animal bond**, and it keeps pets coming to the veterinary hospital. Discuss normal puppy and kitten behaviors with pet owners during their juvenile wellness visits. Technicians are the perfect people to have these educational talks with pet owners, and because we see puppies and kittens several times during their youth visits, we can break up the information into smaller segments for faster visits and to avoid overwhelming pet owners with too much information at once. Table 4.4 shows the behavior topics we suggest

Table 4.4 Puppy wellness visit discussion topics.

Age (wk)	Discussion topics
8–12	Enjoying the veterinary clinic
	Puppy biting and appropriate play
	Housetraining
	Crate training
	Body language of fear, anxiety, and stress
	Positive socialization
	Sensitive periods and normal development
	Environments
	Surfaces
	People (gender, age, size, voice, and clothing)
	Friendly puppies
	Gentle adult dogs
	Other animals
	Leashes, harnesses, and collars
	Choosing a puppy class
12–16	Puppy biting and appropriate play
	Chewing, teething, and appropriate chew items
	Housetraining check-in
	Preventing boredom
	Appropriate physical exercise
	Appropriate mental exercise
	Positive socialization check-in
	Voluntary veterinary home care
	Restraint acceptance
	Home physical exam
	Ear care
	Eye care
	Toothbrushing
	Voluntary grooming
	Nail care
	Coat care
	Choosing an adolescent dog class
16+	Housetraining check-in
	Appropriate play check-in
	Normal adolescent behavior
	Verify adolescent dog class selected.

discussing during puppy wellness visits, and Table 4.5 shows the checklist for kitten wellness visits.

Some of the topics included in the wellness checklist include handling exercises. During the wellness visits, the veterinary team should examine the animal, and also teach the owner how to handle the animal, and when to ask for assistance if fear is noted at home. Teach the pet owner exercises such as brushing the teeth, trimming nails, cleaning and inspecting ears, and tolerating light stabilizing restraint using distractions, desensitization, and classical conditioning. At each visit, provide

Table 4.5 Kitten wellness visit discussion topics.

Age (wk)	Discussion topics
8–12	Enjoying the veterinary clinic
	Stalking, biting, and appropriate play
	Litter training
	Carrier training
	Choosing a scratching post/tree
	Scratching post training
	Body language of fear, anxiety, and stress
	Positive socialization
	Environments
	Surfaces
	People (gender, age, size, voice, and clothing)
	Other animals
	Attending kitten classes where available
12–16	Appropriate play check-in
	Litter training check-in
	Enrichment for indoor cats
	Preventing boredom
	Appropriate physical exercise
	Appropriate mental exercise
	Positive socialization check-in
	Voluntary veterinary home care
	Restraint acceptance
	Home physical exam
	Ear care
	Eye care
	Toothbrushing
	Voluntary grooming
	Nail care
	Coat care
16+	Litter training check-in
	Appropriate play check-in
	Destructive behavior Q&A.

the client with some handling homework to practice between visits. When the puppy or kitten learns to enjoy body handling and husbandry at home with the owner, veterinary care becomes simpler in the clinic, and necessary treatments later in life are much better tolerated at home.

The most common problem home behavior described for both dogs and cats is house soiling [4]. Table 4.6 shows the most common behavior problems that owners describe when surrendering dogs to the shelter; Table 4.7 shows the same for cats. Providing owners with a guide for proper house-training for puppies and kittens will help the owner have realistic expectations and better success during the housetraining process, preventing unwanted house soiling later in life. Other problem behaviors include destructive behavior, and aggressive behavior toward the owner [4]. Destructive behavior can be normal for both puppies and kittens, but it also can be an indicator of a behavioral disorder. Learn the difference between normal and abnormal behavior, and familiarize yourself with local referral options for behavior disorders if your veterinarian does not offer behavioral

Table 4.6   Most common unwanted behaviors according to owners surrendering dogs to the animal shelter.

Owner-defined behavior problem	Prevalence (%)
House soiling	18.5
Destructive outside	12.6
Aggressive toward people	12.1
Escapes	11.6
Too active	11.4
Needs too much attention	10.9
Vocalizes too much	10.7
Bites	9.7
Destructive indoors	9.7
Disobedient	9

Table 4.7   Most common unwanted behaviors according to owners surrendering cats to the animal shelter.

Owner-defined behavior problem	Prevalence (%)
House soiling	37.7
Destructive indoors	11.4
Aggressive toward people	10.9
Does not get along with other pets	8
Bites	8
Needs too much attention	6.9
Unfriendly	6.9
Destructive outdoors	5.1
Requested behavior euthanasia	4.6
Too active	4.6

therapies. Aggression toward people can include normal jumping, vigorous play, mouthing during play, clawing at the owner during play, grabbing clothing, stalking and ambushing, and more. Each of these are normal behaviors for puppies and kittens, and the owner should be advised to use positive reinforcement and negative punishment to help puppies and kittens learn appropriate forms of play and interaction. Positive punishment is not appropriate.

A good training class will cover all of these common topics, and help support owners during what can be a challenging developmental period for both puppies and kittens [5, 6]. Choosing to provide puppy and kitten classes is a good way for clinics to assure these owners are receiving the best information (Figure 4.9). Attending positive reinforcement classes has the bonus benefit of teaching puppies and kittens to love visiting the hospital. If offering classes is not a good fit for an individual practice, referral information for appropriate classes should be provided during the first puppy or kitten checkup. Team members should visit a class prior to referring clients, to assure

Figure 4.9 Puppy classes help build skills such as housetraining to set up patients for success.

the class is using recommended methods and techniques. Puppies and kittens can attend classes starting at eight weeks of age, as long as the classes are structured to be safe and appropriate for that age group. The ideal window of opportunity for socialization closes by 16 weeks for these young animals, so earlier is best when starting classes.

4.4 Hospitalization, Treatments, Diagnostics, and Boarding

Moving through the hospital or having to stay in the hospital can be stressful for both the pet and the client. The same principles of preparing the animal areas to be patient-friendly, and using techniques that are sensitive to the behavioral needs of the patient, apply in the back of the hospital just as they do in the examination room.

4.4.1 Hospitalization

When possible, hospitalized, or boarding patients should be separated by species. If your hospital does not have enough space for separate dog and cat wards, at least keep the species as far apart as possible, and provide visual barriers so they do not have to see one another. Address barking dogs by providing medication to reduce FAS, enrichment to alleviate boredom, and company to reduce separation distress. Harmful experiences in the wards are not restricted to fear: even too much excitement can be harmful to patients in the hospital.

4.4.2 Patient Movements

Moving patients through the hospital in a thoughtful way reduces stress. The foundation behavior of targeting helps simplify patient movements. The handler should face the direction they want the dog to travel, and encourage using a target or lure as needed. Using a long spoon with sticky food as a lure for animals even if they have not previously learned targeting is often effective. Remember: the lure needs to be achievable, and the dog allowed to eat a bit every few steps so he keeps moving. Make sure the route is clear before moving through, so the dog is protected from interactions with other patients. There should be a relaxed "U" in the leash between the handler and the dog whenever possible. If the dog is very reluctant to move, invite the owner to come with you during the movement, as many dogs will move better with the owner. Make sure dogs learn that moving into and through the hospital is pleasant, and changes in the environment predict high-value rewards.

4.4.2.1 For Example
- Dog exits vehicle (change in environment) → 3 treats delivered
- Dog walks through parking lot → Treats delivered approximately every 10 ft
- Dog walks through entrance → 3 treats delivered
- Dog walks through reception area → Treat delivered
- Dog approaches treatment room door → Place 4–6 treats on the floor and let the dog eat them while the door is opened
- Dog moves through treatment room door → Toss 4–6 treats on the floor and allow the dog to eat them while the owner moves back to the reception area.

Figure 4.10 diagrams the use of different treat quantities during a dog's journey through the hospital.

The same target or lure can be used to encourage the dog to enter a kennel. Set up any items in the kennel first, such as bedding and water. Encourage the dog to enter the kennel by facing the direction you want him to go, placing the target or lure of a few treats inside the kennel, and then stepping behind the dog to discourage backward movement. In some cases, you may have to gently lift the dog. Do not drag the dog, or lift him and let him drop onto the floor of the kennel, as this will only increase his fear and make him more difficult to kennel in the future.

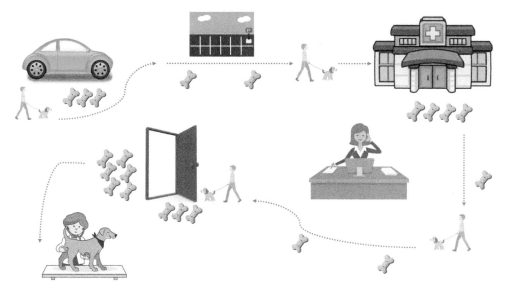

Figure 4.10 Treat flowchart. Each major change in the environment, such as going through a door or into a new room, should predict several treats. Placing several treats on the floor while the dog approaches the door of the exam room, and then four to six treats on the floor inside the exam room, will help create a positive emotional response.

When removing a shy dog from the kennel, approach the kennel with a leash and treats. Stand with your side or back to the door, and crack the door while offering treats at the level of the leash. Control the door with your body to prevent escape, and allow the dog to come to you. If the dog has a good target behavior, using a hand target or spoon will encourage him to come to you and allow leash placement.

If the dog is overly friendly or anxious and bouncing at the door of the kennel, toss a few treats to the back of the kennel so the dog moves away long enough for you to undo the latch and control the door with your body. Offer treats at nose level to encourage him to place his head through the leash, then open the door and allow him to join you outside the kennel.

Video 4.7 shows an excited French bulldog. He leaps out of the cage to greet every team member with joy. The technician uses treats in her right hand to feed the dog as she slips the leash over with her left hand. Notice she placed the leash around her right arm so that the puppy can keep eating the treats without interruption while she loops his leash on. The technician also uses food lures to get the dog to follow her. To return this excited puppy back to his kennel, the technician uses tiny treats to lure him toward and then into the kennel.

Moving cats should use the same low-stress principles, but the techniques are different since cats will most often be transported in a carrier rather than on a leash. When using a carrier, hold the carrier from the bottom rather than the handle for added stability, and cover the carrier with a pheromone-treated towel to avoid the cat seeing people or other animals during transport. Some cats are more comfortable being carried in a towel while eating treats. Choose the method that helps the cat remain the most relaxed, and always check your route in advance to assure you will not be surprised by passing other animals. Verify the ward cage or kennel is set up with any bedding, litter, and water in advance, leaving enough room for the carrier to fit inside the kennel. Place the carrier inside the kennel, and open the door, allowing the cat to come out at his own pace. Once the cat has come out of the carrier, remove the carrier.

Some shy cats will not come out of the carrier on their own when people are around. For these cats, remove the door of the carrier but leave the box itself in the kennel to provide a safe hiding area. When the cat needs to be treated, use the carrier to transport the cat out of the kennel, and gently disassemble the carrier around the cat if more access is needed. Avoid pulling or dumping the cat out of the carrier.

4.4.3 Dog Wards

Mitigating sound is important in dog wards. Preventing stress can help reduce barking. Also, housing barking dogs in a separate, quiet area, if one is available, may decrease the domino effect of one dog initiating a whole ward of barking. If possible, provide sound-reducing acoustic measures such as baffled tiles, acoustic membranes, and an acoustic-muffling ceiling. There are many noise-reducing building materials available, and these can help both dogs and humans have a better quality of life in the dog ward.

Provide acoustic therapy such as music ("Through a Dog's Ear," for example). Pheromone diffusers should be used in the ward, and when possible the bedding can also be treated with pheromones. If possible, the owner can provide bedding such as a towel or familiar mat from home as well as the dog's favorite treats. A nonslip mat or yoga mat should be placed under any slick bedding to prevent the animal from sliding around. Caution pet owners that the mat or bed might become soiled, so they select an appropriate item. Visual barriers across part of the door of the kennel can be helpful for shy or nervous dogs, so they do not see and interact with passing patients. Blankets and towels make good impromptu barriers. Corrugated plastic boards (this looks like corrugated cardboard, but it is constructed from lightweight plastic) can also be cut to fit the fronts of cage doors and affixed to the outside of the door. This plastic can be fully disinfected and used many times before it wears out. For sliding glass doors, an inexpensive privacy film can be applied to the bottom half of the door so that people passing by can easily check on the well-being of the patient, but dogs walking by will not be visible. Food and treats can be provided in a puzzle toy or food dispenser (Figure 4.11). Choose food toys and dispensers that can be easily washed and disinfected. If the dog is not accustomed to using a food-dispensing toy, make sure to record food intake in the record and provide food in a dish if the dog is not using the toy.

4.4.4   Cat Wards

Most cats appreciate having a place to hide while they are in the wards. A carrier without a door can be provided, but a cardboard box, reusable cots or a single step stool covered in a towel, fancy cat condos, or even paper shopping sacks will do. There are commercially available cat ward boxes that provide a place for litter, an enclosed hiding area, and an elevated resting platform (Figure 4.12). A towel or corrugated plastic barrier can be placed over at least half of the cage door so the cat can choose to be visible or hidden, but the team can easily check on the cat at any time (Figure 4.13). Encourage cat owners to bring a towel, mat, or small bed from home that is familiar to the cat, but do caution the owner that the item may become soiled. Pheromone diffusers should be plugged in around the ward, and bedding as well as cage door covers can be treated with pheromones as well.

Instruct cat owners to bring their favorite food and treats from home, and ask what kind of litter the cat prefers. If the litter type is unusual, it is best for the owner to provide litter as well. Most cats prefer unscented, fine-grit litter [7]. Choose a litter of this type for your daily in-hospital use.

4.4.5   Treatment Rooms

If the authors had a magical low-stress genie in a lamp granting three wishes, here are our wishes:

(1) Every pet arrives hungry and with his favorite treats from home.
(2) No-restraint and low-restraint care become standard operating procedures.
(3) Stop taking animals away from their owners, or "to the back" for treatments that can easily be performed in an exam room.

Taking animals to the treatment room without the owner can cause unnecessary stress for both the patient and the client. Each time a pet is relocated to a new area of the hospital, they must re-acclimate to the new area and their stress level will elevate. While some animals may seem "better without the owner," this effect is often caused by learned helplessness rather than true relaxation. Does the animal accept treats in the same eager fashion, have more loose and happy body language, and choose to be closer to the veterinary team in the treatment room without the client? Or does the dog become slower in its movement, stand still, and appear subdued? Use the patient assessment tools to determine if an animal is truly "better" without the owner.

The author understands that some team members are uncomfortable working in front of the owner. As a full-time technician in private practice, I used to be nervous about it, too! With regular practice, this feels normal to team members, confidence grows, and the clients are amazed at what we can accomplish. Some owners may contribute negatively to the patient experience by talking loudly, scolding the animal, or trying rough restraint. Most owners are simply nervous or embarrassed themselves, and will respond well to good instructions from the veterinary team. Coaching the owner on how to talk to the patient, where to stand, and how to give food will help calm the

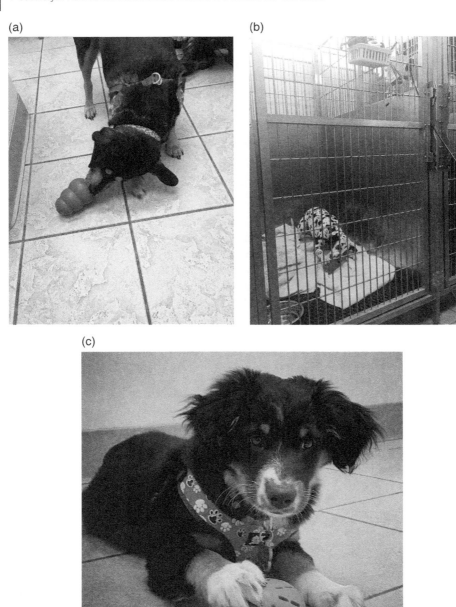

Figure 4.11 (a–c) Dogs using food toys in the hospital.

(a)

(b)

Figure 4.12 Examples of hiding places for cats in the hospital.

Figure 4.13 Partially covering the door of a kennel gives the cat an option to hide while allowing the team to check on the cat as well.

situation. For example, if the owner is nervous, noisy, and touching the animal inappropriately, I may provide the owner with 20 tiny treats and instruct her to deliver one treat per second. Both of the owner's hands will be occupied by the treat-counting task, and her voice will be calmer and counting rather than anxious. If the owner strongly prefers not to be present for injections, nail trims, anal gland expression, blood collection, subcutaneous fluids, or the many other simple procedures performed in the exam room, simply have the owner step into the lobby rather than moving the patient. Before using needles, collecting blood, or performing other procedures, always ask the client if they are comfortable around medical equipment and procedures, and describe the procedure in advance. Good advance communication can avoid unpleasant experiences for the client as well.

When it is necessary to move a patient to the treatment room, check to make sure the treatment area is available, and there are no other patients nearby. Set up everything needed for the procedure prior to moving the patient, including a hospital cage for when you have completed the procedure if you are hospitalizing the patient. Communicate with team members so they know you'll be working in the treatment room, and not to show up with a barking terrier while you are placing an IV catheter in an anxious cat. When moving through the treatment area, prevent social interactions between patients (Figure 4.14). Table 4.8 is a checklist to guide procedural setup prior to moving the patient.

Minimize noise levels in the treatment room, such as boisterous laughter and rapid movements. Keep music levels low, and be considerate with use of equipment such as dental scalers, compressors, vacuum cleaners, suction pumps, and such. These activities can contribute to trigger stacking for patients who are waiting or being treated in the treatment room.

Figure 4.14 Communication between team members and using visual barriers protects patients from social interactions in the treatment room.

Table 4.8 Checklist for procedures outside the exam room.

☐ Plan where to perform procedure
☐ Recon the route: check for other patients before moving
☐ Set up the destination area before moving (patient entered in computer for x-rays, ultrasound machine set up for cystocentesis, etc.)
☐ Explain procedure to client before moving patient
☐ Invite patient to procedure area using luring, targeting, etc
☐ Perform procedure as promptly as possible
☐ Return patient to client or to ward as appropriate.

4.4.6 Radiology

Radiology is a ward where some manual restraint is usually required unless patients are sedated. Sedating patients for radiographs will reduce stress and anxiety, improve the quality of films, decrease the number of reshoots needed, decrease the number of staff members in the room during radiograph exposure, and minimize exposure of the team to scatter radiation. This author advocates sedation for radiographs whenever possible for all of these reasons (some states require sedation for all radiographs; check your practice act). Animals in pain should always receive analgesia prior to radiography, unless the situation is critical and analgesia would present life-threatening complications.

Prior to taking the patient to radiology, make sure the machine and table are fully set up. Input the animal into the computer or make the flash ID card, set the technique, and gather any positioning devices you may need such as a soft V-tray or foam positioning cushions, sand bags, as well as any treats or distractions to be used (Figure 4.15). Collimate the beam, and position the tube head

(a)   (b)

Figure 4.15 Using nonslip surfaces and soft positioning aids increases patient comfort in radiology.

Figure 4.16 Sticky treats delivered in a food toy help this excited patient cooperate for radiographs.

properly. If you are using a film cassette in the tabletop technique, be sure to place a nonslip mat on the table so both the cassette and the patient will be stable and not move. Dress in your gown, other personal protective equipment, and badge if you'll be in the room during the radiograph, then move the patient into the radiology ward.

Many pets will be frightened by noises in radiography such as moving the tube head, activating the rotor with the pedal, and even the swoosh of Velcro® letting go when we remove gowns. Plan to use masking noises and treats during those times to help dogs relax. Use something soft and sticky for healthy pets for getting onto the x-ray table, sitting, lying down, and curling onto a side (Figure 4.16). If you are not sure if the dog will cooperate for positioning, do a luring dry run in the exam room with the owner, and make the client a part of the anxiolytic/sedation decision-making process prior to taking the animal to radiology. Cats will sometimes eat on the x-ray table, and can be positioned and then immediately returned to eating.

Patients who are too sick to eat are often debilitated and easier to handle. Remember to monitor these patients for signs of stress and fear; struggling is not the only way these patients communicate with us. Keep procedures brief, use modified positioning when necessary, and communicate with the team and attending veterinarian if there are problems with obtaining radiographs.

4.4.7 Anesthesia and Surgery

Surgical patients need to be Nil per os (Latin) – Nothing by Mouth (NPO)... Or do they? Some anesthesia studies in both pets and people suggest a small amount of food before surgery is beneficial, particularly for diabetic and pediatric patients, or those with small body mass [8, 9]. That being said, giving water-consistency food such as broth, watered-down baby food, or watered-down canned pet food (either frozen or at room temperature) is a good way to give premedication and collect preoperative lab samples. In general, we suggest collecting preoperative lab work a few days prior to the procedure so that any abnormalities can be addressed without the animal spending excess time in the hospital, and so the blood collection appointment is brief and pleasant for the patient; but sometimes this is not possible based on the patient, the clinic's policies, or the workflow of the hospital.

Pre-anesthesia medications reduce anxiety, provide preemptive analgesia, decrease the volume of induction agent required, and decrease the amount of volatile anesthetic required. Pre-anesthesia medications should be considered for every anesthesia patient [10]. At this author's hospital, all patients are provided anxiety-reducing and nausea prevention medications before elective anesthesia or hospitalization. After pre-anesthesia medications have been given, intravenous (IV) access can be comfortably established in the vast majority of patients (>95% in the author's experience). For dogs who are very nervous even after the premedication, there are several options. Adding to the premedication, placing a standing lateral saphenous catheter, or titrating a portion of the induction agent using a butterfly catheter in the lateral saphenous so that anesthesia and IV access can be established are all options. Using a topical anesthetic cream at the site of IV access can help make the process more comfortable. Remember: increased stress levels prior to anesthesia are correlated with increased anesthesia complications. Reducing stress before anesthesia is associated with better outcomes [10]. For cats who are still anxious after the pre-anesthesia medications, consider giving additional premedication, and using a gentle towel wrap and giving the induction agent with a butterfly in the medial saphenous vein, then intubating and establishing IV access.

Recovery can be a stressful time for animals as well. Assure the animal has a comfortable place to recover, and a dedicated technician during the recovery process. The animal should be gently supported as needed, and if the patient is experiencing significant dysphoria, medical management for dysphoria is appropriate. Postoperative dysphoria represents considerable distress, and should be treated as such.

Patients who have increased anxiety in the veterinary hospital should receive pre-visit medications at home prior to the surgery appointment, and be first in line for surgery to minimize wait times. When possible, schedule the admission appointment so the owner can be with the patient during the pre-anesthetic medication administration. While the patient is in the hospital, try to have one team member be that patient's "person" for the day to offer continuity and predictability. Lastly, schedule a discharge appointment as early in the day as possible; or, for some patients, having the owner be present during the recovery process is best for everyone involved.

References

1 Volk, J.O., Felsted, K.E., Thomas, J.G. et al. (2011). Executive summary of the Bayer veterinary care usage study. *Journal of the American Veterinary Medical Association* 238 (10): 1275–1282. https://doi.org/10.2460/javma.238.10.1275.

2 Rodan, I., Dowgray, N., Carney, H.C. et al. (2022). AAFP/ISFM cat friendly veterinary interaction guidelines: approach and handling techniques. *Journal of Feline Medicine and Surgery* 24 (11): 1093–1132. http://dx.doi.org/10.1177/1098612X221128760.

3 Crowell-Davis, S., Curtis, T.M., and Knowles, R.J. (2004). Social organization in the cat: a modern understanding. *Journal of Feline Medicine and Surgery* 6 (1): 19–28. http://journals.sagepub.com/doi/abs/10.1016/j.jfms.2003.09.013.

4 Salman, M.D., Hutchison, J., Ruch-Gallie, R. et al. (2000). Behavioral reasons for relinquishment of dogs and cats to 12 shelters. *Journal of Applied Animal Welfare Science* 3 (2): 93–106. https://doi.org/10.1207/S15327604JAWS0302_2.

5 Shaw, K. and Martin, D. (2015). *Canine and Feline Behavior for Veterinary Technicians and Nurses*. Ames, IA: Wiley.

6 Overall, K. (2013). *Manual of Clinical Behavioral Medicine for Dogs and Cats*. St. Louis, MO: Mosby.

7 Neilson, J. (2004). Thinking outside the box: feline elimination. *Journal of Feline Medicine and Surgery* 6 (1): 5–11. https://doi.org/10.1016/j.jfms.2003.09.008.

8 Looney, A. (2008). The association of shelter veterinarians veterinary medical care guidelines for spay-neuter programs. *Journal of the American Veterinary Medical Association* 233 (1): 74–86.

9 Manchikanti, L. (2011). Preoperative fasting before interventional techniques: is it necessary or evidence-based? *Pain Physician* 14: 459–467.

10 Muir, W. (2013). *Handbook of Veterinary Anesthesia*. St. Louis, MO: Elsevier.

5

Type One Patients and Training: Distraction Techniques and FAS 0–2 Pets

5.1 Introduction to the Types of Training

Different patients have different needs, and will benefit from individualized training programs. Now that you understand the importance of a clinic culture embracing stress reduction, how animals sense and perceive the environment, how to set up the environment for success, how animals learn, and what the foundation needs are for both trainers and patients, you are ready to start training.

Animals fear veterinary care for a variety of reasons: lack of positive emotional conditioning, negative learning experiences in the past, genetics, socialization, and more. The animal's stress level will dictate which methods are most appropriate to start out. The goal of any training plan is to reduce stress and anxiety, increase compliance, and improve the veterinary experience for the patient, client, and veterinary team. Most animals will respond to training, and will have noticeably decreased stress levels. However, some patients may not progress as we hope. Some animals appear stressed both at home and in the hospital, while others relax more easily. Selecting an appropriate training plan, setting realistic expectations, and adapting to the animal in front of you will improve outcomes.

This guide uses patient assessments to divide patients into three categories: Type One, Type Two, and Type Three. Each type has a tailored training plan template based on that group's stress level and specific needs (Figure 5.1). We will use the same assessment tool introduced in earlier chapters:

(1) Food acceptance, toy acceptance, and tactile acceptance
(2) Body language
(3) Proximity preference
(4) Fear Free (Fear, Anxiety, and Stress) FAS Score.

5.2 Identifying Type One Patients (FAS 0–2)

When assessing patients, it is important to remember that every animal makes decisions, thinks, and changes over time. These changes can be moment-to-moment, or visit-to-visit. Each assessment is a snapshot of an instant in time, and veterinary team members need to be fluid and flexible, changing plans and expectations if the patient's status changes. Type One patients are relaxed or experiencing minimal stress. Table 5.1 provides a checklist to assist with this assessment. Figure 5.2 shows images of a Type One dog.

Cooperative Veterinary Care, Second Edition. Monique Feyrecilde.
© 2024 John Wiley & Sons, Inc. Published 2024 by John Wiley & Sons, Inc.
Companion website: www.wiley.com/go/feyrecilde/cooperative

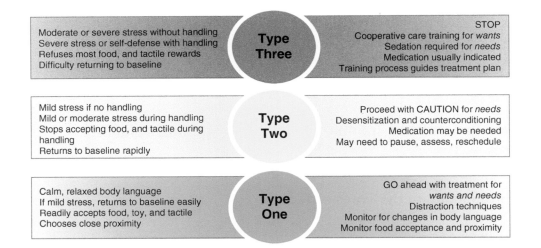

Figure 5.1 The types of training. Type One, Type Two, and Type Three patients will each be assessed and identified, and appropriate training techniques selected.

Table 5.1 Checklist for Type One dogs: each dog assessing at Type One should have each of these attributes.

Stage of visit	Food acceptance	Body language	Proximity preference
Greeting	☐ From any team member ☐ Within 5 seconds ☐ Soft mouth	☐ Relaxed body	☐ Greets immediately ☐ Stays near team member ☐ Solicits attention
Touching	☐ From any team member ☐ Soft mouth ☐ Throughout touching	☐ Relaxed during touch	☐ Does not move away ☐ Remains close when touched
Exam and treatment	☐ From any team member ☐ Soft mouth ☐ Throughout procedures	☐ Relaxed during handling	☐ Does not move away ☐ Remains close during treatments

5.2.1 Type One Dogs (FAS 0–2)

5.2.1.1 Food Acceptance
- Dogs will accept food immediately or after <5 seconds
- Will accept food from any team member
- Takes food with a soft mouth; no snapping or grabbing
- Continues accepting food even when touched
- Accepts food before, during, and after procedures.

5.2.1.2 Body Language
- Relaxed body language (refer to Chapter 2)
- Remains relaxed during touching and handling
- Remains relaxed during procedures.

Figure 5.2 Type One canine patient.

5.2.1.3 Proximity Preference
- On-leash and off-leash, dog immediately greets veterinary team members
- Chooses to remain near team members while they talk to and touch him
- Does not back away or move away when approached
- Does not back away or move away when touched
- Remains near team members during procedures.

5.2.2 Type One Cats (FAS 0–2)

Food acceptance is a less reliable indicator of stress in cats when contrasted against dogs. Many dogs will accept food when stressed, and many cats will refuse a variety of food treats even when they are calm and comfortable at home. However, for cats who will eat in the hospital, changes in food acceptance are a useful indicator of stress levels. In general, kittens who learn to enjoy food treats in the hospital will continue to do so as adults. Many kittens and adult cats will also interact with a toy even if they aren't interested in food, so toy acceptance is also included in the feline assessment. Table 5.2 is a checklist to assist in assessing Type One feline patients. Figure 5.3 shows a Type One cat.

5.2.2.1 Food Acceptance, Toy Acceptance, and Tactile Acceptance
- Accepts food while in carrier, or within 30 seconds of exiting carrier
- Interacts with toy if toy motivated
- Investigates offered food, but may or may not eat depending upon preferences
- Accepts food before, during, and after touching
- Accepts food before, sometimes during, and after procedures
- Accepts tactile rewards before, sometimes during, and after procedures.

5.2.2.2 Body Language
- Relaxed body language (refer to Chapter 2)
- Remains relaxed during touching and handling
- Remains relaxed before, during, and after procedures.

Table 5.2 Checklist for Type One cats: each cat assessing at Type One should have each of these attributes.

Stage of visit	Food acceptance	Body language	Proximity preference
Greeting	☐ From any team member ☐ Shows strong interest ☐ May eat within 30 seconds ☐ May prefer toy ☐ May prefer tactile	☐ Relaxed body	☐ Exits carrier willingly ☐ Explores exam room ☐ Solicits attention
Touching	☐ From any team member ☐ Not diminished by touch	☐ Relaxed during touch	☐ Does not move away ☐ Remains close when touched
Exam and treatment	☐ From any team member ☐ Not diminished by procedure	☐ Relaxed during handling	☐ Does not move away ☐ Remains close during treatments

Figure 5.3 Type One feline patient.

5.2.2.3 Proximity Preference

- Chooses to exit carrier
- Explores exam room willingly
- Approaches team members within 30 seconds of exiting carrier
- Will rub against team members' legs
- Will head bump and allow touching and facial rubbing
- Remains near team members during touching and handling
- Remains near team members before, during, and after procedures.

Patients who are appropriate for Type One training are largely comfortable with the environment and procedures from the start. Type One training is a combination of **distraction techniques**, luring, and classical conditioning to maintain this relaxed state (Figure 5.4). Treating fear is much like treating pain: it is far easier to prevent than it is to reverse. By using Type One training techniques for relaxed patients, we teach the patients to remain relaxed and develop positive emotional

Figure 5.4   Type One patient assessment.

responses while also rewarding desired behaviors and participation in care. Type One training should be basic hospital policy for relaxed patients to keep them relaxed in the long term and build a positive and trusting relationship. Rewarding patients for "doing nothing" while they are being treated will teach them how to cooperate for procedures, and how to enjoy veterinary visits.

Individual patients may also assess as different types based on their health status and the procedures required. For example, some dogs may be Type One dogs for everything except nail trimming, and assess as Type Three when a nail trim is attempted. A normally relaxed cat may assess at Type One for an annual examination and vaccinations, but as Type Two when she is presented for limping. As always, we must remain flexible during our assessments, and adjust to work with the patient in front of us in real time.

Video 5.1 shows a dog who has been presented for nail care training. It's important to realize that Types and FAS levels fluctuate continuously due to a variety of factors. This dog has a history of FAS 5 behaviors at home for attempted nail care including a growl and an air snap. This video shows the initial evaluation visit where Monique was investigating and observing the dog to make a detailed training plan specifically for him. Because of health and safety requirements at the time the video was made, the appointment was conducted without the client present. In this video, the dog shows stress levels varying from Type 1 FAS 0–2 up to Type 3 FAS 4. He is learning to come onto the bench when he is ready to interact, and to leave the bench when he is uncomfortable. Monique is working on rewarding the dog for choosing to move away. Look for the body language signs of leaning closer, leaning away, moving closer, moving away, lip licking with the presentation of food, lip licking without the presentation of food, ears held up, ears folded, looking at the handler and glancing away from the handler. This puppy moves very quickly through his body language cues: see if you can spot all the different things he is saying here. You might be surprised at how subtle his body language cues are while still receiving a score of Type 3/FAS 4.

Every interaction is a training opportunity, whether we are choosing to train or not. Understanding classical conditioning, operant conditioning and the value of positive reinforcement, the fundamentals of training, and the foundation behaviors every patient should learn is a great start to making training plans. Training plans need not be complicated, but the more complex the goal behavior, the more complex by necessity the training plan will be.

Making a training plan for any type patient starts with the patient assessment. What is the patient's stress level? Regardless of the type of training needed, the basic flow for creating a training plan will remain the same:

(1) Identify the patient's stress level and how it is being measured (panting, lip licking, moving away from the veterinary team, etc.).
(2) Identify a non-stressful starting point for training. This includes when, where, who, what, and how much you will train.
(3) Identify stopping points in advance. For example: Moving away from the station, avoiding touch, or body language changes such as expression, position, and muscle tension.
(4) Develop a reinforcement hierarchy. What does the pet prefer, and in what order?
(5) Identify the training goal. Determine what method(s) you will use. If DS/CC/CCC (desensitizing and counter conditioning), design the exposure ladder for desensitization. If OC (operant conditioning), make a shaping plan including a variety of approximations to look for.
(6) Identify the point of consent. How will the animal tell you he is ready to interact?
(7) Identify how the animal can withdraw consent, and be ready to stop if they do.
(8) Identify the desired cue or cues for the completed behavior.
(9) Make a plan for how to fade prompts, lures, and modeling if they will be used.
(10) Determine how to introduce duration and release cues for the behavior if appropriate.

5.2.2.4 Criteria and Fundamentals for Distraction Techniques

Type One training consists largely of the use of distractions, lures, and rewards during care. Distraction techniques rely on the animal staying engaged with the distraction to facilitate handling or a procedure. The distraction is presented before, or at the exact same time as, the handling and needs to last throughout the event. It can be helpful to have a dedicated person providing the distraction, separate from those who are handling the pet or doing a procedure.

The most common distractions are food and tactile stimuli, with toys and other distractions such as verbal and visual being less common. Interactive distractions include things like toys, games, and participating in a training session of cued behaviors. For example, a dog might hold his tennis ball while he is being examined, or watch it be bounced during auscultation. Kittens may chase a toy and capture it, then receive a vaccination once they have caught the toy.

Fundamentals:

- The animal shows a strong interest in the distraction.
- The animal has no history of guarding or protecting food items or resources (gulping, freezing, hovering, growling, etc.)
- The patient is nonpainful.
- The animal finds the distraction pleasurable.
- The distraction does not rely on aversion (head tapping or pinching are aversion-based distractions).
- The distraction protects the safety of the team and pet, and is compatible with support and stabilization where appropriate.
- The distraction is feasible – meaning it can be presented to the pet in the correct body position, physical procedure location, will last the duration of the procedure, and does not create problems during the procedure itself.
- The procedure will not be serial: it will be a single or infrequent procedure. Repeat or frequent procedures carry a higher risk for emerging fear when distraction techniques are used.

Communication is key for all the people who are involved. Setting up for success means making a plan for how and where to deliver the distraction, talking with your team members to establish language for starting and stopping the distraction or the procedure, and assigning monitoring tasks. Phrases like "treat start" and "treat stop" are easy to understand and implement, but anything the team agrees on will work.

The person presenting the distraction or another team member needs to be responsible for monitoring how the pet interacts with the distraction. What is the animal's body language? Any interruption in interacting with the distraction? Suddenly gulping food or grabbing it roughly? Discuss before any procedure who will communicate what, and how to pause the procedure as needed.

Testing out a few different types and methods for delivering the distraction in advance is a good idea. The person giving the distraction may need coaching, especially if it is the client, on how and where to give food or treats, or other distractions.

Determine if a long lasting or lickable treat is best, or multiple individual bites or swallows is better. Is it ok if the pet is chewing something crunchy? Would a scatter or a line of treats be better? Testing in advance helps assess the pet's interest in and behavior around the distraction and make the best possible plan for how to incorporate the distraction into the treatment plan.

Safety of the team is paramount, regardless of which technique is selected. Careful ongoing pet assessment is needed before, during, and after the procedure. Make sure there is a way to pause the procedure and move away from the pet safely and swiftly if the need arises.

In some cases, protected contact such as a muzzle or Elizabethan collar is appropriate.

Sometimes, pets will engage with the distraction even though their FAS is above 2, as with Type two and Type three patients. Sometimes food can be coercive: the pet does not truly feel they have a choice to opt out of the interaction because the pull of the food is strong. These pets would prefer to avoid the procedure but also have a difficult time refusing the distraction. They are motivated to engage the distraction while also motivated to move away. When two motivations are at odds, we call this motivational conflict. Distractions are simplest to use, but can carry risks, so be alert to changes in the pet.

When pets are licking or eating a high value food, they may not be able to show changes in body language to communicate fear or stress. They may allow more invasive handling than they normally would, then appear to suddenly lash out or run away. This happens when the desire for the distraction is strong and it artificially changes the pet's threshold of tolerance.

Distractions can be impractical if the positioning needed is not compatible with the specific distraction. In small pets, using tactile distractions like scratching or rubbing may cover the area of interest. If a pet is very excited for a toy, using the toy may cause the pet to move too much. Feeding easy cheese or peanut butter while a pet is in dorsal recumbency may be unsafe for the animal. Feeding crunchy treats causes a lot of noise which can inhibit auscultation, and causes movement in the pets jaw and throat area, which would make it incompatible with jugular venipuncture but feasible for peripheral venous access.

Is there something you would do, even if you were afraid, if you knew you would receive a $1000? One example would be someone who is afraid of heights. I show the person a stack of ten 100-dollar bills. I clip them together and then tie them to the top rung of an extension ladder. I extend the ladder 30′ into the air, and let them know they can have the $1000, no strings attached, if they just climb to the top and retrieve it.

Think about how this person's body language looks while they are climbing. White knuckles, shaking knees, and sweat beading on their brow. Their respiratory rate and heart rate increase, their pupils dilate. They may creep their way to the top of the ladder, snag the 1000 bucks, then descend as quickly as possible and standing panting at the bottom from the emotional experience.

This person is now a $1000 richer! But did their feelings about heights change? Are they less afraid? Maybe, but very probably not. Their feelings of fear and anxiety about heights will continue in the future, even though they received a high value "treat" this time.

5.2.2.4.1 General Handling and Stabilization

Stabilization and general handling are a key for safe veterinary care, especially for patients without in-depth trained skill-specific behaviors. Type one training for stabilization means pairing any stabilization of the animal's body with a valued distraction they truly enjoy. It can be easy to skip this step because the animal is cooperative or "easy" to handle. That would be a missed opportunity! Pairing the animal's preferred distraction with stabilization handling will help maintain those "easy" Level one pets at a nice low FAS score. Remember to reach for the treats for every pet, not just the ones you worry may be higher in FAS score.

5.3 Type One Training: Dog Exam Room and Examination

Remember: every interaction is a training opportunity, because patients are always learning while they are in the hospital. For each training type, we will present common scenarios that veterinary teams encounter in the hospital every day. For each scenario, training suggestions will be provided. Use these training suggestions as a scaffold to build a training plan appropriate for the individual patient. Most patients will respond favorably, but remember to constantly assess and reassess the patient's responses for the comfort and safety of the patient and the veterinary team. In later chapters, detailed training plans for specific skills and veterinary behaviors will also be provided.

5.3.1 Reception, Weight, and Moving to the Exam Room

Dogs can learn to walk with a team member from the moment we greet them in the reception area. Type One dogs will greet the team member in a relaxed or happy and excited way, and will not move away when greeted. Teaching these dogs to walk with the team member is usually a combination of luring and targeting.

A treat trail is one way to lure a Type One dog to accompany a handler. Place a series of treats on the floor, showing the path the dog should take through the lobby, onto the scale, and into the examination room. Treats need to be close enough together so the dog stays interested, but far enough apart so that the dog is motivated to continue moving. As discussed in Chapter 4, if the lure is too difficult because the treats are too infrequent or too difficult to reach, the animal may lose desire to follow. A sticky spoon is another good luring strategy. Coating a large cooking spoon with sticky treats such as spray cheese, cream cheese, canned food, nut butter, or baby food makes a desirable lure. Hold the spoon at nose level, and allow the dog to take a few licks every few steps as he walks along with the handler.

If the dog stops moving, slow the lure down, try a different kind of lure, or select a different training strategy. Do not drag the dog forward by its leash, as this will increase fear and stress, and decrease trust.

If the dog knows a foundation target behavior such as a nose target to a hand, going to a mat, or a nose target to a spoon or other marker, moving through the hospital becomes simple. Face the direction you want the dog to go, and present your hand or the target item at nose level a few steps ahead of the dog. Allow the dog to touch the target, then reinforce with a click or verbal marker and one small treat. Advanced dogs will be able to travel numerous steps for a single reward, while more novice dogs should only be asked to walk a few steps for each click and treat.

In many cases, the owner can be trained in these methods, and the dog and owner can learn together how to move through the lobby, onto the scale, and into an examination room. Once the dog has entered the exam room, toss 5–10 treats onto the floor, spread out around the exam room as a small **jackpot** for going into the room and to encourage exploration.

Video 5.2 shows some key aspects of successful luring. Choosing the right kind of treat, the right way to deliver that treat, and delivering treats frequently enough will help handlers show the animal how to move in the desired way. Handlers proficient at luring can use a treat trail, individual treats, a lickable spoon, and later even targeting without a lure to move pets through the hospital and into a variety of body positions to facilitate treatment.

5.3.2 The Exam Room

Relaxed dogs will approach the technician during the history. Technicians can multi-task while taking the history and work through greetings and behavioral assessments while asking medical questions. Practice feeding happy dogs for every "hello" they offer. Every time a dog approaches the technician, he should be rewarded with his favored reward at the moment (probably food) in an effort to make approaches pleasant and repeated. When the dog approaches and has received a treat, begin greeting the dog. Some dogs will be comfortable with a face-to-face greeting, but most prefer a 45° angle for greetings (Figure 5.5). Once the dog is comfortable staying nearby during the greeting, we can attempt some touching. Most dogs prefer to be stroked along their sides or scratched low on the chest. The dog should respond by leaning into the touch. When you move, you may find the dog moves away for a brief period (<5 seconds for a Type One dog), but he should adjust to your movement and rapidly return to baseline, approaching again for a reward.

Figure 5.5 Many dogs prefer an angled greeting rather than face-to-face.

> **Training Tip: Welcome All Greetings!**
>
> Every happy greeting, even jumping up with excitement, is welcomed in the veterinary setting. Encourage dogs to keep four paws on the floor by offering treats low or dropping them on the floor, then greeting the dog closer to his level. Never punish dogs for excited greetings, as it can increase stress.

Work where the dog is comfortable during the examination and treatments. In many cases, this will mean working on a nonslip mat on the floor, but in some circumstances the dog will need to be lifted to the table. Just because a dog approaches and is comfortable with touching and petting, this does not mean he will be comfortable with being picked up.

When picking up a large dog, two team members should work together to assure the dog is secure and well-supported, and to distribute the load evenly so team members are not injured while lifting. A third team member or the owner can be offering food while the dog is gently lifted. If the dog stops eating, continue the lift until the dog is safely on the table. If the dog begins to struggle, he is no longer assessing as Type One, and a new plan will be needed. The goal is to pair the thing the dog likes (treats) with the lifting event. It will act as a distraction, and also may offer some stimulus pairing to promote positive feelings in the future. The dog should remain engaged with the distraction throughout the handling. If they disengage, this is a sign the pets FAS score may be increasing.

Video 5.3 shows a team using Type one distraction methods for lifting a dog onto the table. First, they verify the dog finds the distraction interesting and pleasurable. Then, they gradually introduce the kind of touch the dog will feel when lifted, taking a moment to assess the dogs response at each stage. Finally, two people work together to lift the dog while a third provides treats throughout. Communication is key so everyone knows when to move, when the feed, and when it's safe to remove their hands and arms.

Providing an intermediate step, stairs, or a bench is another great option for helping dogs onto tables. Lure for one step, then roll a treat away. Two steps and treat, then roll a treat away. Repeat the loop until the dog is comfortable going up and down the steps or bench.

When picking up a small dog, the dog should be well-supported and secure. The technician can squat next to the dog and offer treats, scratching and touching in a similar way as during the greeting. While giving treats with one hand, the technician can stabilize the dog against her leg and hip with the other, then carefully lift the dog onto the table by straightening her legs. In some cases, the dog may be more comfortable being lifted by the owner. The technician should coach the owner on proper lifting technique and assist with treat delivery to assure the dog has a good lifting experience even if the owner is the one doing the lifting. (Some clinics stipulate clients are not allowed to lift animals. Make sure you are familiar with your clinic's policy.) Figure 5.6 shows supportive body positioning for picking up a small dog. A second person can provide a food distraction.

Video 5.4 shows a small dog who has been trained to allow lifting. Her training plan included being rewarded to come to the client's feet, allow the client to place one arm and then two arms around her, and then lifted with a food treat delivered afterward. This particular dog does not prefer to eat while she is being lifted, but some dogs will prefer to be fed throughout the lift rather than afterward.

Once a dog is on the table, she should learn the table is a place where good things happen. Frequently deliver small treats or a few licks of a sticky treat throughout the time period the dog is on the table. Giving plenty of small treats may assist in classically conditioning the dog to like the table, and operantly conditioning the dog to remain on the table through positive reinforcement. If

Figure 5.6 (a–d): A technician safely stabilizes and supports a small dog while lifting. A second person can give treats during the lift. The dog in the photo was given treats on the floor and after lifting because she prefers not to eat while being lifted.

the dog is taking treats with too much excitement, or is a mouthy puppy, try using a food delivery toy or lick mat to prolong the treat delivery period and save your hands.

Video 5.5 shows Monique working with her puppy Quill at home. It is Quill's sixth day in his new home and his first time having a training session about body handling and care equipment. Quill is learning a lot in this session. Where treats come from and may appear, a variety of skills such as stillness, hand targeting, and pairing the stimulus of touching with hands and equipment with the stimulus of delicious treats. These kinds of early stimulus–stimulus pairs can really contribute to setting up a pet for a lifetime of success.

Video 5.6 shows using Type One training by pairing delicious treats as a distraction with being on the table, examination, and vaccination. (Bonus grooming content at the end.) There is no contingency for the dog to receive these treats, all that he needs to do is exist in the environment. Each touching event is paired with food treats. A long-lasting lickable distraction is given for vaccination and the grooming demonstration. For this puppy, canned cheese on a silicone lick mat was a very effective distraction.

5.3.3 Physical Examination

In veterinary and technician school, we are taught to perform a physical exam in the same order every time. Having a system is helpful. Systems decrease the chances we will miss something or forget a step. In most cases, we are taught to perform the exam from nose to tail. As discussed in earlier chapters, many patients may find touching of the face and oral cavity stressful, and would prefer not to greet the veterinarian or technician face-to-face. Developing a plan for examining a pet that saves the potentially painful, unpleasant, and socially stressful portions for last will decrease anxiety and increase cooperation. We suggest the following order for physical examination for most patients: general appearance, skin (excluding feet), auscultation, abdominal palpation, lymph nodes, musculoskeletal except paws, neurologic, ears, eyes, oral, paws, rectal/genital. Of course, individual preferences and variations as well as the presenting complaint will modify this order, as they do with any standard examination protocol. Lastly, we should remember wants versus needs. For a healthy patient, the entire exam is a want and can be postponed, modified, or rescheduled when necessary due to patient stress.

During the examination, the patient should always be free to move away if he or she is feeling uncomfortable. The veterinary team will be assessing and reassessing food acceptance, body language, and proximity preference throughout the exam to assure the patient is remaining at Type One/FAS 0–2.

The technician's role is to provide food treats and keep the veterinarian safe. When giving food, the technician should choose a strategic posture and location where it is easy to observe and assess the animal, and where a bite can be safely prevented if the animal's stress level increases unexpectedly. The technician will also communicate with the veterinarian about changes in food acceptance and body language, alerting the veterinarian to possible increases in anxiety.

Each stage of the examination should predict a small, wonderful food reward. Food should be given freely and frequently enough for the dog to stay interested and cooperative, but rationed in such a way the dog will not become full or satiated prior to completing all the day's procedures.

The skin exam looks like modified petting to the owner, and should feel this way for the dog. As with the greeting, it is usually best to begin by stroking low between the front legs and assessing the patient's response. If the patient remains relaxed, glide the hands over the trunk from ventral to dorsal, examining the skin for abnormalities, masses, and so on. Treats should be given during touching, but withheld between touches. Alternating between examining the skin and giving normal petting will help dogs relax and accept the skin exam as normal.

Auscultation for Type One dogs is generally a smooth process. While maintaining contact from the skin exam, the stethoscope can be removed from the neck, placed in the ears, and introduced to the chest. When changing sides, reach under or over the dog depending on which reach will disturb the dog least. Each of these steps should be paired with a small delicious treat. Some dogs are afraid of the stethoscope and may require Type Two training to accept it.

Palpate the abdomen from beside or behind the dog. When replacing the stethoscope, try to do so with one hand so you can maintain tactile contact without restraining the dog. By maintaining contact, we decrease the effect of startling the dog each time we reestablish contact during the exam. The team member who is feeding and providing stabilization in case of unexpected reactions should also be beside the dog rather than face-to-face with him. The technician who is offering treats and stabilizing the dog should monitor and reassess the patient continuously, alerting the veterinarian or person performing the exam to any changes.

Palpation of the lymph nodes and the musculoskeletal examination can often be combined for good efficiency and to increase patient acceptance. Remaining beside the dog, the veterinarian can palpate the cranial lymph nodes, then the shoulders and neck, prescapular and scapular lymph nodes, then the elbows and forelimb range of motion; and glide down along the spine and ribs, inguinal and popliteal lymph nodes, and then the pelvic limb joints and range of motion. Reflexes such as conscious proprioception may also be appropriate to check at this time.

Once the rest of the body has been examined, it is time to move to more sensitive areas. Some dogs will prefer to look at the veterinarian for the ear, eye, and oral examination, while others will feel more comfortable with the veterinarian approaching from the side. Monitor the patient and select the least stressful approach based on the animal's preference.

For the ear examination, begin touching in a less sensitive area such as the shoulder or neck, and glide up toward the ear. Inspect the ear visually, and lift the ear flap to examine the pinna and canal. Avoid grasping the pinna by its tip or using the ear as a handle. Throughout this procedure, the technician will be offering small treats. If there is visible inflammation and debris, an otoscope exam may be warranted. Consider placing a topical anesthetic cream on the skin inside of the pinna and vertical canal, then complete the remainder of the physical examination. Placing topical anesthetic will not compromise cytology results and will improve patient comfort during later otoscopic examination. If the ear is infected, Type One training is not appropriate because the patient is in pain.

Targeting or using a food lure can ease examination of the eyes. The technician or veterinarian can help the animal hold still and direct her gaze using treats in different ways: either using a treat spoon to have the animal hold still and the veterinarian moves around to look at the eye, or holding the treat beside your nose to encourage the animal to look at you. Holding a treat near your own nose, and drawing a line between the dog's nose and your own, can help the dog look into your eyes to facilitate examination. Holding a treat beside a light source or ophthalmoscope may help the dog look toward the light source for pupillary light reflex **(PLR)** and further ophthalmic evaluation. Cranial nerve responses can also be tested at this time if appropriate for the patient. For tests such as tear tests and corneal staining, Type Two training is usually more appropriate.

Video 5.7 shows using a spoon with lickable cheese as both a lure and a distraction to facilitate puppy examination and vaccination. The technician introduces the food distraction, then takes several seconds to move through the handling leading up to the injection. Since the dog is relaxed and remains interested in the distraction, the injection is administered. The dog continues eating throughout the injection process, and shows relaxed body language. Notice that the lure is kept in the correct position so the puppy can easily reach it to eat while maintaining the body position the veterinarian prefers for examination and vaccination.

Oral examination for Type One dogs is generally well-accepted. Since the dog has been accepting treats throughout the exam, he has had a chance to become comfortable with fingers and hands near and in his mouth. From one side, lift the lips to see the teeth and gums, and insert a treat. Repeat this process on the opposite side. Stand beside the dog rather than face-to-face when opening the mouth. To open the mouth, use a pretzel rod with a sticky treat, or a sticky treat on your fingers right behind the canines. The dog will generally reach to lick the treats, opening the mouth. You can then gently support the open mouth to see inside.

Some veterinarians like to examine the toenails, toes, and bottoms of the paws with each checkup. Remember that the paws and toes have a high concentration of nerve endings, and are more sensitive to touch. Begin touching in a less sensitive area such as the shoulder or hip, glide a hand down, and gently lift the paw in a normal ergonomic walking position. Monitor the dog for food acceptance and proximity preference. Many dogs will stop eating while you are touching the foot, but will resume as soon as the foot is put down. If the dog tries to move away or struggle, allow him to move away and reassess the situation to make a new plan.

Last should be the rectal and genital exam. Temperature measurement can be performed at this time, or during the history, depending upon patient preference. To examine the external urogenital and rectal area, begin touching in a less sensitive area such as the shoulder. Glide a hand along the back, and gently displace the tail laterally or lift it. For breeds who carry the tail over the back, Type One dogs have already raised their own tails. For other breeds, avoid raising the tail higher than the level of the spine (parallel with the floor in a standing dog). Excessive elevation of the tail requires a firm grasp and is uncomfortable or painful for some patients. Avoid raising the tail unless it is medically necessary.

5.4 Type One Training: Cat Exam Room and Examination

Type One cats should be comfortable entering and exiting the cat carrier at home and in the veterinary clinic. Pet owners should be instructed in how to condition cats to like the cat carrier rather than avoiding it. Teaching a cat to like her carrier requires a bit of planning combined with a bit of training. First, the carrier should be a normal part of the household furniture at home. The carrier should be placed in an area the cat likes to rest, such as at the base of the cat tree or in a comfortable corner. Place a comfortable bed inside the carrier. The door should be removed or fastened open so the cat does not become accidentally trapped inside. Many cats will choose to rest in the carrier when one is provided as part of the living quarters. Cat owners can place tasty treats inside the carrier, deliver a treat anytime they find the cat resting in the carrier, and place things like catnip inside to encourage the cat to enter and exit the carrier regularly. Cats who understand targeting a spoon or stick will often follow the target into or out of the carrier both at home and in the clinic.

As discussed in Chapter 4, the cat owner should be escorted to the exam room as soon as possible to decrease stressors experienced in the reception area. Carry the kennel from the bottom for a smoother ride. Depending upon patient preference, place the kennel on the floor or an elevated surface in the exam room, opening the door. Allow the cat to acclimate, and offer treats such as lickable paste, canned cat food, cream cheese, butter, fish paste, or cat treats (Figure 5.7). Allow the cat to explore the exam room and approach you to say hello. Every time the cat comes to a veterinary team member, she should be offered a treat, toy play, or pleasurable touch such as stroking the cheeks or chin. Some cats will be more comfortable remaining in the bottom of their carriers (Figure 5.8). Observe the cat during the history and determine which forms of reward the cat prefers, as these will be used during the examination.

Video 5.8a shows a variety of luring strategies for helping a cat get on the scale. Video courtesy of Mikkel Becker and Fear Free Pets.

Relaxed cats can be lifted gently to the table, assuring they are well-supported. Some cats will follow a lure of treats or a toy onto the table and scale. Most cats will not eat while being lifted, but Type One cats will resume interest in treats, toys, or tactile rewards when they are on the table.

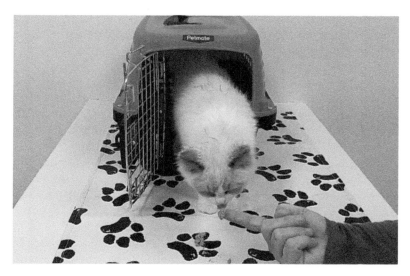

Figure 5.7 Cat following food treats while coming out of the carrier.

Figure 5.8 Feline patient allowed to remain in the bottom of her carrier for ultrasound.

Examining cats on the floor, a bench, or a lap is another excellent option if this feels safe to the team based on the pet's body language signals. If the cat chooses not to exit the carrier, the carrier can be placed on the table and the top of the carrier gently removed. As with dogs, the cat should be encouraged to stay on the exam table by the technician who is offering the preferred reward (treats, toys, or tactile) for remaining there. Frequent rewards help to form a positive emotional association with being on the table, and positively reinforce the choice to stay still on the table.

5.4.1 Physical Examination

The same principles of physical examination for Type One dogs apply for Type One cats. The examination should be performed in order from least invasive to most invasive, saving the oral exam, rectal exam, or any painful areas for last. We need to remember needs versus wants, and that for a healthy cat, a physical examination is a want rather than a need. In some cases, medical management of fear and anxiety is needed, additional training is indicated, and the exam or appointment can be postponed and rescheduled if appropriate.

For physical examination, consider completing the entire examination prior to discussing findings with the owner. Narrate the exam, but avoid pausing for discussion so the examination period is as brief as possible. Most cats also prefer when the veterinarian stands beside rather than face-to-face, as this position is less socially intimidating. When examining the skin, begin by stroking the cheek, chin, and then the neck and shoulders. Begin on the **midline** over the spine, and work downward. Most cats prefer to be touched dorsally rather than ventrally, which is different from dogs. Each touch should predict treats or tactile rewards, which will be given by the technician. The technician should stay ready to provide additional stabilization if the cat has an unexpected reaction, but assessing and monitoring the cat's food acceptance, body language, and proximity preferences will catch stress responses before they manifest as self-defense. For cats, lymph node and thyroid evaluation can be combined with the skin and coat exam.

Next, auscultation can be performed. Stand beside the cat and maintain contact with the cat with one hand while placing the stethoscope in your ears with the other. Introduce the stethoscope dorsally, then slide ventrally to auscult. Cats tend to startle more than dogs when touch is stopped and started, so maintaining contact with at least one hand between touches is often helpful for cats. The technician should be offering preferred rewards throughout this process, and monitoring the cat for changes in food acceptance, body language, and proximity preference.

Abdominal palpation is the next step in the physical examination. Pressure should be applied gradually during palpation, and only to the point where the cat remains comfortable. The technician will continue to provide small treats and tactile rewards during this exam, while being ready to provide stabilization if the cat responds unexpectedly. Abdominal palpation is a good segue into musculoskeletal examination including range of motion of the limbs if indicated, and signs of spinal discomfort. An estimated 90 percent of cats over age 11 years have osteoarthritis and degenerative joint disease on radiographs, and few owners are aware of the pet's pain. Keep in mind an unexpected pain response can occur sometimes more commonly in cats because of their tendency to hide pain exceptionally well.

Saving the most sensitive areas for the end of the exam, the face, feet, and rectogenital examination should be done last. While standing beside the cat, touch is introduced in a less sensitive area such as the shoulder and glides up to the base of the pinna. Many cats have open enough ears so that the pinna does not need to be manipulated. If there is visible otic inflammation or infection, Type two training and handling will be more appropriate. The eyes can be examined in much the same fashion as for dogs, using a food treat or toy to encourage the cat to gaze in the desired direction. Hold a treat or toy, even something as simple as a moving cotton ball, next to your own temple or nose so the cat will look at you for ocular examination. Type One cats will generally watch this distraction even while an ophthalmoscope or indirect handheld lens is used. More restraint tends to make cats close their eyes or try to escape, compromising the quality of the exam.

Oral examination is crucial for cats whenever possible without causing increased stress levels. Because so many cats (>70 percent of cats aged 7 and older) have painful tooth resorption, the oral exam should be gentle but thorough [1]. The American Veterinary Dental College states annual dentistry with radiographs is indicated for senior cats even when the visual oral exam is normal because the risk for this silent and painful condition is so high. Stand beside the cat and offer treats if he has been accepting them. Something sticky such as cream cheese or butter is often useful. Offer the treat near the commissure of the lips, then press gently inward to lift the lip and examine the teeth. Repeat from each side. To open the mouth, use a finger with a treat, or a pretzel rod or

Table 5.3 Least invasive first: One possible examination order.

Least invasive first: one possible examination order
General appearance
Skin (excluding feet)
Auscultation
Abdominal palpation
Lymph nodes
Musculoskeletal
Neurologic
Ears
Eyes
Oral
Paws
Rectal/genital
Any known painful areas should be reserved for last

tongue depressor with treats, directly behind the canines. Insert the sticky treat, and the cat will generally open. Support the open mouth with your fingers while the cat is licking the food. Never use hair or whiskers as a handle when examining a pet's mouth.

Plan physical examination from least invasive to most invasive, saving any painful areas for the end of the exam. Individual preference may require changes to the examination order, depending upon what a specific patient considers to be invasive.

Video 5.8b shows feline physical and oral examination. Notice the exam is gentle and moves at the pace the cat is comfortable; the use of food encourages him to open his mouth. He stops eating briefly during the middle of the exam, but returns to his treats after the exam is complete.

Lastly, examination of the paws if indicated, and the rectal area. Paw examination is similar to that for dogs. Begin touch in a less sensitive area such as the shoulder or hip near the dorsal midline, then glide down the leg to the paw, lifting the paw in a natural walking posture. To examine the rectal area, begin touching over the shoulder or neck, glide your hand down the dorsal midline, and, using one or two fingers, displace the tail to the side. Rather than grasping the tail, use your fingers in the "OK" sign around the tail to move it aside or minimally lift it. Avoid lifting the tail above the level of the spine, which is parallel with the floor in a standing cat. Many Type One cats will elevate the tail on their own in response to stroking along the spine, or already have the tail elevated when standing simply because they are relaxed, simplifying the genital exam considerably. Table 5.3 summarizes a suggested order for physical examination starting with the probable least stressful portions, and saving the most concerning parts of the exam for last. Individual patient preference will affect the examination order as well.

5.5 Type One Training: Injections and Sample Collection

For Type One animals, the training process is very similar for dogs and for cats for routine procedures. Type One essentially combines luring and distractions with aspects of Touch Gradient and desensitization to form positive associations with medical procedures, and to decrease the amount of restraint or physical stabilization required to accomplish the procedure.

Plan physical examination from least invasive to most invasive, saving any painful areas for the end of the exam. Individual preference may require changes to the examination order, depending upon what a specific patient considers to be invasive.

5.5.1 Subcutaneous and Intramuscular Injection

Subcutaneous injection is the most common route used for injectable agents in small-animal medicine. Both dogs and cats will often remain stationary and cooperative for subcutaneous injection when a distraction such as food treats is provided. **Intramuscular** is another route often used for injections in the veterinary hospital, distraction methods can help some animals with this type of injection.

For both dogs and cats, follow the same basic steps. First, determine what treats or distractor the patient prefers. Assure all materials and treats are ready prior to beginning the injection process. To assess the animal's comfort level with the procedure, begin offering the preferred treat, then touch the injection area lightly. Gradually stroke the injection area more firmly, then tent the skin. Pinch lightly, then firmly, with a fingernail. If the animal continues to remain interested in the distraction and does not move away, give the injection. After the injection, remove the food distraction. For any needle sticks, applying a topical anesthetic product can sometimes help. Prilocaine 2.5 percent/ Lidocaine 2.5 percent cream is readily available and affordable. Apply the cream to the area making sure to work it into the skin (against the grain of the fur is helpful) and allow it to sit for 5–30 minutes before injecting. Be aware animals can become sensitized to any part of the injection process if the needle stick ends up causing distress, even in spite of our best efforts. Touching an injection area, tenting skin, the sight of the syringe, application of numbing cream, and more can all become antecedents to a painful experience. Monitor the patient closely for any signs of fear through the process, and be ready to pause and make a new plan using Type two or Type three training plans if the animals FAS level increases.

Video 5.9 shows two Type One kittens being vaccinated. The technician first checks to assure the kittens are interested in the food distraction, which is canned kitten food. She reaches toward the injection site, tents the skin, pinches with her fingers, and then gives the injection. The first kitten never stops eating and seems not to notice the injection process. For the second kitten (a littermate to the first), she is interested in the food distraction throughout the preparation for injecting. When the technician begins the actual injection, the kitten moves away a few inches and stops eating briefly, but the injection is almost completed so the technician floats along with the kitten to finish the vaccination. As soon as the injection is finished, the kitten returns to relaxed body language and eating her treats. The second kitten is a better candidate for Type Two training discussed in later chapters.

Video 5.10 shows two different adult cats from the same household. These cats are a good example of choosing the right reward for the right patient. The first cat does well for vaccination with food rewards. She eats throughout the procedure. When we offer food for the second cat, he is less interested, but he likes tactile rewards. He remains relaxed for his injection while tactile rewards are given.

Video 5.11 shows Skittles, a black Labrador retriever, receiving an intramuscular injection using a distraction technique. The technician lightly stabilizes Skittles while another person provides baby food from a syringe. The veterinarian touches the injection area lightly, then pinches it, then administers the injection. Skittles notices the injection (it stings), but returns to eating right away. This dog is a good match for distraction techniques to maintain her low FAS level in the future.

5.5.2 Venipuncture

5.5.2.1 Cephalic

Cephalic venipuncture is common for both dogs and cats. Many dogs and cats will remain stationary for a food distraction during cephalic venipuncture. Some animals may experience increased stress for this procedure if they dislike nail trimming or paw handling, so consider the animal's individual preferences prior to selecting cephalic venipuncture.

To allow cephalic venipuncture, the animal must allow stabilization of the forelimb, occluding, or holding off the vein, alcohol or other preparation solution applied to the skin, palpation of the vein, and needle puncture, and must remain stationary for long enough for the sample to be collected.

First, verify what treat or distraction method the animal prefers. One technician or assistant will be stabilizing the patient and providing food distractions, while the second collects blood. The technician who is stabilizing will invite the animal to sit close to her, and begin offering treats. If you are stabilizing the patient, place your arm gently between the dog's or cat's head and the person drawing blood to protect against any unexpected reactions to the needle puncture, and provide treats with the opposite hand. Once the patient is stabilized, the person who is feeding will monitor the patient's food acceptance, body language, and proximity preferences.

The person drawing blood will touch the shoulder, then the elbow, and then occlude the vein, or the person who is stabilizing may also occlude the vein depending upon the phlebotomist's preference. Prior to drawing blood, the technician will stroke the limb, gently hold the limb, apply alcohol, pinch the injection area, and then finally perform venipuncture (Figure 5.9). If the patient shows an increase in fear or anxiety, using a different blood collection site or a Type Two training plan may be more appropriate. In some hospitals and with certain patients, practitioners may choose to have the pet owner administer the food distraction during sample collection, but this varies by hospital policy.

Figure 5.9 Positioning for cephalic venipuncture using a food distraction.

Video 5.12 shows a Type One kitten cephalic venipuncture. The assistant who is stabilizing the kitten gets her interested in the canned food on the tongue depressor, then holds the limb at the elbow and occludes the vein. The technician who is drawing blood palpates the vein, places alcohol, tests the venipuncture site, then collects the blood. The kitten remains interested in the food distraction throughout the procedure.

Video 5.13 shows this same procedure with a senior cat.

Video 5.14 shows a Type One feline cephalic venipuncture. This cat is a very quick eater! Observe the cat's body language. It changes to moderate stress when the food is gone. This error caused the cat to experience more stress than preferred during the procedure. Make sure you have plenty of treats at hand before you begin to assure the distraction lasts through and after the procedure.

5.5.2.2 Lateral Saphenous (Dogs)

The **lateral saphenous** is an excellent place to collect a sample from a dog who is comfortable standing or lying down on a hip. When collecting from the lateral saphenous, there are several positioning options shown in Figure 5.10. For the three-person option, one person provides treats and stabilizes the dog's front end, while the second occludes the vein and the third draws blood. In the two-person option, the first person provides treats and stabilizes the front of the dog, while the second person both occludes the vessel and collects the blood.

When collecting from the lateral saphenous, remember to have the dog on a comfortable nonslip surface. The dog should be standing or lying down rolled onto a hip. It is not necessary or appropriate to restrain these dogs in lateral recumbency. Offer the treat distraction at nose level, holding it still so the dog remains still. Place an arm near the dog's neck to prevent him from turning around if he is startled by the needle stick. The person who is occluding the vein (whether this is a dedicated team member or the person drawing the blood) should start touch higher on the leg near the hip, then glide down to the back of the stifle to occlude the vessel (Figure 5.11). The person who is offering treats should monitor the dog's body language and food acceptance, and communicate any changes to the rest of the team. Stroke the area where the blood will be drawn, then pinch, apply alcohol, and collect the sample. For patients who tend to move slightly, a butterfly catheter can simplify blood collection as the patient can move a bit and the blood draw can continue.

5.5.2.3 Medial Saphenous (Cats)

Type One cats will often give blood from the **medial saphenous** while calmly sitting sternal on a table. Please do not scruff and stretch cats for this sample. The cat should be positioned on a comfortable nonslip surface. One person will offer treats and stabilize the cat while occluding the vein, while a second technician collects the blood. Allow the cat to sit in sternal recumbency, rolled onto a hip. While the cat is eating his treats, gently hold off the vein using a few fingers. A whole-hand "karate chop" is not necessary; try to apply the minimum required pressure in the correct location to raise the vein. The person who is stabilizing the cat will monitor body language and food acceptance. When collecting the sample, stroke the sample area, apply alcohol, palpate the vein, pinch to test for reaction, then collect the sample. A butterfly set can be extremely useful in slightly wiggly patients.

Video 5.15 demonstrates this technique with a feline patient and using a tactile distraction. The tactile stimulus is pleasurable for the cat and provides both support and distraction during blood collection.

5.5.2.4 Jugular

The **jugular vein** is a preferred site for venipuncture for rapid blood collection because the sampling time is far shorter and if the peripheral veins need to be conserved for some reason (e.g.

(a)

(b)

(c)

Figure 5.10   (a–c) Several options for lateral saphenous venipuncture using food distractions.

Figure 5.11 Begin touch near the hip, then glide to the venipuncture or injection area.

chemotherapy, or an IV catheter anticipated within the next week). Further, the distribution of nerve endings in the jugular region is less dense than over the peripheral veins resulting in less skin sensitivity in some patients. If a volume of blood larger than 3 ml is required, the jugular vein will supply this sample size more easily than peripheral veins. However, jugular access may be slightly more socially invasive from the animal's perspective.

For both dogs and cats, assure the patient is sitting or standing on a comfortable nonslip surface. One person will be helping the patient sit stationary and offering food, while a second person collects the sample. Assure the patient is accepting food or tactile rewards, and gently position the chin using both the location of the treats and a hand under the chin for stability. Do not stretch patients over the end of the table. Once the patient is comfortable, occlude the vessel, palpate, apply alcohol, pinch the area lightly, then collect the sample. The technician who is stabilizing the patient should communicate any changes in food acceptance and body language. If the dog or cat struggles, pause the procedure and evaluate the handling plan.

Video 5.16 shows a black Labrador retriever, Skittles, participating in a jugular blood draw while eating baby food from a syringe. Monique invites Skittles onto the mat by luring her with the treats, then gently stabilizes under her chin. Skittles eats the baby food before, during, and after her blood draw.

Video 5.17 shows a low-restraint jugular blood draw with an older Chihuahua, and we use minimal stabilization for her head. Before the blood draw positioning was attempted using a food distraction, but the dog was so eager to reach the food she was moving around too much to safely collect the blood sample. Instead, the dog was provided with a tactile distraction during her blood collection, and food rewards immediately before and after the blood draw. A good example of choosing the right strategy for each individual patient and assessing if a specific distraction is feasible to position each specific pet for each specific procedure.

5.5.3 Blood Pressure Measurement

For blood pressure measurement using a Doppler or self-contained noninvasive blood pressure unit (NIBP), it is important to reduce stress as much as possible to obtain an accurate reading.

Restraining the pet and causing anxiety or struggling will increase the patient's blood pressure reading, and can lead to false high readings.

Allow the patient to assume a comfortable position. This may be standing, sitting down, or lying down depending upon the pet. When possible, have the owner nearby to help the patient relax and cooperate, and even offer the treats. Once the patient is in a comfortable position, allow the patient to keep his limbs in the preferred position and apply the blood pressure cuff. Assess the patient for changes in food acceptance and body language. If the patient appears comfortable, hold the Doppler crystal to the artery. Use headphones to listen for the signal so the sound does not upset the patient. Once the signal is acquired, continue offering food and tactile rewards through the measurement and while the crystal and blood pressure cuff are removed.

Traditionally, blood pressure has been measured in forced lateral recumbency. If the animal is even mildly uncomfortable with restraint, the blood pressure measurements will be elevated by stress, invalidating the result. A balance must be found between the pet's emotional state and the ideal physical positioning of the blood pressure cuff to establish a plausible test result.

Video 5.18 shows a Type One cat having her blood pressure measured while sitting in an owner's lap. This cat is not interested in food, but enjoys stroking and the owner speaking softly to her. The technician tries to disturb the cat's preferred position as little as possible during the measurement, and the cat remains relaxed through the procedure.

5.5.4 Cystocentesis

Cystocentesis is the gold standard for urine sample collection, but it may not be right for every patient. Positioning for cystocentesis can be stressful for patients, so choosing a plan appropriate to the patient is important. For patients who are stressed by cystocentesis, consider a sterile free-catch sample as a reasonable alternative [2]. If a free-catch culture is positive and there is a question of contamination, confirmatory cystocentesis can be scheduled if medically necessary, using appropriate anxiolytic or sedative medications.

Type One cats will often allow cystocentesis standing or in sternal recumbency rolled onto a hip in the same position used for medial saphenous venipuncture (Figure 5.12). The cat must have an easily palpated bladder for this procedure to be safe and simple. If the bladder is small or difficult to palpate, select another position for cystocentesis, or collect the sample at a better time when

Figure 5.12   Positioning for Type One feline cystocentesis.

the bladder is more full. One technician should stabilize the cat, offering food and tactile distractions depending upon the cat's preference. The technician performing the cystocentesis will begin touching in a less sensitive area, such as over the back, then move to abdominal palpation. Isolate the bladder and move it laterally toward the flank, smoothing the skin over the bladder with your thumb. Assure no other intra-abdominal structures are between the bladder and the body wall. Once the bladder is well isolated, apply a small amount of alcohol, and perform the cystocentesis. Type One cats generally stand or sit nice and still throughout this procedure. If dorsal recumbency is selected, have two people available to stabilize the cat and provide distractions rather than a single person attempting to do so.

Cystocentesis for dogs requires slightly different positioning because the bladder is not as freely palpated and moved compared with cats Ultrasound guidance is encouraged for canine cystocentesis.

For large Type One dogs with a full bladder, standing ultrasound-guided cystocentesis can be a low-stress procedure (Figure 5.13). One technician will stabilize the dog standing on a nonslip

(a)

(b)

Figure 5.13 Positioning for Type One canine standing cystocentesis.

surface and offer treats, monitoring the dog's body language and food acceptance. A second technician can approach from beside the dog, sitting or kneeling on the floor. Begin by stroking the dog on his side or back, then touching the abdomen with a hand and then the ultrasound probe. Verify the bladder is full, and there are no other intra-abdominal structures between the bladder and the body wall.

Introduce the needle and perform cystocentesis. Small and medium dogs may be gently placed in lateral or dorsal recumbency. Using similar strategies to those seen in the radiograph positioning examples, gently establish recumbency while offering pleasant food and tactile distractions. Using ultrasound, verify the bladder is full and appropriately positioned, then perform cystocentesis. If the dog is struggling or fearful about positioning or scanning, stop and allow the dog to move away, then make a new handling plan. Medical treatment of anxiety and stress is generally the most expedient means for obtaining cystocentesis for fearful animals. This is rarely a frequent or serial procedure, so investing the time and effort training specifically for cystocentesis may have diminishing returns.

5.6 Administering Medications and Grooming

5.6.1 Medication Stations

Often, we perform treatments in the hospital such as eye medication, ear medication, or oral medication, and then prescribe these same treatments to be continued in the home. Training a medication station will simplify treating pets at home. It is crucial, whenever we prescribe a treatment, that the method for how to complete the treatment is part of the prescription. The medication station is introduced in Chapter 4. The patient should be taught to target the desired location, be it a mat, a cushion, a bed, or another area. The station should be easy for the pet to recognize and a location of much fun and reinforcement. Once the medication station has been taught, we can sometimes take "training shortcuts," relying on the positive power of the station to avoid having to desensitize every type of medication.

Video 5.19 shows using a medication station for nail care. Notice how excited this dog is to get to the station! Watch her body language when she sees the nail clipper cue that the station is available for work and reinforcement. Building on her positive association and enjoyment of the station behavior we were later able to construct a number of functional and useful veterinary care behaviors. For this dog, using the station she is so enthusiastic about has facilitated really rapid training of her easier skills such as blood collection and physical examination.

Video 5.20 shows the use of food distractions to facilitate eye drops for a feline patient. Notice the food is positioned strategically to allow the easiest possible application of the eye drops.

5.6.2 Oral Medications

Imagine you are sitting on a blanket at a lovely summer picnic, with a bowl of beautiful berries in your lap. As you eat the delicious berries, you encounter a lip-puckering eye-squinting sour berry. Ick! But the rest of the bowl beckons, and you try another berry even though one was sour. This is how we would like pets to think of oral medications. If they notice the "sour berry" at all, it happens infrequently enough compared to the delicious ones they will try again. However, if every time we give a special treat, there is a sour pill in the center the patient may learn that the special food predicts the bitter pill, and will become wary of special treats.

For Type one oral medication administration, teach owners to disguise a pill in a food treat. Do not give pills in an entire meal, as this is just an invitation to eat around the pill and skip taking the medication. Clever pets will quickly make this decision. Before using treats to hide a pill, teach the skill of eating five treats in rapid succession. When the pet accepts the first treat, immediately offer the second, and so on until all five treats are gone. A simple exercise like this builds fluency in the swallowing behavior, and prepares the pet for the eventuality when pills may be needed in the future. When preparing a pill, the client will then prepare three to five treats rather than just one. Select a treat the patient enjoys such as canned food, small meat pieces, cheese, cream cheese, or even commercially available pill-hiding treats. Offer one or two plain treats, then the medicated treat, and immediately offer one or two plain treats. Rapidly offering the plain treats will encourage the animal to eat the medicated treat rapidly to make room for the next food being offered just like they did in the five treat exercise.

Video 5.21 demonstrates the multiple-treat method for giving a pill to a dog. Notice the technician gives the treats rapidly, encouraging the dog to swallow right away and not spend a lot of time thinking about what might or might not be hidden in them. When one treat is presented and the dog accepts it, the next is immediately offered. The goal is to reinforce the behavior of rapid swallowing.

Liquid medications can usually be mixed with delicious soft food. Starting young animals out accepting food from a syringe will prepare them to accept liquid medications in the future. If it is a small volume of medicine, it can be mixed with a small amount of food and administered simply as a treat. If the volume of medicine is a bit larger, use an alternating syringe method, just as the three to five treat method is explained above. Load one syringe with delicious food, and one syringe with the medication mixed with a bit of delicious food. Begin by offering the syringe with the delicious food. Once the animal is licking the syringe well, change syringes and administer the medication, then change back right away to the plain delicious treat syringe. Going back to our analogy, the delicious sweet berries should outnumber the sour ones in any bowl.

This may sound like a lot of work! Consider how much time will be saved when patients willingly show up for medication rather than the owner having to chase pets all over their homes. Filling and washing two syringes is much more efficient than getting the medication ready, hunting down Fluffy who has run off and is hiding under the bed, dragging Fluffy out from under the bed, wrapping her in a blanket, prying her mouth open, spraying the medicine in, and then cleaning up the towel, the medication mess, putting the bed back where it belongs, and washing out the syringe.

Puppies and kittens can be taught from an early age to accept treats manually like a pill, and to eat treats from a syringe. Often when we give liquid treats in the clinic, we will administer them using a syringe because of the helpful effect it has of teaching animals how to enjoy accepting liquids from syringes.

Video 5.22 shows a puppy's first introduction to accepting treats in the same fashion as a pill, and accepting liquid food from a syringe simulating oral medications. Notice the puppy stays near the technician, has relaxed body language, and continues accepting food throughout the training session.

Video 5.23 shows a young kitten learning to accept liquid medications from a syringe. Notice the technician switches between the syringe holding only delicious food and the syringe with the mixture of medicine and food to keep the kitten engaged and willing to participate.

5.6.3 Ear Examination, Medications, and Cleaning

Type One dogs and cats will often allow ear cleaning and placement of medication using a distraction method without restraint. *If the animal has a painful infected ear, please use a different plan. Sedation is recommended for all treatments of painful ears.* Using distraction methods for animals with painful conditions will often poison the distraction. The food begins to predict something painful occurring, so the animal learns not to take food in that circumstance, rather than learning to tolerate and enjoy handling and treatment.

Use a distraction such as sticky treats on a spoon, a toy or bowl with canned food, or treats smeared on a vertical surface. Help the animal stand, sit, or lie down comfortably. Once the animal is eating, touch a less sensitive area such as the shoulder. Glide up to the base of the ear, then lift the ear flap. Using a wet cotton ball or cleansing pad, apply cleanser and then massage the ear canal. The animal will generally stop eating during this moment, and then shake his head. If the animal returns to eating right away, continue with the ear cleansing. If the animal's body language, food acceptance, and proximity preference indicate increasing stress levels, change to Type Two training described in Chapter 6.

Video 5.24 shows Monique using a combination of the station and food distractions to examine a puppy's ears. The puppy has a history of sensitivity to handling but has progressed dramatically in her training after learning her station. She shows sensitivity when her infected right ear is examined compared to the left ear. She was subsequently given pain medication and mild sedation so her ear could be treated without causing extra stress.

5.6.4 Nail Trims

Nail trimming is a fact of life in the veterinary hospital, but why? We are not groomers, and this is a basic part of animal husbandry just like feeding or brushing. Nail trims are almost never a medical emergency, but they can permanently damage the relationship between the veterinary team and the pet. Animals have sensitive paws, and often they have had negative experiences where a huge wrestling match predicts a nail trim, and perhaps even pain when a nail is trimmed too short. Remember, even dogs and cats who have never had a painful nail trim can find nail trims stressful, so prevention and Type One training are important to get this grooming procedure started out on the right paw. Type One training is only appropriate if the patient has no previous unpleasant learning history and negative emotional response. To reverse an existing problem, please refer to Type Two and Type Three. No dog ever "needs" to be put into lateral recumbency for grooming. No cat "needs" to be scruffed and stretched for a nail trim. These animals deserve medical and behavioral treatment of fear and anxiety prior to grooming, rather than to be subjected to a non-emergency, nonmedical procedure that can damage the trust between veterinary team and patient forever.

Training Tip: Remember the 2-2-3 Rule!
Two gentle stabilizing arms Two seconds of struggling for cats Three seconds of struggling for dogs Any more than this requires a pause, assessment, and new training plan.

For Type One patients, allow the dog or cat to choose a comfortable position. Standing is generally the easiest position to access all the paws and provide food distractions. Very small dogs sometimes prefer to be held in someone's arms or sit on the owner's lap during nail trims. Some cats prefer to sit in a carrier bottom. One technician (or the owner, depending upon your hospital policy) should provide food distractions while a technician works to provide the grooming. Begin touching in a less sensitive area such as the shoulder, then glide down to the elbow, carpus, paw, toe, toenail, and

(a)

(b)

Figure 5.14 (a) Correct paw positioning for a standing canine nail trim. The paw should be held low in a comfortable walking position. (b) Incorrect paw position.

then clip. Raise the paw into a natural walking or reaching position, avoid lifting the leg too high or off to the side (Figure 5.14). If the patient struggles, has an increase in anxious body language, or stops accepting food, pause the procedure. If pausing the procedure does not result in an immediate return to baseline, consider changing to Type Two or Type Three training.

Preventive desensitization and classical conditioning can also be used for Type One dogs and cats, especially puppies and kittens. Desensitization and classical conditioning have an advantage over distraction techniques because the food distraction is unlikely to begin predicting the nail trim, so the patient will not become wary of food offered in the hospital if their FAS suddenly increases with nail care. The primary difference between the distraction method and the classical conditioning method is timing. For the distraction method, the food is offered before, during, and after the procedure. With desensitization and classical conditioning, touch *predicts* the food, so it is provided during or after each step in the process, but not before the handling.

Uncomfortable tail position and
handling

Comfortable tail position and
handling

Figure 5.15 Correct and incorrect tail position for temperature measurement or anal gland expression.

Video 5.25 shows two different Type One pets receiving nail trimming with distraction techniques. Notice the pet stays engaged with the distraction before, during, and after each clip. The
pet is allowed to choose the body and paw position that feels comfortable to them. If the pet shows
decreased interest in food or moves away, a new plan will be made.

Video 5.26 demonstrates preventive desensitization and classical conditioning. The goal of nail
trimming is broken down into numerous small steps as discussed in Chapter 3. Each small step
predicts a click and treat. The puppy begins offering his paws and impatiently trying to participate
in the nail trim while the owner watches, learning how to replicate the technique at home with her
puppy.

5.6.5 Anal Gland Expression

Anal gland expression is sometimes medically necessary, but often a grooming request from the
owner. This means it is almost always a want, and rarely a need. Using lidocaine jelly as lubri-
cant can assist in making anal gland expression more comfortable, but this procedure understandably provokes strong responses in many patients. As with temperature measurement, assure the
tail is lifted mildly, and not excessively, to reduce patient discomfort (Figure 5.15). Because of
the strong response many patients have, Type One training is almost never appropriate for anal
gland expression. Refer to Type Two and Type Three for strategies to condition pets to accept this
procedure.

5.7 Conclusion

Type One training should be the basic standard of care for most patients who do not have a pre-
existing fear response, do not have a painful condition, and will not require repeated treatments.
The proper application of distractions and gentle support allows many relaxed patients to receive
care with little or even no physical restraint for both traditional and complementary therapies (see
feline acupuncture using this method in **Video 5.27**). If the patient is anxious, stressed, or fearful;
has a painful condition such as otitis or arthritis; or will require the treatment repeatedly, such as
insulin injections; Type Two and Type Three training are more appropriate choices.

References

1 Reichart, P. (1984). Periodontal disease in the domestic cat: a histopathological study. *Journal of Periodontal Research* 19 (1): 67–75.

2 Weese, J. (2011). Antimicrobial use guidelines for treatment of urinary tract disease in dogs and cats: Antimicrobial Guidelines Working Group of the International Society for Companion Animal Infectious Diseases. *Veterinary Medicine International* (2011): 263768. https://doi.org/10.4061/2011/263768.

6

Type Two Patients and Training: Conditioning Plans for FAS 0–3 Pets

6.1 Type Two Training: Desensitization, Counterconditioning

Training for Type Two patients goes beyond using distraction techniques. Type Two training is appropriate for Type Two and Type One patients (FAS 0–3), but is usually not a good *starting* point for Type Three patients who display FAS 4–5. Remember: setting up the environment for success is still crucial. Check the medical record for individual preferences, set up the working area in a relaxing way from the pet's point of view, and remember to consistently assess and reassess the patient throughout the visit, pausing to make a new plan if necessary.

Referring to Chapters 3 and 4, you will recall the procedures of desensitization, classical conditioning, and classical counterconditioning. Type Two patients will benefit from these techniques because they are already showing signs of FAS which are contraindicated for distraction techniques using the criteria established in Chapter 5. Some Type Two patients are naturally shy or wary of new experiences, may be naturally fearful of restraint, or have had a learning history of fear-provoking veterinary procedures in the past. Rather than prevention, as is the case with most Type One patients, Type Two patients need intervention to reverse their fear and anxiety, and prevent it from worsening over time. When making a training plan for a Type Two patient, we will need to identify the assessment protocol for Type Two patients and determine if desensitization and classical conditioning or counterconditioning procedures are the tools of choice. We can then make a desensitization hierarchy and classical conditioning or counterconditioning plan to improve the patient's ability to tolerate the procedure, remain in a positive emotional state, and cooperate during medical treatment.

Some Type Two patients will need to have training visits prior to the completion of a service, such as a physical examination. The methods described in this chapter can be used during a primary visit, during training preparation visits, or both. Veterinary technicians with the right skills are extremely valuable, because we can provide training visits to prepare patients for better care from the veterinarian. Many of the videos in this chapter are from training visits used to ready the patient for more in-depth veterinary care.

6.2 Identifying Type Two Patients (FAS 2–3)

Patient assessment requires us to be flexible as observers. Patients may switch between Types at any time in the process, and there is fluidity in their behaviors. The structure of these assessments is a basic guideline. In general, Type Two patients are experiencing mild or moderate stress as described in Chapter 2. These patients often find the environment or the procedure mildly fear provoking,

Type Three
- Moderate or severe stress
- Severe stress or self-defense with handling
- Refuses most food and tactile
- Difficulty returning to baseline

STOP
Cooperative care training for *wants*
Sedation required for *needs*
Medication usually indicated
Training process guides treatment

Type Two
- Mild stress if no handling
- Mild or moderate stress during handling
- Stops accepting food and tactile during handling
- Returns to baseline rapidly

Proceed with CAUTION for *needs*
Desensitization and counterconditioning
Medication may be needed
May need to pause, assess, reschedule

Type One
- Calm, relaxed body language
- Returns to baseline easily
- Readily accepts food, toy, and tactile
- Chooses close proximity

GO ahead for *wants and needs*
Distraction techniques
Monitor body language
Monitor food acceptance and proximity

Figure 6.1 Evaluation guide for Type Two patients.

but not severely. When patients are experiencing moderate stress, it is difficult for them to learn new skills or form positive emotional responses. If the fight-or-flight response gets triggered, the patient will move into self-defense or self-preservation mode, and the good window for learning will close. Part of Type Two training will be to interact with the patient in a way that improves their emotional status and decreases anxiety and fear, so they can learn the veterinary skills more effectively (Figure 6.1).

Many patients with FAS 2–3 will benefit from medical management of fear and stress. From nutraceuticals and pheromones to anxiety-reducing pharmaceuticals, many options are available for the medical treatment of veterinary anxiety. For truly stress-free care, consider using event-based treatments prior to veterinary visits. Over time, if the owner pursues training, the dosage can often be decreased or the medication weaned entirely away; but the patient experience should be a top priority for the veterinary team, and for some patients, "Medicine is the best medicine."

Training Tip: Drugs Not Hugs!

Medicine is often the best medicine, not more restraint. Be sure to provide medical intervention for fear, stress, and anxiety whenever indicated. Early intervention treating fear is always more effective than attempts to reverse severe anxiety once it has already begun.

6.2.1 Type Two Dogs: FAS 0–3

6.2.1.1 Food Acceptance
- Dogs will accept food immediately or after <5 seconds
- Will accept high-value food from any team member
- Will accept lower value food from trusted or preferred team members
- Takes food with a soft mouth; no snapping or grabbing when no handling is occurring
- May begin taking food roughly when handling or procedures begin

- May continue taking food or may stop taking food during procedures
- If stopped accepting food during the procedure, may accept a higher value food
- If stopped taking food during handling or procedure, immediately begins taking food again when the handling or procedure is completed.

Table 6.1 provides a quick reference checklist for assessing Type Two dogs. Figure 6.2 shows a Type Two dog.

Table 6.1 Checklist for Type Two dogs: each dog assessing at Type Two may have a combination of these attributes.

Stage of visit	Food acceptance	Body language	Proximity preference
Greeting	□ High-value from any team member □ Low-value from preferred people or owner □ Within 5 seconds □ Soft mouth	□ Relaxed body	□ Greets immediately □ Stays near team member □ May or may not solicit attention
Touching	□ High-value treats only □ May take treat roughly	□ Mild tension during touch	□ Moves away □ Moves toward owner
Exam and treatment	□ High-value treats only □ May take treat roughly	□ Mild tension during procedures □ Returns to baseline <10 seconds	□ Does not move away □ Remains close during treatments □ Returns to baseline <10 seconds

Figure 6.2 Type Two canine patient.

6.2.1.2 Body Language
- Relaxed body language in the hospital when not being handled (refer to Chapter 2)
- May show mild stress markers during handling:
  - Looking or leaning away
  - Mild pupil dilation
  - Closed mouth or increased respiratory rate (refer to Chapter 2)
  - Moving away when procedure begins or is attempted
  - Attention seeking from the owner but not veterinary team members
  - Tense muscles or exaggerated panniculus response when touched
  - Tail is tense or held abnormally low for the breed
- May show mild to moderate stress markers during procedures
- When the handling and procedure are stopped, returns to baseline relaxed state within 10 seconds.

6.2.1.3 Proximity Preference
- When unrestrained, dog immediately greets veterinary team members
- Chooses to remain near team members while they talk to and touch him
- May retreat closer to the owner, back away, or move away when approached
- May choose to stay near team members when approached, but show other signs of stress simultaneously
- Will retreat closer to the owner, back away, or move away when touched
- Tries to move away during procedures
- Will return to baseline proximity preference within 10 seconds of stopping procedures.

6.2.2 Type Two Cats: FAS 0–3

As mentioned in this book, food acceptance is a less reliable indicator of stress in cats when contrasted against dogs. However, for cats who will eat in the hospital, changes in food acceptance are a useful indicator of stress levels.

6.2.2.1 Food Acceptance, Toy Acceptance, and Tactile Acceptance
- Investigates or accepts food while in carrier, or within 30 seconds of exiting carrier
- Interacts with toy if toy motivated
- Investigates offered food, but may or may not eat depending upon preferences
- Accepts food before touching, but ceases eating or eats more roughly during touching
- Stops eating during procedures
- May return to eating after procedures, or show interest in food and then choose not to eat
- May show interest in tactile rewards such as chin and cheek rubs
- May stop tactile acceptance during procedures, but rapidly returns to baseline after procedure.

6.2.2.2 Body Language
- Relaxed body language after exiting carrier and before handling (refer to Chapter 2)
- Mild stress markers during handling, such as:
  - Moving slowly and cautiously
  - Whiskers pulled forward
  - Ears to the side
  - Increased respiratory rate (refer to Chapter 2)

- ■ Purring without soliciting attention
- ■ Slightly tense muscles when touched; exaggerated panniculus response
- ■ Tail tucked close to body
- ■ Paws concealed when lying down
- Mild stress markers during procedures
- Returns to baseline body language within 30 seconds of completion of procedure.

6.2.2.3 Proximity Preference

- Chooses to exit carrier within one minute of arrival
- May explore exam room but cautiously, crouching or following walls
- May choose to sit stationary near the owner or in a neutral location
- May approach team members, but may not
- Does not retreat when team members approach without attempting handling
- Allows facial petting and stroking before handling or procedures
- Attempts to move away when handling begins
- Attempts to move away during procedures
- Returns to baseline proximity preference within 30 seconds of completing procedures.

Table 6.2 provides a quick reference checklist for assessing Type Two cats. Figure 6.3 shows a Type Two cat.

Figure 6.3b Shows a visual representation of these delivery strategies. Experiment with different timing strategies to determine if the patient shows an individual preference.

Patients who are appropriate for Type Two training are either relaxed or mildly stressed in the veterinary environment. Their stress level generally increases slightly during handling and procedures, but they are capable of returning to baseline after handling and procedures. Type Two training is a combination of helping the animal to relax, and then teaching the patient that the veterinary procedure is nonthreatening and is associated with pleasurable things.

Remember: health status and individual preference influence assessment and training Types. Any patient known to have a painful condition such as an ear infection, lameness, or gastrointestinal (GI) upset should be assumed to need Type Two protocols at minimum. A little extra proactive planning for these patients will increase success and decrease unwanted outcomes over time. Often,

Table 6.2 Checklist for Type Two cats: each cat assessing at Type Two may have a combination of these attributes.

Stage of visit	Food or tactile acceptance	Body language	Proximity preference
Greeting	□ Shows some interest □ May eat within 30 seconds □ May prefer tactile	□ Relaxed body	□ Exits carrier willingly □ Explores exam room □ Solicits attention
Touching	□ Desire diminished by touch □ Return to baseline <30 seconds	□ Moderate stress markers	□ Moves away □ Return to baseline <30 seconds
Exam and treatment	□ Desire diminished by touch □ Return to baseline <30 seconds	□ Moderate stress markers	□ Moves away □ Return to baseline <30 seconds

Figure 6.3 Type Two feline patient.

Type Two patients can have their exam and procedures done during a single visit. In some cases, these patients need to be rescheduled to allow either medical management of stress and anxiety, or training prior to proceeding with nonvital treatments. When attempting Type Two training with patients, notify the veterinarian right away if the patient's fear and stress seem to be worsening rather than improving, so the patient can be reassessed and a new plan formulated.

6.2.2.4 Treats, Treatments, and Timing

When handling animals, we are always teaching and training them. As we go through the examples in this chapter, we will break down some possible desensitization and Touch Gradient approaches to common procedures. Each step in the exposure process should be paired with something the animal likes as part of the conditioning or counterconditioning procedure.

The timing of when we give the treat or other preferred item matters. Different pets will prefer different treat delivery timing, and different treat timing may be helpful for certain procedures.

The basic types of timing for food delivery are:

Distraction: Food first, then procedure and food happen together, then food stops. This was covered in Chapter 5.
Simultaneous: Food and procedure start at the same time and stop at the same time.
Touch-then-Treat: Touch starts, food starts, both continue together, both stop at the same time.
Treat-after-Touch: Touch starts, touch stops, food is delivered.

Figure 6.3b shows a visual representation of these delivery strategies. Experiment with different timing strategies to determine if the patient shows an individual preference.

6.3 Type Two Training: Dog Exam Room and Examination

Type Two dogs may show mild to moderate stress in the reception area and on the way to the exam room. Signs can change rapidly, so be watchful, and continue to do things like offering treats repeatedly even if the dog refuses them. Often dogs who initially refuse food will decide to accept it as time passes. Also, offering different treats and using different approaches can enhance food acceptance. Type Two dogs may not feel comfortable taking treats from your hand or a spoon, but may follow a treat trail or accept treats from the owner's hand. As these dogs are slightly more stressed, they are more susceptible to trigger stacking. The more stressed an animal is, the less emotional energy they have available to tolerate time and events within the hospital. We need to plan to provide services in order of importance to make the best use of the patient's ability to cooperate.

6.3.1 Reception, Weight, and Moving to the Exam Room

The team member should calmly greet the dog, allowing the dog to approach if he chooses to. If the dog chooses not to approach, dropping a few treats onto the floor and turning away may promote movement and approaches. If the dog will follow a treat trail onto the scale, collect a body weight. If the dog is too nervous to be weighed easily, consider postponing the weight until after the examination at the end of the visit.

To invite the dog into the exam room, try using a treat trail or a lure as described for Type One patients in Chapter 5. If the dog is too nervous to accept food, stops moving, or begins backing up, stop trying to move the dog and instruct the owner how to make a treat trail or how to hold the lure. Move out of the way, preferably to a point behind the dog so the entrance to the exam room is clear, and see if the owner can invite the dog into the exam room. Coach the owner to keep the leash loose, and observe the dog's ability to follow the lure. If the dog is reluctant to follow, try having the owner offer higher value treats, give treats more frequently or place treats closer together, or toss the treats so they are exciting to chase. Figure 6.4 shows an example of using treat placement on the floor of the exam room to promote patient movement.

If this plan fails, do not drag the dog into the examination room. This dog may be best examined in the lobby, the parking lot, or the car for today, and signed up for happy visits or Type Three training for moving into the exam room in the future. Stressing the dog excessively over trying to enter the exam room may sabotage your ability to provide an exam or other treatments by using up the dog's emotional reserves before they ever step into the room.

Some dogs who are moderately fearful approaching the scale or examination room may be nervous about the texture or sheen of the floors. Rolling out a few rugs or yoga mats to make a good-traction trail into the exam room sometimes makes all the difference for dogs who are sensitive to slick or shiny floors. If you're not sure, ask the owner. Many owners are aware their dogs fear slippery floors, but it doesn't occur to them that this is the reason the dog is reluctant to move through the lobby or exam room.

Video 6.1 shows a dog who is too nervous to enter the exam room. The technician shows the owner to use food lures to move the nervous dog forward. Notice the technician uses a jackpot of several treats once the dog is in the exam room as a reward.

6.3.2 The Exam Room

Mildly stressed dogs will still usually approach the technician. Greeting these dogs in a nonthreatening way is crucial. Sit in a chair next to the owner, or on the floor with your side to the dog. Begin by tossing treats away from you to encourage the dog to move around the room. Each time he approaches you, mark with a click or a verbal marker, then toss the treat away. By feeding away from where we are sitting, we are resetting the dog to practice approaches several times and giving him

(a)

(b)

Figure 6.4 (a) A treat trail on the floor and (b) having the owner move can encourage fearful dogs to explore.

Table 6.3 Desensitization and counterconditioning worksheet: a basic template for setting up a DS/CC/CCC plan for a patient.

Training plan: desensitization and counterconditioning	
Trigger:	Exposure ladder:
Foundation behaviors required:	
Preferred rewards to generate positive emotional response 1. 2. 3.	
Medications:	Working area:
Nonstressful starting points:	
Distance	
Duration	
Pressure	
Volume	
Other	
Homework	
Plan for next visit	

Source: Available for download in the Online Resources.

a chance to relax in between approaches. Usually these dogs will approach closer and closer, and after only a few repetitions will try to take food from a hand held low, below their nose level. Once the dog is taking treats from a hand held low, gently reach and offer to touch the dog on his chest between his front legs, as with the Type One greeting. Once you've initiated touch, immediately treat. Repeat the touch–treat, touch–treat, touch–treat process several times. If using a clicker, the order is touch, click while touching, stop touching, treat. The goal is to establish that *touch* **predicts** *food*, rather than using food as a distraction or to convince the dog to stick around for touching. Type Two dogs are often suspicious if food is offered and then we try to reach out with a second hand to touch. Use the principles of classical conditioning rather than distractions for these Type Two patients. Table 6.3 shows a worksheet for planning and tracking the desensitization and counterconditioning (DS/CC) process.

While questioning the owner regarding the medical history for the day's visit, and greeting the Type Two dog, the technician should begin to assess where the dog will be most comfortable for the examination. Most large Type Two dogs will respond negatively to team members trying to lift them onto the table and should be examined on the floor. Many small Type Two dogs will allow lifting to the table with a rapid desensitization protocol.

6.3.2.1 Table Training and Stabilization Training

To desensitize and countercondition the table, we need to make a desensitization hierarchy, or exposure ladder. For a small dog, the completed sequence will be "A technician picks you up and places you on the table." To make the exposure ladder, we need to break down the pick-up event into its component parts. For counterconditioning, we need to make sure every baby step up the ladder predicts something wonderful from the dog's point of view: something that evokes a pleasant emotional response (Figure 6.5).

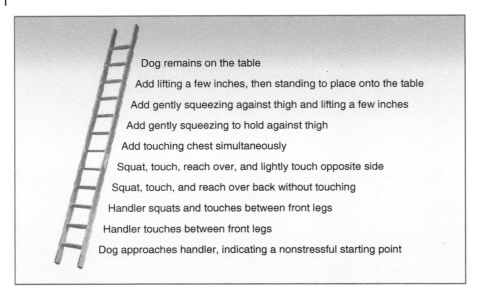

Dog remains on the table

Add lifting a few inches, then standing to place onto the table

Add gently squeezing against thigh and lifting a few inches

Add gently squeezing to hold against thigh

Add touching chest simultaneously

Squat, touch, reach over, and lightly touch opposite side

Squat, touch, and reach over back without touching

Handler squats and touches between front legs

Handler touches between front legs

Dog approaches handler, indicating a nonstressful starting point

Figure 6.5 Example exposure ladder for table training.

Example exposure ladder for placing a small dog on the table:

- Dog approaches handler, indicating a non-stressful starting point
- Dog allows handler to touch between the front legs
- Dog allows handler to squat beside while touching between the front legs
- Dog allows handler to squat, touch, and reach slightly over the back
- Dog allows handler to reach over the back and touch the opposite side
- Dog allows handler to reach over, touch, and then reach under the chest
- Dog allows handler to reach over, reach under, and squeeze dog against her thigh
- Dog allows handler to squeeze against her thigh and lift a few inches
- Dog allows handler to lift a few inches, then stand up and place on the table
- Dog remains on the table.

Every one of these baby steps should *predict* a *wonderful* treat the dog wants and willingly accepts. Remember: if the patient's stress level increases, pause the process and let the animal rest for a moment, then try again from the most recent nonstressful rung on the ladder. Of course, this description includes plenty of operant behaviors: approaching, standing still, individual body language behaviors. *Delivering the treat is not contingent on the animal's behavior*: the treat will happen regardless of what the animal does. Remember, operant conditioning and classical conditioning are happening all the time simultaneously. We discuss them separately to better understand what is occurring, but neither process happens discretely.

Training Tip: Exposure Ladders are Always Under Construction!

Remember: exposure ladders are not set in stone. They are flexible and can be deconstructed, modified, or reconfigured at any time.

You might go up the ladder and down the ladder in a few repetitions, you may have to add rungs if an approximation causes stress, or you may be able to skip rungs if the patient is comfortable and relaxed.

Video 6.2 demonstrates how to rapidly desensitize and countercondition a small dog to allow lifting onto the table. This process took about 30 seconds, and the dog had a pleasant experience. Notice the technician makes sure the dog will approach; breaks down the process of lifting into a series of baby steps, with each step predicting a tasty treat; then makes sure the dog will remain on the table for treats.

This dog has been presented for a nail trim. After the table training and pick-up training, the puppy is still showing signs of moderate stress. The technician takes the time to educate the owner about what she is seeing, and the owner asks if it would be better to do the nail trim another day after some training. What a terrific interaction!

Stabilization and Gentle Control is worth conditioning. So many pets are fearful of being held, even gently. When we introduce any stabilization technique, it is helpful to take a desensitization-minded approach. Stabilization techniques vary on the position the pet needs to assume and the procedure being performed, but there are some similarities across all stabilization techniques. Here is an example of some of the aspects of stabilization which can be broken down into controlled exposures for enhanced success:

- Handler is at a non-stressful distance to the pet
- The distance is gradually decreased until close together
- If two people will be working with the animal, both people are present and at a non-stressful distance
- The distance is gradually decreased until both people are close to the pet
- Once the pet is comfortable with proximity, one person reaches out toward the pet while the other person remains at a distance
- One person touches the pet
- One person glides their hand over the pet in a number of repetitions until their first arm is around the pet in the desired position
- One person touches with their opposite hand only and the process is repeated with each hand
- One person touches the pet with both hands and simulates stabilization for one second
- Duration is gradually added
- The second person approaches and is closer
- The touching exercise is repeated with the second person closer
- The second person begins exposures for the specific procedure while the first person stabilizes the pet (see specific procedures later in this chapter)
- If examination gloves, loupes, or other equipment will be worn, put it on and then diminish the intensity of handling, returning to a series of less intense exposures to evaluate the patient's response.

Many pets perceive "one hand is petting and two hands is vetting." Also, "one friend, two foes." Changing from touching with one hand to two hands and adding a second person are common points where pets will instantly show a higher stress level. Putting on examination gloves is another exceptionally common trigger for pets to experience escalating FAS. Watch for these, and plan in advance to introduce them gradually to set pets up for success.

6.3.3 Physical Examination

Communication is vital. Either during the history, or when the veterinarian comes into the room to greet the client and patient, time should be taken to educate the client about the patient's stress level, and how this will guide the handling plan for the day. Keeping a copy of the Fear Free^sm

FAS Spectrum posted in the exam room is excellent for facilitating conversation. Consider the following script: "Mrs. Smith, I see Fluffy is a bit nervous to be here today. We will do our best to help her feel comfortable by teaching her the exam is nothing to fear. If she becomes too nervous, we will stop what we are doing, but we are going to try and complete her exam as efficiently as possible. Once we are done with her exam, we can discuss our findings while Fluffy has a chance to relax."

The order of the physical examination should be much as it is in Chapter 5, with the least invasive touches performed first, always starting in a less sensitive area first and moving to more sensitive areas. The oral exam, paw handling, rectal exam, and any painful areas should be examined last. The position of the veterinarian to the side of the patient most of the time should also remain the same, avoiding face-to-face potentially confrontational body language unless the dog clearly prefers this approach. The main difference between a Type One and a Type Two examination is the change from distraction training to desensitization and counterconditioning.

For a Type Two exam, the process will need to be broken down into small steps. Each small step should predict or be paired with a wonderful treat. Recall that for desensitization, we control the intensity of the trigger. Controlling intensity of the exam portions can include softening touches getting gradually more firm, small touches such as with a finger covering a larger surface area with more fingers or a whole hand, brief touches becoming more lengthy, or gliding a touch from a less sensitive to more sensitive area.

The role of the veterinary technician is to monitor the patient's response, provide well-timed treats in coordination with the veterinarian's examination to facilitate desensitization and counterconditioning, and alert the veterinarian to changes in the dog's stress level during examination. It is important that each step on the exposure ladder is linked with or predicts something wonderful. Also, *each exposure ladder example we provide is simply an example.* Steps may need to be done in a different order, divided into even smaller approximations, or modified in difficulty or duration depending upon the needs of the individual patient. With practice and good patient observation, modifying exposure ladders can become second nature.

Example exposure ladder for a Type Two physical exam:

- Allow the dog to find a comfortable position as the non-stressful starting point
- Touch shoulder
- Touch shoulder, glide along spine
- Glide along spine, down **flank**
- Glide down flank, examine ventrum for two seconds
- Extend to five seconds
- Present stethoscope
- Place hand on auscultation location
- Approach touch point with stethoscope
- Auscultate for two seconds, then for five seconds
- Auscultate for gradually longer periods until completed
- Glide one hand to the abdomen
- Add a second hand to the abdomen
- Palpate gently
- Palpate deeply for two seconds
- Palpate deeply for progressively longer intervals
- Palpate lymph nodes
  - May need to make subsets of one to two lymph nodes at a time

- Palpate limbs one at a time, each one counting as a step on the ladder
  - The limbs may need to be subsets of a joint at a time
- Examine the external ear
  - Divide the ear exam into **pinna**, visual outer canal, opening canal with a finger
- Examine each eye
- If necessary, reach toward the upper eyelid on one side
  - Touch the upper eyelid
  - Repeat steps for the second side
- Oral exam
  - Touch the nose
  - Touch the lateral aspect of the upper lip
  - Raise the lip to expose the canine tooth
  - Raise the lip to expose the canine tooth, then stretch the lip backward to expose caudal teeth
  - Repeat for the second side
  - Gently add a second hand to the muzzle
  - Carefully open the mouth if patient is relaxed enough
- Examine limbs by touching the shoulder or hip first, then:
  - Elbow/**Stifle**
    - **Carpus/Hock**
    - Paw
    - Toe, Toenail
- Rectal and genital visual exam.

Remember: approximations should *predict* a wonderful treat. If the patient's stress level is increasing through the examination, consider postponing part of the examination to provide medical management of anxiety and training visits before trying again. Veterinary technicians with the right skills can desensitize the dog to portions of the (or the entire) physical examination over a series of visits, then the examination skills can be transferred to the doctor.

6.4 Type Two Training: Cat Exam Room and Examination

Type Two cats are mildly stressed, but still accepting food or toys, and tactile rewards such as facial grooming. Often, Type Two cats will benefit from medical treatment of anxiety prior to visits.

If a cat has a conditioned response to the cat carrier, desensitization and counterconditioning (DS/CC) are indicated. Using a combination of desensitization and operant conditioning, cats can learn to enter their carriers and enjoy the cat carrier (Figure 6.6). Sometimes, an aspect of habituation (the intensity of the stimulus stays the same rather than being modified) is also required at the beginning of the training process.

Training a cat to like and enter the carrier involves determining something the cat likes, such as canned food, cream cheese, butter, tuna flakes, or semi-moist cat treats. As with dogs, cats can learn the clicker predicts a wonderful food treat. We can then use the clicker to mark desired behavior, following up with the treat. Here are examples of multipurpose approximations for desensitization, classical counterconditioning, and shaping using operant conditioning to enter the carrier voluntarily.

Each approximation listed in this section, and any progress toward the carrier, earn a click and a treat. Give one treat near the carrier, then give a second treat 12–18 in. away from the carrier to

Figure 6.6 This cat is relaxed in the presence of her carrier.

reset the cat for a new opportunity to try the approach. Each step should be repeated a few times before criteria are increased. The length of this process depends upon the previous conditioned emotional response, how eager the cat is, the skill of the trainer, and the duration the cat chooses to remain engaged and working. The more intense the existing negative emotional response, the more patience and time will be required for desensitization. If there is a considerable negative response already, consider using a different carrier or dismantling the carrier and only using the bottom half to begin the training process. Try to stop training sessions before the cat chooses to opt out, instead ending on a positive note when the cat is still interested and happy.

Examples of approximations to desensitize, countercondition, and shape a carrier entrance:

- Establish a non-stressful starting point where the cat doesn't notice the carrier
- Remain in room where carrier is located
- Glance at carrier
  - Short glance, longer glance, look >3 seconds
- Glance at carrier, and then take one step toward it
  - Two steps, three steps, and so on until next to the carrier
- Sniff the carrier, or explore it by touching it
  - Sniff or touch the half with the door
  - Sniff or touch the end with the door
  - Sniff or touch the door opening
- Place nose in door opening
- Place head in door opening
- Place one paw inside carrier
  - Place two paws, then three paws, then four paws inside carrier
- Walk entirely inside the carrier and remain there for two to three seconds
- Walk into the carrier and remain there while the door is closed briefly
- Exit the carrier when the door is opened without increase in anxiety or flight.

Video 6.3 demonstrates using a combination of desensitization, classical conditioning, and shaping to teach a cat to voluntarily enter the carrier.

Cats who have been trained to enter the carrier will be happier and more relaxed when they arrive at the hospital. As with Type One, escort cats to the exam room promptly to avoid stressors in the reception area.

6.4.1 The Exam Room

For success, the cat needs to be relaxed enough in the hospital to accept food, toys, or desired tactile interaction. If the cat is too fearful or anxious to accept food, toys, or tactile interactions, or will not approach team members nor allow handling without trying to move away or escape, consider providing medical management for anxiety before continuing. Every interaction with a patient is a learning experience, and we want them to learn not to fear us!

For Type Two cats who are accepting food, follow a similar procedure as for greeting dogs. For cats who are not accepting food, continue to offer it. Smelling the delicious food can serve as reinforcement, and food acceptance may improve over time. When the cat approaches, toss a small piece of food a few feet away (about two cat body lengths). With each subsequent approach, the cat will likely come closer and closer. When the cat chooses to greet, offer attention by stroking the cheek or along the spine, avoiding the top of the head or the sides and flanks. Reach out with one hand to pet, and then follow the touch with a treat. Each brief touch should *predict* a tiny delicious treat, to begin classically conditioning the cat to accept and enjoy touch in the exam room. If the cat prefers to sit with the owner, or remain in the bottom of the carrier, offer treats periodically and watch for signs of relaxation. Attempt a brief touch of the cheek or along the spine, and immediately provide a small delicious treat. If the cat chooses to remain stationary, continue. If the cat moves away or shows body language signs of increasing stress, stop touching at that time. If the cat is actively trying to hide, make sure to provide a hiding place such as a towel, a box, carrier lid placed back over the cat, or a bed with high sides.

While taking the history, assess where the cat seems most comfortable, and plan for the examination to be performed there. This may be on the exam table, on the floor, in the owner's lap, in a team member's lap, on a bench beside the owner, or the like. Comfortable cats are more cooperative.

6.4.2 Physical Examination

The physical examination can be broken down for desensitization and classical counterconditioning for cats in the same way as for dogs. Explain to the owner the importance of a rapid examination to decrease stress and increase the positive aspects of the patient's visit, and plan to discuss findings once the exam is completed and the patient is more comfortable. Each step of the physical examination should *predict* delicious food, a few seconds of toy play, or preferred tactile rewards such as cheek or chin stroking. Remember: most cats prefer to be approached from the side rather than face-to-face. A similar exposure ladder as what is suggested for dogs can be effective for cats as well.

Training Tip: Pause, Rewind, Playback in Slow Motion

During desensitization and classical conditioning or counterconditioning, the patient should look calm and relaxed. If you see a change in food acceptance, body language, or proximity preference, hit the pause button. Rewind the process to the most recent non-stressful point, and proceed in slow motion through the approximations, adding rungs to the exposure ladder if needed and assuring the patient remains comfortable and relaxed.

Example examination exposure ladder:

- Find a nonstressful starting position
- Stroke the cheek to establish touch
  - Stroke neck
  - Stroke chin; evaluate thyroid gland
  - Stroke shoulders
  - Follow midline along the spine
  - Stroke from the spine ventrally
- Evaluate lymph nodes while stroking the body
  - Each body region should be considered an approximation
- Touch the spine over the shoulders; glide laterally and ventrally to the sternum
- Touch the side of the chest where the stethoscope will touch the patient
- Place the stethoscope next to the hand touching the chest
  - Auscult for three seconds
  - Auscult progressively longer until complete
- Remove stethoscope, and glide hand to the abdomen
- Add a second hand to the abdomen if two hands are used to palpate
  - Alternatively, add a stabilizing hand elsewhere if single-hand palpation is used
- Palpate limbs one at a time, each one counting as a step on the ladder
  - The limbs may need to be subsets of a joint at a time
- Examine the external ear
  - Divide the ear exam into pinna, visual outer canal, opening canal with a finger
- Examine each eye
  - If necessary, reach toward the upper eyelid on one side
  - Touch the upper eyelid
  - Repeat steps for the second side
- Oral exam
  - Touch the nose
  - Touch the lateral aspect of the upper lip
  - Raise the lip to expose the canine tooth
  - Raise the lip to expose the canine tooth, then stretch the lip backward to expose caudal teeth
  - Glide finger to the lower lip to expose mandibular premolars and canine
  - Repeat for the second side
  - Gently add a second hand to the head
  - Carefully open the mouth if patient is relaxed enough
- Examine limbs by touching the shoulder or hip first, then:
  - Elbow/Stifle
  - Carpus/Hock
  - Paw
  - Toe, Toenail
- Rectal and genital visual exam.

6.5 Type Two Training: Injections and Sample Collection

For Type Two patients, again dogs and cats are similar. Ultimately, there's nothing we can do to make a needle not be a needle: it is reasonable to expect animals will show some kind of response or take notice during actual needle pokes. We can however make the entire experience better for the patient by using thoughtful techniques which hold space for the animal's emotional welfare. With any patient, observe the pet closely for changes in food acceptance, body language, and proximity preference. If the pet's stress level is increasing during the visit, pause and assess the situation. Assure the treatment being performed is truly a want and not a need. If it is a need, notify the veterinarian that the patient is stressed, and obtain permission to give anxiety-relieving medications. If the procedure is a want, discuss a handling plan with the veterinarian for later in the day or another visit.

For procedures involving injections or needle sticks, consider topical anesthesia such as lidocaine–prilocaine prior to the procedure (also great for skin scrapings, ear treatments, rectal exams, and so much more!).

6.5.1 Subcutaneous and Intramuscular Injection

Type Two patients benefit from DS/CC for subcutaneous injections. The process may take as little as a few seconds, or as much as a few visits for the pet to be truly comfortable. Desensitization always progresses at the patient's rate. If we allow the animals to communicate with us, and we pay attention to what they are trying to say, we can gain trust and form positive emotional responses to injections as well as other procedures. Desensitization and classical conditioning or countercondi-tioning should not only be practiced in the hospital, but also be demonstrated to every pet owner when an injectable medication is prescribed such as insulin.

As with the exam, table training, carrier training, and more, desensitization for injections begins with finding a non-stressful starting point. Next, each step along the exposure ladder will *predict* a wonderful treat, toy, or tactile reward. If the patient's stress level is increasing, stop and reassess the situation. The exposure ladders presented in this chapter may take a few seconds, a few minutes, or a number of visits spread out over time to implement. If the process takes more than a moment or two, consider whether the patient is actually a better candidate for adding in Type three training as discussed in the next chapter.

If the patient has a prior history of fear of injections, be mindful of antecedents to injections. For example, the pet may be comfortable with petting around the flanks but respond strongly and suddenly when common injection sites are stroked. They may be comfortable with petting of injection sites, but have a sudden increase in FAS if the skin is lifted or tented. The sound the needle cap being removed is another common trigger, along with the actual needle piercing the skin. Done properly, desensitization should not elicit a stress response but you may still notice a skin twitch or small anticipation of the actual painful stimulus.

Example exposure ladder for subcutaneous injection:

- Patient remains stationary while approached, or chooses to approach veterinary team member, establishing a non-stressful starting point
- Reach toward a non-sensitive area near the injection site
- Glide toward the injection site
- Pick up the syringe in your other hand, and reach toward the non-sensitive area
- Tent the skin to the degree required for injection
- Approach the tented skin with the capped syringe
- Approach the tented skin with the capped syringe, and pinch the skin mildly
- With the capped syringe near the skin tent, pinch firmly to simulate a needle stick
- Touch the capped syringe softly to the injection site

- Touch the capped syringe firmly to the injection site
- Rehearse the injection with a training needle (depending upon the patient)
- Remove the syringe cap, and perform the handling steps
- Administer injection.

Figure 6.7 shows a diagram of this exposure ladder. Table 6.4 provides a worksheet example for one training session using DS/CC for injections.

For patients who show a high sensitivity to needles, using training needles is often extremely helpful. Training needles are blunt cannulas or trimmed needles or butterflies used to simulate an injection as closely as possible. Training needles allow us to add additional splits or approximations to bridge the gap between a capped needle or finger pinch and the actual feeling of a needle. You will see training needles used in a variety of the videos.

Video 6.4a shows examples of training needles and how to create them. For patients with a strong existing fear of needles, Type three training is probably more appropriate.

Video 6.4b shows two different dogs.

The first is a puppy being presented for vaccinations. Monique takes a moment to break down the stimulus of the injection into a number of approximations to conduct a rapid preventive desensitization and classical conditioning procedure during the vaccine visit. Notice each touch predicts a treat. When it's time for the actual injection, the order is touch → treats appear → injection and treats occur simultaneously. This method is often super effective, but it requires some practice with respect to mechanics, hand coordination, and remembering touching is like the on-switch for the treats. The timing of this exercise is different from the distraction methods shown in Chapter 5.

The second dog in Video 6.4b is an adult dog with a history of fear of all new indoor environments and locations as well as a fear of injections. The way her fear manifests is through crouching, hugging walls, or lying down and being unable to walk or move. She closes her eyes and folds her ears entirely flat, as if she can become invisible. This video shows a longer interventional desensitization and counterconditioning protocol which is still completed in a single visit. The dog is able to sit up on the mat rather than crouching and lying down, accept treats, periodically raise her

Administer injection
Remove the syringe cap and perform the handling steps
Touch the capped syringe firmly to the injection site
Touch the capped syringe softly to the injection site
Hold capped syringe near the skin tent and pinch firmly
Approach tented skin with the capped syringe; pinch skin lightly
Approach tented skin with the capped syringe
Tent the skin to the degree required for injection
Tent the skin slightly
Touch the injection site lightly
Glide toward the injection site
Pick up the syringe in your other hand and reach toward nonsensitive area
Glide toward the injection site
Reach toward a nonsensitive area near the injection site
Patient chooses to approach, establishing a nonstressful starting point

Figure 6.7 Example exposure ladder for injection training.

Table 6.4 Desensitization and counterconditioning worksheet for subcutaneous injection.

Training plan: desensitization and counterconditioning	
Trigger: Subcutaneous injection, owner needs to begin giving insulin at home Session 1	Exposure ladder: Choose to approach; allow contact Reach toward nonsensitive area Glide to injection site
Foundation behaviors required: Orient/attention to team member Station helpful but not required	Repeat steps, with syringe in hand Touching of injection site Tenting skin at injection site Approach with syringe Tap skin with capped syringe Simulate injection while pinching skin Handling steps and pinch Actual injection
Preferred rewards to generate positive emotional response 1. Baby food 2. Canned cat food 3. Tactile of cheeks	
Medications: none required	Working area: exam room 3, owner's lap
Nonstressful starting point: patient sitting in owner's lap soliciting for treats	
Distance	Close proximity throughout procedure. No change when syringe is closer to patient.
Duration	Initial interactions 2–3 seconds, simulated injection ~5 seconds, actual injection ~1 second
Pressure	Starting pressure light petting, gradually worked up to strong pinch, and finally actual injection. Pinch was noticed more than the injection.
Volume	N/A
Other	Patient comfortable with complete progression of touch. Repeated the capped syringe injection twice when cat did not show interest in food after the first attempt. Interest in food returned for the next approximation.
Endpoint	Injection
Homework	Administer first 3 days of insulin injections using the full progression shown today. This should take about 60 seconds per injection. Then over the next 3 days, begin shortening the process so the final behavior is prepare injection, patient shows up, touch, glide, pinch, inject for a total time of about 15–30 seconds.
Plan for next visit	None needed unless questions; complete DS/CC protocol completed during first visit

ears, and interact with Monique. She is still showing moderate FAS, but is dramatically improved compared to her prior appointments. The types of touch needed to vaccinate, the sight and smell of the syringe, the tactile feeling of a capped needle and training needle, the duration and firmness of the touch required, and the smell of the actual vaccine are all broken down into multiple exposures. The word "Yes" is used to communicate that food is coming but there is no required behavior the dog must perform to "earn" a "Yes." If she moved, turned, or responded in any other way Monique would still mark the end of the touch and give the food, then decrease the intensity of the touching on the next repetition based on the helpful information the dog provided about her threshold for tolerance. Remember, however, that all learning is happening simultaneously. There is no contingency for the dog to receive the food, but she is still likely operantly associating the food with behaviors such as interacting, sitting, stillness on the mat, and orienting toward the food. This dog is a candidate for ongoing training and medical management of her fear.

Video 6.5 shows a complete desensitization and classical conditioning start-to-finish for a cat to subcutaneous injections. The cat is assessed first for food acceptance which is good. His body language is loose and comfortable. The injection stimulus is broken down into many approximations, including the sound of preparing the injection, the sight of the syringe, and all the kinds of touching needed to give the injection. Partway through the video notice the cat swallows after the touch begins, a good sign he is anticipating food!

Video 6.6 shows conditioning for an intramuscular injection. The dog is already comfortable with being stabilized. If the dog was fearful of stabilization, conditioning for handling would need to be done before conditioning for injection. In the video, one person is stabilizing the dog, one person (Debbie Martin RVT, VTS [Behavior]) is performing injection approximations and indicating to a third person when a treat should be given and when treats should stop. The third person presents food when asked, and stops when asked. Before training, the team discussed how the communication would work regarding starting and stopping the food, and also what the pause and exit strategy would be if the dog responded with fear or avoidance during the training session.

6.5.1.1 Venipuncture

6.5.1.1.1 Cephalic

Cephalic venipuncture for Type Two patients uses desensitization and classical conditioning to walk the pet through the process relying on learning principles rather than primarily on physical restraint, and without causing an increase in fear or stress. With blood collection, each step in the desensitization process should predict something wonderful. Sometimes, it makes sense to allow the animal to keep eating throughout the process, while other patients will do better with the touch–treat–touch–treat rhythm. Experiment to see which method works best for each specific patient.

The team member providing the treats and support or stabilization will be monitoring the animal's body language throughout the procedure, and alerting the person collecting blood to any important changes or the need for a pause and regroup. If the animal struggles or tries to move away, stop, and add more rungs to the exposure ladder. Also, with peripheral venipuncture in general, butterfly catheters can make procedures easier, because a small amount of patient movement will not spoil the sample collection.

A sample exposure ladder for cephalic venipuncture could look like:

- Allow one technician to approach and feed; nonstressful starting point
- Technician with food reaches over or under and provides a stabilizing hand in case of unexpected responses from the patient
  - Break down into reaching over and touching as two to three steps, if needed
- Technician collecting blood approaches
- Touch the limb where blood will be collected at the shoulder
  - Glide touch to the elbow
- Use hand touching elbow to apply a "hand tourniquet" lightly
  - (Other tourniquets require adding rungs to the ladder here)

- Occlude the vessel
  - Leave the limb in a natural position when feasible
  - If picking up the limb, lift it from the elbow rather than the paw and break down the lift into a few exposures
- Palpate
- Apply alcohol or other prep liquid (no spray bottles, use a cotton ball or squeeze bottle)
- It may be necessary to countercondition the odor of any products used
- Approach with syringe
- Mimic venipuncture with capped syringe
- Add approximations with training needles depending upon patient response
- Pinch the area with a fingernail to assess response to sharp stimulus
- Collect blood
- Apply pressure or bandage after venipuncture is complete.

Video 6.7 shows an example of when to pause and make a new training plan. Monique experiments with trying a desensitization and classical counterconditioning plan with this Irish Setter puppy. His owners report it is difficult to groom him, and he is due for a heartworm test. Notice his body language. He inches away periodically and is wiggly. This patient's FAS level is too high for this training procedure. A new training plan was made teaching him to use the mat to opt in and out of handling, and breaking down the touching into much smaller increments. These methods are shown in more detail in Chapter 7.

6.5.1.2 Lateral Saphenous (Dogs)

For Type Two dogs, consider the use of a butterfly catheter as previously mentioned. One technician will stabilize the patient and provide the food, while a second collects the sample. For very large dogs, a third person may be needed to help stabilize the dog's rear, as demonstrated for Type One dogs.

Sample exposure ladder for lateral saphenous blood collection:

- Dog stands comfortably and does not move away when technician approaches, establishing a non-stressful starting point
- Technician stabilizes the dog and pets the neck in case of unexpected responses
- Second technician touches the hip
- Glide hand down to stifle
- Glide hand to back of stifle
- Apply mild pressure where vein will be occluded
- Occlude the vessel
- Touch the injection area
- Apply alcohol
- Touch the area firmly
- Touch firmly with capped needle, or pinch to assess response to sharp stimulus
- Add approximations with training needle if appropriate
- Perform venipuncture
- Apply pressure or bandage after venipuncture is complete.

Figure 6.8 illustrates an exposure ladder for venipuncture.

Video 6.8 shows a dog named Holly with Monique and her colleague technician Kayla. In this training session, a series of approximations are shown which can be used to desensitize and

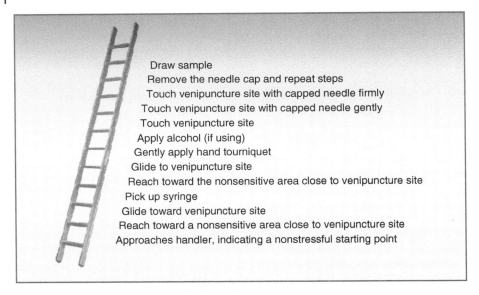

Draw sample
Remove the needle cap and repeat steps
Touch venipuncture site with capped needle firmly
Touch venipuncture site with capped needle gently
Touch venipuncture site
Apply alcohol (if using)
Gently apply hand tourniquet
Glide to venipuncture site
Reach toward the nonsensitive area close to venipuncture site
Pick up syringe
Glide toward venipuncture site
Reach toward a nonsensitive area close to venipuncture site
Approaches handler, indicating a nonstressful starting point

Figure 6.8 Example exposure ladder for venipuncture.

countercondition lateral saphenous venipuncture. This dog has foundation training and is already comfortable with: coming to the mat, two people being present, general touch gradient, and body handling on the mat. She has not been exposed to venipuncture training, so this shows her first session. Her foundation knowledge and skills make the session look easy, because it is! Before the training began, Monique and Kayla discussed the training plan, and how to communicate best about food delivery, starting handling, and stopping handling. The person touching the patient should be the one to indicate when food will start and stop.

6.5.1.3 Medial Saphenous (Cats)

Type Two cats are still relaxed enough to allow support and gentle manipulations, and accept food and/or tactile rewards intermittently during handling (Figure 6.9). For medial saphenous

Figure 6.9 Positioning for medial saphenous blood collection with a Type Two feline patient.

collection, the positioning is the same as for Type One, with the cat sternal or voluntarily lateral, lying on a hip with the back legs extended. For Type Two cats, progress through each step of the blood collection in a gradual fashion, with each step predicting something the cat enjoys such as a treat or facial petting. It is sometimes helpful to have a third person available to offer treats during this process.

Example exposure ladder for medial saphenous blood collection:

- Cat allows gentle positioning into a down position, establishing a nonstressful starting point
- One technician gently stabilizes the head
- Occlude vessel gently with only the necessary pressure to raise a vein
- Second technician strokes the inner thigh
- Touch the venipuncture site
- Apply alcohol
- Palpate the vein
- Use a capped syringe or butterfly to simulate injection
- Pinch the venipuncture site firmly to simulate a sharp sensation
- Add approximations with training needle if appropriate
- Perform venepuncture
- Apply pressure or a bandage to the venipuncture site.

6.5.1.4 Jugular

Dogs are better candidates for DS/CC to jugular venipuncture than cats, because the positioning is more natural. Type Two dogs are likely to prefer to stand or sit, while Type Two cats will usually prefer to lie down with their paws retracted. It is easy to collect jugular blood from a dog who is standing or sitting, but challenging to collect from a cat who wants to lie sternally with her paws pulled in.

Example exposure ladder for jugular blood collection for dogs:

- Dog approaches handler or allows handler to approach, establishing a nonstressful starting point
- Handler gently touches under chin
- Handler raises chin slightly
- Technician collecting blood approaches
- Stroke between the front legs
- Glide up to the thoracic inlet
- Lightly touch the jugular furrow
- Occlude the vessel
- Palpate the vessel with the opposite hand
- Pinch the skin to simulate a sharp stimulus
- Simulate blood collection with a capped needle
- Add approximations with training needle if appropriate
- Perform venipuncture
- Apply pressure to the venipuncture site.

6.5.2 Blood Pressure Measurement

We should question the validity of the test results for blood pressure measurements when a patient is showing Type Two signs of mild to moderate stress and anxiety. While DS/CC to this procedure are relatively simple, if the patient is nervous enough to require desensitization, the test results will likely be inaccurate. For patients who will require serial blood pressure measurements, DS/CC is likely worth-while. For a single measurement, anxiety-reducing medications can be considered prior to the measurement.

Example desensitization exposure ladder for blood pressure measurement:

- Patient approaches handler, or allows handler to approach without moving away, establishing a nonstressful starting point
- With the patient in a natural position, select the limb to be used
- Begin touch of the limb high on the leg at the shoulder or hip
- Glide to the next distal joint
- Glide to the area where the cuff will be applied
- Approach with the cuff; allow animal to investigate if they show interest
- Touch the limb with the cuff
- Wrap the cuff halfway around the limb
- Close the cuff around the limb
- Glide touch to the paw
- Touch the artery
- Place some gel on your finger and apply it to allow the pet to experience the gel tactile
- Using plenty of gel placed on the crystal, approach the paw
- Touch the crystal lightly to the paw
- Hold the crystal to the paw, and acquire the signal using headphones
- Inflate the cuff one-half pump
- Deflate the cuff
- Inflate the cuff one full pump
- Deflate the cuff
- Inflate the cuff until the signal is ceased
- Measure Doppler blood pressure
- Use a paper towel to remove the crystal and wipe away any gel
- Remove the cuff, minimizing Velcro closure sounds.

6.5.2.1 Cystocentesis

Cystocentesis is a procedure that can have very rare but serious adverse events associated if the patient is too tense or moves too much during the puncture. To avoid these unwanted outcomes (e.g. laceration or rupture of the bladder, peritonitis, vasovagal response, abdominal vessel perforation, and GI injury), help patients be as comfortable as possible during this procedure [1–3]. For Type Two dogs and cats, consider providing medical management of anxiety, and then following the procedures described for Type One patients. If the patient is still too nervous to participate without excessive stress and struggling, sedation should be provided, or a sterile free-catch sample considered.

6.6 Administering Medications and Grooming

6.6.1 Medication Stations

Type Two patients can benefit from medication stations just as Type One patients can. The medication station is a powerful tool, because it allows the patient to give consent for the procedure by remaining at the station, and withdraw consent simply by leaving. Because so many rewards are given to reinforce the stationing behavior, the patient should have a highly positive emotional response to being at the station. This positive emotional response helps to establish a nonstressful starting point for desensitization and classical counterconditioning for Type Two pets.

6.6.2 Oral Medications

Type Two dogs are not comfortable being held to manually give a pill. When provided with a pill wrapped in a treat, they will often find the pill, eating around it and spitting out or avoiding ingesting the pill. These patients will quickly learn they are only being given a certain special food when it contains a pill, and will begin to avoid that special food entirely because it predicts a "sour berry" if we revisit the analogy from Chapter 5. When oral medications are prescribed, provide the client with enough education to successfully administer the medications at home, and make sure the client understands to call the clinic for help if there are problems giving the medication.

To administer a pill, use treats the animal receives at other times, such as for training and during medication time. Have at least five total treats, one containing the pill. Invite the patient to the medication station. Click and treat rapidly and repeatedly for the stationing behavior, using the pill treat as one of these rewards. When these patients go into "training mode" mentally, they will often be more focused on the task at hand than on investigating the treats for concealed pills. If the patient is not trained for a medication station, ask for a group of other trained behaviors or tricks, such as sit, down, shake, spin, or any other tricks the patient knows. Click and treat for each trick, with the pill treat being one of the ones used during the clicking and treating session. Another approach is to use the meatball-to-meal method. Instruct clients to prepare the animal's meal, making a production of the event. Then, a pill should be concealed in a meatball of canned pet food or sticky treats. Hold the meatball in one hand, and the meal in the other. Give the meatball, and as the pet is swallowing the meatball, immediately follow by offering the remainder of the meal.

For liquid medications, the same guidelines apply. Prepare the liquid medication as described in Chapter 5, and then use the syringes to administer treats when clicking and treating at the medication station or in response to cued behaviors. Either hold both syringes and rotate the medicine syringe into the mix, or set the syringe down each time, changing which syringe is picked up so that the patient receives a few plain treats from a syringe, then the medicine treat, then a few more plain treats to finish up.

For particularly discerning patients, compounding medications is a great option. Many medicines can be made into a flavored liquid or a flavored chewable treat to at least partly disguise the medication. Some medicines may not make a good liquid or chewable treat, but can be compounded into a capsule that is at least flavorless on the outside, and has no medicine taste unless the capsule is bitten and punctured. Keeping some plain gel capsules in the clinic to dispense with bitter medications such as metronidazole and tramadol can ease administration. The pill or fragment can be placed inside the gel capsule by the owner prior to administration. It is important not to handle the gel capsule if there is powder from the pill on your hands, as this will flavor the outside of the capsule, defeating the purpose of decreasing the unpleasant taste.

6.6.3 Ear Medications and Cleaning

Type Two patients may start out allowing ear cleansing and medications with distractions, but may escalate, become nervous, stop eating, or try to move away even though food is being offered. These patients will benefit from desensitization and classical counterconditioning to break down the process and help build a positive cooperative response. If the animal has a painful ear, pain medication should be provided prior to working with the ear, and applying a topical anesthetic cream to the pinna and external ear canal can make the procedure more comfortable. This product should *not* be inserted deep into the ear.

Break down the ear-cleansing and ear-medicating process into an exposure ladder, making sure to find a non-stressful or least-stressful starting point. Each step on the exposure ladder should predict wonderful treats, and the patient needs to be comfortable enough to eat for each approximation. Monitor food acceptance, body language, and proximity preference throughout the procedure. If the patient's stress level is increasing, try adding more rungs to the exposure ladder, breaking the process into smaller steps. If that does not help, stop the procedure, and provide improved medical management of pain, stress, and anxiety prior to continuing. Please do not add assistants restraining the patient to the mix. If it takes two or more people to physically restrain a patient for any kind of treatment, we are doing harm to that patient, and need to stop and make a new plan.

Example exposure ladder for ear medication:

- The patient approaches, or remains still while approached, establishing a nonstressful starting point
- Touch a less sensitive area, such as the shoulder
- Glide toward the ear
- Touch the base of the ear
- Touch the pinna lightly
- Place a finger and thumb on either side of the pinna, preparing to position it
- Pick up the ear medication, swab, or the like
- Touch a less sensitive area
- Glide toward the ear
- Touch the base of the ear
- Touch the pinna lightly
- Place a finger and thumb on either side of the pinna, preparing to position it
- Touch the ear canal opening with a finger
- Move the medicine vial closer to the patient: this may require several incremental movements
- Touch the medicine vial to the ear
- Insert the medicine applicator into the ear
- Dispense medication
- Massage the ear canal to distribute medication
- Touch a less sensitive area to finish.

Table 6.5 is an example of a possible worksheet from a desensitization and counterconditioning session for ear cleansing. Figure 6.10 shows a possible exposure ladder for ear treatment.

Training Tip: Touch It

If there is an existing negative response to a piece of equipment such as nail trimmers, the ear cleanser bottle, or eye drops, considering using the object for a game of targeting. Use shaping to encourage the patient to target the object with a nose or a paw, and reward frequently for this behavior. Making a game out of interacting with potentially scary items can decrease fear and improve conditioned emotional responses as well. Monitor the pet for signs of motivational conflict (wanting to both approach and avoid the object) – if you see conflict, decrease shaping criteria or choose a different raining approach.

Table 6.5 Desensitization and counterconditioning worksheet for ear cleansing.

Training plan: desensitization and counterconditioning	
Trigger: Ear cleansing, routine Owner needs to clean ears at home for maintenance and grooming Session 2	Exposure ladder: Patient chooses to approach Touch nonsensitive area Glide to ear Short duration touch, longer duration Hold ear cleanser and repeat steps
Foundation behaviors required: Approach/attend handler Station helpful but not required	Touch ear Base, mid, pinna, lift/open Touch with dry cotton ball Touch with wet cotton ball brief Increase duration with wet cotton ball Cleanse ear
Preferred rewards to generate positive emotional response 1. Bacon 2. Cheese 3. Tennis ball	
Medications: none required	Working area: exam room 1, mat on floor
Nonstressful starting point: dog approaches handler and chooses to interact	
Distance	Patient comfortable with close proximity
Duration	Began with 1–2 seconds of ear handling with dry cotton. Gradually progress to 15 seconds of swabbing and massage with dry cotton.
Pressure	Started with a gliding touch, progressed to firm massage with fingers and cotton.
Volume	N/A
Other	Progression through exposure ladder was cautious and gradual. Endpoint during session 1 was approaching with dry cotton; patient tolerated this within two approximations and made significant progress.
Endpoint	Dry cotton tactile for 15 seconds; external manual massage of ear canal
Homework	Dry cotton tactile for 15 seconds; external massage of ear canal
Plan for next visit	Increase from dry cotton to wet cotton tactile for 15–30 seconds

Remember: if the animal has a decrease in food acceptance, shows more stress markers in his body language, or tries to move away, it does not mean the method is ineffective. Allow him to opt out and take a break when needed, and watch for him to return and show he is ready to try again. He is simply giving us great information about what he needs: more rungs on the exposure ladder, more medical management, different treats, a break from training, or to be moved to a Type Three training protocol as described in Chapter 7.

Video 6.9 shows an excellent example from Debbie Martin RVT, VTS (Behavior), KPA-CTP of checking a dog's preference for when and how to deliver food for ear cleaning. Debbie shows gradually controlling the stimulus of ear cleaning while communicating clearly with her helper how and when to deliver food. Notice if the dog shows a change in body language, the handler pauses

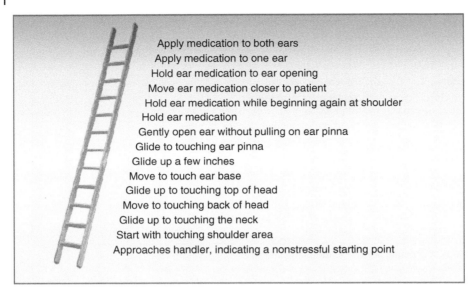

Apply medication to both ears
Apply medication to one ear
Hold ear medication to ear opening
Move ear medication closer to patient
Hold ear medication while beginning again at shoulder
Hold ear medication
Gently open ear without pulling on ear pinna
Glide to touching ear pinna
Glide up a few inches
Move to touch ear base
Glide up to touching top of head
Move to touching back of head
Glide up to touching the neck
Start with touching shoulder area
Approaches handler, indicating a nonstressful starting point

Figure 6.10   Exposure ladder example for ear treatment.

handling until the dog is ready to try again. This particular dog prefers if the handler keeps her hands on between repetitions rather than repeatedly initiating touch.

Video 6.10 shows Amanda Schwartzwalder LVT, VTS (Behavior), CVPM demonstrating a desensitization and counterconditioning protocol with a feline patient for ear treatment. Each touch predicts the delivery of salmon paste via a syringe. (Bonus: Positive syringe conditioning!) The ear handling is broken down into a series of small tolerable exposures, and the patient is free to move away at any time should he feel uncomfortable.

6.6.4   Eye Medications

For patients who will need lifelong eye drops, such as those with dry eye, allergies, or glaucoma, consider Type Three training as described in Chapter 7. For Type Two patients, DS/CC should be sufficient. Use regular saline or a plain eye rinse for the training period, then move to medicated drops when appropriate (Figure 6.11).

Example exposure ladder for eye drops:

- Patient approaches or does not move away when approached, establishing a nonstressful starting point
- Touch a less sensitive area, such as the shoulder or dorsal neck
- Glide toward the head, avoiding the ear
- Glide toward the upper eyelid
- Pick up the saline drop bottle
- Touch a less sensitive area
- Glide toward the head, avoiding the ear
- Glide toward the upper eyelid
- Touch just above the upper eyelid
- Apply light pressure just above the upper eyelid, as if to hold the eye open

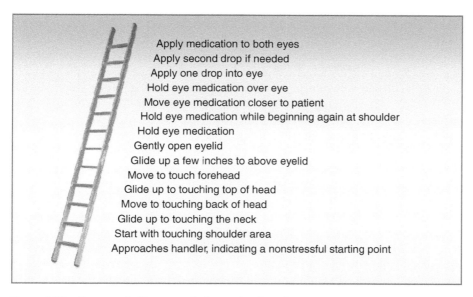

Apply medication to both eyes
Apply second drop if needed
Apply one drop into eye
Hold eye medication over eye
Move eye medication closer to patient
Hold eye medication while beginning again at shoulder
Hold eye medication
Gently open eyelid
Glide up a few inches to above eyelid
Move to touch forehead
Glide up to touching top of head
Move to touching back of head
Glide up to touching the neck
Start with touching shoulder area
Approaches handler, indicating a nonstressful starting point

Figure 6.11 Exposure ladder example for eye treatment.

- Approach with the saline drops
- Hold the saline drops over the head
- Dispense a drop onto the fur of the head or muzzle, *not* into the eye
- Repeat the drop-dispensing step until the patient is comfortable with a few locations
- Place a drop into the eye
- Finish by touching a less sensitive area
- Repeat, using actual eye medication.

Video 6.11 shows an eyedrop procedure for needed eye drops for a patient. The puppy is generally concerned about all handling, and particularly handling from the front and above his head. However, he has an eye injury and absolutely must receive eye drops. He also has food guarding behavior, so providing him with lickable food while applying the drops is not a safe training plan. He can follow food but if he is licking he becomes very tense. This video shows a series of handling experiments Monique conducted to rapidly introduce eye drops to the reluctant but excited puppy. It uses a combination of luring, distraction, desensitization, classical and operant countercondi-tioning. Notice there is a warm up and a cool down, so the actual eye drop is not the final sensation the puppy experiences.

Video 6.12 shows type two eye medications for an adult dog.

Training Tip: Harness The Power Of Medication Stations

Pets who understand the medication station will love to visit it. It is an antecedent for fun, treats, and handling games. We can use the positive emotions and excitement linked with the medication station to encourage patients to enjoy treatments like eye drops. Remember to maintain fun at the medication station, so the patient trusts it and finds experiences there to be predictably pleasant.

6.6.5 Nail Trims

Many patients have a negative emotional association with nail trimming. This could be due to personal preference; increased sensitivity of the paws (natural differences or due to illness); history of fear-provoking nail trims involving excessive restraint; history of nails trimmed too short, causing pain; or nail trims during another stressful event (e.g. a dog is barking in another room), causing a lasting emotional impression. As discussed in Chapter 5, grooming is never a good reason to permanently damage the relationship between the veterinary team and the patient, poison the veterinary clinic as a good place, or put team members and the patient at risk for injury. More restraint is not the right answer for grooming. Train the pet, instead!

Type Two nail trim patients are reluctant to take food as a distraction, or stop eating when they are touched, but do not show any defensive or aggressive behaviors and will return for numerous repetitions by choice. If the patient is showing opting out repeatedly or showing any signs of defensive aggression, provide medical management and move to Type Three training techniques. Patients should not be subjected to strong restraint for nail trims: choose another strategy for safety and to build a functional long-term care approach.

Some of the more common triggers within the nail care process are encircling the paw with a hand, isolating a toe, the squeezing sensation of clippers on a toe, and the sound of nail clippers snipping the nail. If the pet is concerned about the sound, practice snipping a piece of dry pasta, cocktail straw, or skewer and pairing the sound with treats. When coaching clients how to trim nails, assure they are comfortable using the equipment before starting training. Clients can practice on pasta, straws, or skewers as well to assure they have good dexterity and can operate the clippers quickly and confidently.

Example exposure ladder for nail trims (this example is for a front paw, but can be adapted for rear paws as well) (Figure 6.12):

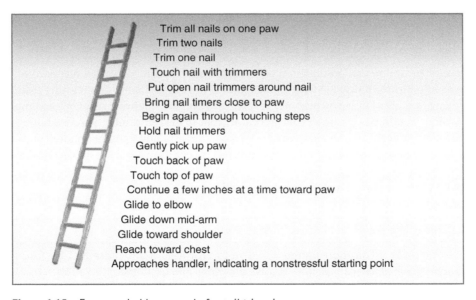

Trim all nails on one paw
Trim two nails
Trim one nail
Touch nail with trimmers
Put open nail trimmers around nail
Bring nail timers close to paw
Begin again through touching steps
Hold nail trimmers
Gently pick up paw
Touch back of paw
Touch top of paw
Continue a few inches at a time toward paw
Glide to elbow
Glide down mid-arm
Glide toward shoulder
Reach toward chest
Approaches handler, indicating a nonstressful starting point

Figure 6.12 Exposure ladder example for nail trimming.

- Patient approaches technician, or chooses not to move away when approached, establishing a non-stressful starting point
- Touch a nonsensitive area, such as the shoulder
- Glide toward the elbow
- Glide toward the carpus/wrist
- Glide toward the paw
- Lift the paw an inch*
  - Gradually lift the paw higher with each approximation until a comfortable height for clipping

    *Some patients' conformation allows nail clipping without raising the paw
- Pick up the nail trimmers
- Touch the shoulder
- Glide toward the elbow, then the carpus
- Glide toward the paw
- Lift the paw a small distance
- Lift to comfortable nail trim height
- Isolate a toe
  - Hold the toe for one second
  - Gradually hold the toe for longer periods of time
- Approach the toenail with clippers
- Surround the toenail with clipper
- Tap the toenail, making a clicking sound
- Clip one toenail
- Clip multiple toenails
- Finish by touching a less sensitive area.

Table 6.6 shows a worksheet example for a DS/CC session for nail trimming.

For some patients, this process can be accomplished by one person in less than one minute. For other patients, the process can take several visits, even with anxiety-reducing medications. Remember: grooming is virtually never an emergency need, and if it is, simply use sedation rather than risking lasting emotional trauma to the animal.

Video 6.13 shows a preventive desensitization and counterconditioning protocol for nail care with Border collie puppy Quill. This method is most appropriate for pets without an existing fear of nail care. The handling is set up so each touch predicts a treat, and the touching is presented in a series of controlled exposures. One particularly important point is when the nail clippers are added to the scenario: notice adding the clippers means the handling exposure level is decreased considerably for several repetitions to assure the animal is comfortable before proceeding. In most cases, choosing Type three training strategies for nail care is preferred.

6.6.6 Anal Gland Expression

Anal gland expression is an invasive procedure. Many patients are fearful for this procedure, and those who aren't initially, often become so. Using a topical anesthetic cream can help ease the process, decreasing tactile sensitivity for the patient. For this example, one person stabilizes the dog, while another expresses the anal glands.

Table 6.6   Desensitization and counterconditioning worksheet for nail trims.

Training plan: desensitization and counterconditioning	
Trigger: Nail trim Session 3	Exposure ladder: Session 3: Orient and allow approach
Foundation behaviors required: Orient to handler Stationing helpful but not required	Paw lift starting at shoulder Touch trimmer to nail Make noise of trimmer near nail Encircle nail with trimmer Tap nail with trimmer Clip one nail
Preferred rewards to generate positive emotional response 1. Steak 2. Chicken 3. Cheese	
Medications:	Working area: rubber mats Exam Room 3
Alprazolam night before and 2 hours prior	
Nonstressful starting point: orient to handler on rubber mats, allow shoulder touch	
Distance	Nail trimmer distance was 12″ from front paw, gradual approach until contact with nail
Duration	Initial duration: 10 seconds per touch; final duration: 10 seconds, including trimming one nail
Pressure	Initial pressure was no contact, gradual increase to tapping, pressing, and clipping nail
Volume	Sound of nail clippers introduced when clippers were 6″ away, then gradually closer to increase sound influence
Other	Tactile increase from no contact gradually up to trimming one front nail
Endpoint	Trimming one front toenail
Homework	Trim front nails one at a time
Plan for next visit	Begin training for rear paws

Example exposure ladder for anal gland expression (Figure 6.13):

- Patient does not move away when technician approaches from the side, establishing a non-stressful starting point
- Technician reaches in front to stabilize the patient
- Technician reaches across the patient's body
- Technician begins stabilizing the patient
- Second technician approaches from the side
- Touch a less sensitive area, such as the dorsal rump, lateral thigh, or hip
- Glide toward the rectal area
- Place a hand between the tail and the rectum
- Use a flat hand to raise the tail without grasping it
- Apply anesthetic cream or jelly.

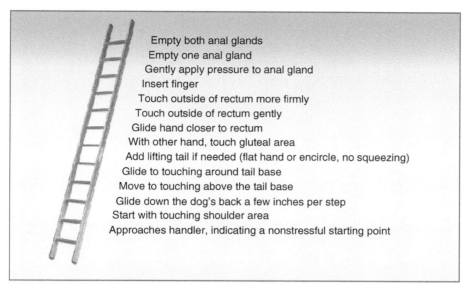

Figure 6.13 Exposure ladder example for anal gland expression.

- Palpate the rectal area lightly
- Touch the anus with a finger lubricated with anesthetic gel
- Insert the finger; palpate the gland
- Express the gland
- Reposition for the second gland
- Palpate
- Express
- Cleanse the area with a damp paper towel and odor-reducing product.

When possible, work with the owner present. Owners often underestimate how invasive some pets perceive this procedure to be, and the skill level of the technicians performing the procedure. If the patient shows increasing signs of stress and is struggling, pause the procedure and consider a new plan.

6.7 Conclusion

Type Two patients are generally mildly anxious and concerned about veterinary care. These patients may become wary during distraction techniques, or avoid handling when the progression of handling is too fast. Using systematic desensitization and classical conditioning or counterconditioning improves patient care. Remember: training is a patient-directed process. The patient is allowed to opt in or opt out of training, and the desensitization and counterconditioning process should look boring or happy, rather than increasing the patient's stress level. If the patient opts out, rewind the process to a nonstressful point, and begin again, adding more rungs to the exposure ladder; or stop training for the day and try again when the patient is more relaxed, using even more finely controlled exposure steps during the next session. By empowering our patients to direct their treatment plans, we can earn lasting trust and provide a higher standard of care. When we show empathy for patient stress and make efforts to reduce it, the veterinary care experience is improved for patient, client, and the entire veterinary team.

References

1 Brown, C. (2006). Diagnostic cystocentesis: techniques and considerations. *Lab Animal* 35 (4): 21–23.

2 Buckley, G. (2009). Massive transfusion and surgical management of iatrogenic aortic laceration associated with cystocentesis in a dog. *Journal of the American Veterinary Medical Association* 235 (3): 288–291.

3 Odunayo, A., Ng, Z.Y., and Holford, A.L. (2015). Probable vasovagal reaction following cystocentesis in two cats. *Journal of Feline Medicine and Surgery Open Reports* 1 (1): 1–4. https://doi.org/10.1177/2055116915585021.

7

Type Three Patients and Training: Incorporating Operant Techniques, FAS 0–5 Pets

7.1 Type Three Training: Incorporating Operant Techniques

Type Three training has many applications. Type Three methods should be considered for *any* patient, but they require a time investment and some training skills for success. Some clients, especially if they are sophisticated trainers, may express interest in learning Type Three skills even for relaxed, cooperative patients. These owners are highly motivated to build great experiences for their pets.

Relying on a combination of desensitization and classical conditioning paired with operant conditioning, Type Three training establishes a language of consent for the patients while conditioning them to accept and even enjoy care. Remember to take the time to set up the environment to be as non-stressful as possible, and review the medical record for success notes and individual preferences before you begin.

Patients with fear, anxiety, and stress (FAS) scores of 4–5 may have unwanted behaviors in the veterinary clinic due to negative past experiences, intrinsic fears, or a combination of both. Type Three dogs and cats are experiencing severe emotional distress. These patients require intervention to try to reverse the fear response, and then instruct the patient how to cooperate for care. The first training goals for Type Three patients usually involve devising a sedation strategy so needed care can be administered, then a training plan so both wanted and needed care are more successful in the future. Some of these patients will require sedation for some procedures permanently – and that's perfectly alright!

When working with Type Three patients, use the same patient evaluation tool as for Type One and Type Two (Figure 7.1). Unless the patient has a true need for immediate veterinary care, Type Three patients should be slated for medical management, training visits, and attempting care once these services have been offered. Training visits can be provided by technicians, veterinarians, or trainers who are comfortable with the techniques and skilled in the application of desensitization, classical conditioning, and operant conditioning. Sometimes, as few as one to three visits are required, while in other circumstances five or more preparatory visits are needed. The client should be counseled in advance about the anticipated time required for training, the costs associated, and how to build realistic expectations. In general, the more fearful the patient is during initial assessment, the longer the training process will take.

The time investment for Type Three training may seem overwhelming for some owners. A few owners may be hesitant to invest the time and money required to achieve the goal of training all behaviors, including full examination, sample collection, and so on. It might not take as much time as the owner thinks. Once an animal has learned to train for their first voluntary behavior,

Cooperative Veterinary Care, Second Edition. Monique Feyrecilde.
© 2024 John Wiley & Sons, Inc. Published 2024 by John Wiley & Sons, Inc.
Companion website: www.wiley.com/go/feyrecilde/cooperative

Figure 7.1 Assessment of Type Three patients: FAS 0–5.

subsequent behaviors are easier to train because the animal understands the process. For owners with Type Three patients who consider their options and still decide they don't wish to pursue full cooperative procedure training, teaching the dog or cat to allow low-stress sedation protocols will be a realistic goal. Many of these techniques mirror the handling methods used for wild animals housed in zoos and aquaria. How would we obtain blood from a killer whale? How many people would be required to manually restrain the animal? Would sedation be appropriate and safe? The answer: we collect blood from a killer whale by training cooperative husbandry and veterinary care behaviors. If a goldfish can learn agility, or a shark can cooperate for abdominal ultrasound, a dog or cat can certainly learn to cooperate for sedation, and possibly even physical examination, blood collection, and injections with the proper training.

Training Tip: Life in a Perfect World

In a perfect world, training combining operant procedures layered along with touch gradient, considerate approach, and desensitization procedures would be the option selected for *every* patient, because it allows complete voluntary and cooperative care. The patient directs how care is administered, and the veterinary team communicates clearly and respectfully what the animal needs to do to be successful.

7.2 Identifying Type Three Patients (FAS 4–5)

As mentioned, some Type Three patients are calm and cooperative, but have owners who are interested in less invasive and better trained veterinary care. The remainder are those who are too fearful to permit care without medical management and training. The goal with Type Three patients is to maintain low stress levels in calm patients, and to decrease stress levels in high FAS patients to the point where they can constructively learn new skills, and then train the necessary skills to allow care. Type Three patients may display some or all of these signs. As with Type One and Type Two, we need to be flexible and monitor the patient continuously. Many patients will display aspects of all three types and have fluctuating FAS levels during the same assessment. *Even one Type Three marker is enough to score a patient as Type Three.*

7.2.1 Type Three Dogs

7.2.1.1 Food Acceptance
- Dogs will accept food from the owner or pick it up off the floor, or may refuse all food
- Will not accept high-value food from most or all team members
- Rarely may accept high-value food from trusted team members
- Takes food with a hard mouth, even when not being handled
- May take food quickly, then retreat ("snakebite")
- If accepting some food at any point, food acceptance stops or becomes frantic during any handling attempts
- Difficulty returning to baseline food acceptance, even from the owner, after handling attempts.

7.2.1.2 Body Language
- Mild, moderate, or severe stress body language in the hospital when not being handled (refer to Chapter 2)
- May show moderate and severe stress markers during handling:
  - Dilated pupils with widened eyes; sclera may be visible
  - Scanning the environment; hypervigilance
  - Increased respiratory rate; possible stress panting
  - Ears held flat or pulled back
  - Tail held low or tucked up against the abdomen
  - Piloerection
  - Tries to escape when handling attempted
  - May freeze when handling attempted
  - Possible defensive aggression during handling attempts
  - Vocalization
  - May void bladder, bowels, or anal sacs
  - Possible signs of learned helplessness
- When the handling and procedure are stopped, difficulty returning to baseline.

7.2.1.3 Proximity Preference
- Dog chooses to stay near the owner or hide (e.g. under a chair)
- Looks away and leans away when team members make social contact
- Will approach team members only for very high-value food or when the team member is looking and facing away
- Is reluctant or completely unable to come out from hiding places
- Actively tries to avoid or escape handling efforts

Table 7.1 is a quick reference checklist for assessing Type Three Dogs. Figure 7.2 depicts a Type Three Dog.

7.2.2 Type Three Cats

Type Three cats present unique challenges to the veterinary practitioner. Many owners of Type Three cats are unable to bring them to the veterinary clinic. Capturing the cat to place it in the carrier may be dangerous for the owner, because of defensive aggression. Also, the client's perception

Table 7.1 Checklist for Type Three dogs: each dog assessing at Type Three may have a combination of these attributes.

Stage of visit	Food acceptance	Body language	Proximity preference
Greeting	☐ Rarely accept food ☐ Will eat from floor but not from hand ☐ Hard mouth or rapid retreat	☐ Tense with mild, moderate, and/or severe stress markers	☐ Does not greet ☐ Hides ☐ May interact with owner
Touching	☐ Refuses food ☐ Difficulty returning to baseline	☐ Tense, fearful	☐ Avoidance ☐ Self-defense
Exam treatment	☐ Refuses food ☐ Difficulty returning to baseline	☐ Tense, fearful ☐ Difficulty returning to baseline	☐ Avoidance ☐ Self-defense ☐ Does not return to baseline

(a)

(b)

Figure 7.2 (a) Type Three canine patient. (b) Type Three feline patient.

of stress may be so upsetting that the client avoids making appointments because they don't want their beloved pets to have such frightening experiences.

Because Type Three cats are in severe distress, and often the owner is very stressed as well, you will see more training for dogs than for cats in this chapter. The techniques used for dogs can be applied to cats, if the cat is in a good mental state for learning new skills. Most pet cats are more environmentally sensitive than dogs. Their social lives are considerably different. The expectations of skills and social experiences presented to dogs are much more varied than those presented to pet cats by most owners. The author firmly believes cats are capable of learning to cooperate for veterinary behaviors! However, the unique challenges of the veterinary–client–patient relationship with cats and their owners make training cats in the veterinary clinic substantially more difficult. These methods can be applied in the home, via house calls, with the assistance of a veterinary behaviorist, or with the assistance of a skilled trainer.

7.2.2.1 Food Acceptance, Toy Acceptance, and Tactile Acceptance
- Does not investigate or accept food or toys
- May allow gentle petting/tactile by a team member for periods <3 seconds
- May allow petting by owner
- May or may not allow any petting/tactile

7.2.2.2 Body Language
Moderate or severe stress markers are present in the hospital.

- Moderate stress markers in the carrier or during handling attempts, such as:
  - Widened eyes with dilated pupils
  - Whiskers pulled forward; mouth tight
  - Ears held back or flat
  - Increased respiratory rate
  - Hypervigilant; scanning the environment
  - Tense muscles; flinches if touched
  - Tail tucked close to body or twitching/slashing
  - Piloerection
  - Elimination
  - Vocalization
  - Defensive aggression
- Difficulty returning to baseline after handling attempts
- Difficulty returning to baseline after arriving home.

7.2.2.3 Proximity Preference
- Chooses to hide in the carrier
- Chooses to exit the carrier, but hides elsewhere
- May explore exam room but cautiously, crouching or following walls
- Retreats when team members approach without attempting handling
- Moves away when handling is attempted
- Difficulty returning to baseline when handling attempts are ceased.

Table 7.2 is a quick reference checklist for assessing Type Three cats. Figure 7.3 shows a Type Three Cat experiencing severe stress.

Table 7.2 Checklist for Type Three cats: each cat assessing at Type Three may have a combination of these attributes.

Stage of visit	Food or tactile acceptance	Body language	Proximity preference
Greeting	☐ Refuses food ☐ Rarely allows brief tactile <3 seconds	☐ Tense with mild, moderate, and/or severe stress markers	☐ Hides in carrier ☐ May show self-defense when approached
Touching	☐ Refuses food and tactile ☐ Difficulty returning to baseline	☐ Tense, fearful	☐ Avoidance ☐ Self-defense
Exam treatment	☐ Refuses food and tactile ☐ Difficulty returning to baseline	☐ Tense, fearful ☐ Difficulty returning to baseline	☐ Avoidance ☐ Self-defense ☐ Does not return to baseline

(a)

(b)

Figure 7.3 Canine patient choosing to move onto the station (a) and choosing to move off the station (b).

7.3   Preparing to Train

For any training to work, the environment needs to be conducive to stress reduction and positive learning. Refer to Chapter 4 for ideas on setting up the examination room to maximize success. Training should be done with the owner present in most cases. The technician, veterinarian, or trainer (each are described as "trainer" in this chapter) will need to give clear instructions to the owner about how to participate, where to sit, what to say, etc., but the eventual goal will likely include the owner's participation, and the owner may also be enlisted to do homework between sessions.

In some circumstances, the patient may be a candidate for day training, in which the pet is dropped off at the hospital for a series of training sessions throughout the day. Day training candidates need to be relatively relaxed in the hospital environment for this strategy to succeed. Another option for some clients may be to cooperate with a qualified trainer outside the clinic, and with the help of the trainer, transition these skills to the clinic environment.

Make sure the appointment is scheduled to allow enough time. I suggest 30–60 minutes for initial appointments and 15–30 minutes for follow-ups. The client should be instructed to give all pre-visit medications at the correct interval, to fast the patient for at least four hours prior to the visit, and to come prepared with the patient's very favorite foods and toy.

Choose a room that can be set up the same way each time at first. Patients who are nervous in the hospital will be suspicious of change. Minimize change at first to maximize patient trust and comfort. Small changes to the environment should intentionally be introduced later in the training process. After escorting the pet into the exam room, sit down and explain the goals of the training process to the owner. The discussion, history, and explanation portions can also be done in advance via telemedicine, which carries the advantage of zero stress for the animal if they find the veterinary environment stressful even in the absence of any handling or treatments. Does this patient need to cooperate for examination, vaccination, ear or eye care, or sample collection, or simply to allow sedation to go more smoothly? Invest a moment and discuss the plan and the goals with the client to assure everyone is on the same page (a phone interview prior to the visit can also serve this purpose). During this time, assess the patient's food acceptance, body language, and proximity preference while you're preparing to get started training. If the patient is too stressed to train, formulate a plan to improve the patient's response to the environment (home plan prior to transport, transport, environmental setup, medical management, etc.) prior to attempting Type Three training strategies.

The owner can be helpful by explaining what potential reinforcers they think the animal will like best, and what methods have been used in the past. Dogs who have been trained using punishment-based methods may be anticipating something unpleasant happening. Those who have been trained using lure-reward training may be waiting for a lure or treat to be presented prior to trying new skills. Type Three training relies heavily on shaping, and shaping requires the patient to be willing to explore the environment and try new things in an effort to earn clicks and treats. If the pet already has experience with shaping, training will progress more quickly. For patients who are new to shaping, we will first have to teach them the fun process of this game, and then how to apply the shaping process to acquiring new skills.

Training Tip: Telemedicine Can Help!

At the beginning of the treatment and training process, you will need to take a detailed history, discuss the needs and wants for the family, and lay out a training plan. Offering the preparatory visit via telemedicine or with only the client can prevent unnecessary stress for the patient.

7.3.1 Establishing Consent and Operant Conditioning

Type Three training stresses voluntary, cooperative veterinary care. *Voluntary* means the animal is free to participate, or choose not to participate if they are feeling stressed. *Cooperative* means the patient understands to perform a certain behavior, or allow a specific touch, to earn a desired reward. To allow the animal to make this choice, the trainer needs to establish a consent point: a point at which the animal understands training and handling will start and stop at his or her request. Type Three training is different because there is a **contingency** the animal must satisfy to earn a reward. For desensitization and counterconditioning, the animal received the food, toy, or tactile pleasant stimulus regardless of what they were doing while gradually being exposed to the handling scenario. The goal was to create a conditioned positive emotional response, prevent stress, and reward desired behaviors. While the animal was *also* likely operantly learning how to stay in proximity to handlers, how to remain still for treatments, how to move through the hospital, etc. there was no contingency placed on receiving the treats: it was not required the animal do a specific behavior. Type Three introduces cued behaviors for specific skills, positions, movements, and procedures as an additional layer of training. The patient is learning to give consent and is opting in for training. The trainer can then begin requiring certain criteria to be met before a click and treat result. Remember, classical conditioning is always happening even when we are discussing skills using operant conditioning language.

The point of consent will be unique to each patient, and perhaps to each procedure. To communicate the idea of consent to the animal, the trainer will begin training and handling when the desired consent point has occurred, and will immediately pause if the consent behavior is withdrawn. By consistently starting and pausing in this fashion, we can teach the animals how to control their own care and how to communicate if they are ready to continue or if they are feeling overwhelmed.

For example, we will use stationing as a consent point for some behaviors in this chapter. By choosing to go to the station, the patient is giving his consent to train for the procedure. To pause the session, the patient can simply move off the station (mat, table, rug, etc.). When the patient moves away from the station, all training, and therefore all reinforcement, pause (Figure 7.3). Any discomfort the patient may have been feeling during the training process will pause. Roll or toss a treat away from the station and wait to see the animal's response. Many will immediately opt back into the session, in which case the trainer can begin again. The temptation for "one more repetition" or "I'm going to just put the drops in quickly" might be strong, especially as you near completion of a trained behavior. Remember: it takes only one bad experience to damage trust but many good experiences to gain it. Respect the point of consent, and retain the animal's trust.

There is a notable exception to the pause training guideline: patients who don't move away when they feel uncomfortable. Most animals will have learned through prior experience that moving away from a stressful situation will reduce their stress. However, some animals will choose to stay on the station or near the handler even when they are stressed. These patients usually fit into two categories: either they find the rewards so valuable it's not actually a choice for them to move away, or they stand their ground and escalate through a sequence of distance-increasing signals.

For patients who do not immediately move away, but rather stay closer to the trainer and show body language signs of discomfort, pause handling and toss or roll a treat away to lure the animal to a more comfortable distance. The animal should be rewarded for moving away: the desired behavior is movement away when the pet feels uncomfortable. Reward several times at the comfortable distance and observe between rewards if the animal chooses to come closer. Watch for any signs of mild hesitation or ambivalence when the animal approaches. You may even be able to detect an invisible "bubble" or "boundary" the animal feels when they approach you. In those circumstances, always lure the animal away by tossing or rolling a treat when you see the body language signs of hesitation. The goal is to build the behavior of moving away when the animal experiences a specific feeling. *Moving away when stressed is an extremely functional behavior and worthy of reinforcement because it keeps handlers safe.* Some animals need to be taught how to move away rather than to stay in an uncomfortable situation.

The goal loop for this animal initially would look like:

A: Internal feeling of discomfort (inferred based on observed body language FAS >2)
B: Moving away from the stressor
C: Treats delivered at a comfortable distance, then a second treat delivered further away to create more distance and allow a new repetition
A: Internal feeling of comfort (inferred based on observed body language FAS 0–2)
B: Moving toward the trainer
C: Treats delivered at the closest comfortable distance, then a reset treat tossed further away to begin again.

Gradually you will find these animals start to relax and become more comfortable approaching. For animals with a strong desire for food, use medium or lower value treats during this kind of training in an effort to avoid coercing them to come closer with food they can't refuse. For animals with a fear of approaching, they will learn to trust that you will not trick them or try to grab them. When they feel free to move away, they will voluntarily approach with greater confidence more frequently.

7.3.1.1 Training Loops
Training loops are sequences where the A–B–C can repeat multiple times, and part of the C builds in an opportunity to start a new repetition again with A. Loops are useful because they allow the trainer to be trustworthy and predictable, they keep duration low during the early parts of training, and they help the animal learn what is expected.

7.4 Making a Training Plan

Prior to starting training, get in the habit of making a training plan. The training plan is your roadmap to accomplishing the goal behavior. To make a simple veterinary procedure training plan, follow these steps:

(1) Define the completed behavior.
    If there are multiple behaviors, each behavior needs its own smaller plan. For example, injections need a different plan from blood collection, which will both be separate from nail trims.
(2) Determine the patient's preferred potential reinforcers and how to deliver them. Identify at least three options, and rank them in order of preference.
(3) Decide where to work.
(4) Identify the point of consent.
    There are a number of simple ways to establish consent points. Location is one method, such as choosing to move toward and stay on the station (mat, rug, and table). Another option is body position. If the procedure is to be done in a sitting position, the patient can

withdraw consent by moving into a stand. Targeting, such as maintaining a chin rest or hand target, is another way to establish consent. The patient's preference, practicality of training, owner preference, and procedure to be performed will all dictate what the consent point will be. In some cases, each separate behavior may also have a separate point of consent.

(5) Decide which foundation behaviors, if any, will be needed, and train foundation behaviors in advance.

(6) Verify medications needed, if any.

(7) Imagine approximations.

Shaping is all about *approximations*, or baby steps or building blocks toward a goal behavior (see Chapter 3 for a review of shaping techniques). Consider what the building blocks may be for your behavior, and then split them down as small as you can. The better you are at splitting behaviors into small approximations, the better you will be at shaping!

(8) Establish criteria for reinforcement for approximations.

(9) Determine advancement points where the patient is ready for criterion increases to earn reinforcers.

(10) Plan to chart your progress using detailed notes or video.

(11) Record the ending point for the training session.

Table 7.3 is an example training plan worksheet for Type Three training. In the Appendix, you will find training plan worksheets to help you build your own training plans. A few example training plans are included in this chapter to get you started. Remember: each patient is different, and will benefit from customizations to the training plan.

Table 7.3 Type Three training plan worksheet: this is a basic template for the steps of creating a Type Three training plan.

Training plan: Type Three training	
Completed behavior: Goal A, B, C:	Component behaviors:
Consent point:	Consent point:
Preferred reinforcers 1. 2. 3.	
Medications:	Working area:
Foundation behaviors required:	Known cues needed: Additional DS/CC/CC needed: Yes No
Starting criteria	
Progression	
Ending criteria	
Observations	
Homework	
Plan for next visit	

Available for download in the Online Resources.

7.5 Getting Started: Reinforcement, Stillness, Approaches, Target, and Station

We will be using mostly dog examples for these training videos, but remember: any animal can learn these behaviors with proper training and the right reinforcement.

Training Tip: Make a Movie

Videotape your training sessions. Reviewing the video will help you catch errors and improve your training skills. The videos are also excellent for tracking patient progress, and posting on social media.

7.5.1 Reinforcement Procedures

To participate in training, pets need to understand how reinforcement will be delivered. In previous chapters, we have talked about giving treats using spoons or pretzel rods, lick mats, and placing treats right near the pet as well as handing treats to their mouths. Where we place rewards and how they are delivered are an important part of training. Do I want the animal to sit, stand, or lie down? Do I want them to be still or to move? Which direction should they move? Does the animal like to be able to watch the treats, or is that unimportant? To use placement of reward to best advantage, I need to be able to deliver rewards in a variety of different ways.

Before introducing contingencies where the animal needs to perform a specific behavior to receive a reward, we need to verify the different ways the animal knows how to receive treats! Some reinforcement procedures come naturally for the animal, some may have already been trained in the past, and some may need to be taught before cooperative veterinary care training can be undertaken. Not every pet needs to know every single reinforcement procedure, but having at least three different reinforcement procedures available is extremely helpful. How to train every single reinforcement procedure is beyond the scope of this text, but don't be afraid to play, get creative, and branch out to other resources for teaching these general skills!

Ideally, I like to have animals understand all of these:

- Follow and pick up a rolled or tossed treat in front of the pet
- Follow and pick up a rolled or tossed treat behind the pet
- Accept a treat from my hand quickly
- Wait while I deliver a treat slowly to the animal's mouth
- Lick a treat from a squeeze tube or syringe
- Eat a treat from a dish
- Focus on a fist holding multiple treats and accept one treat at a time when pinched out of the fist to be delivered
- Be near a dish containing food and wait for me to pick up a piece to give it to them
- Wait while looking at a treat then on cue move to take the treat
- Wait while looking at a bowl with a treat in it then on cue move to take the treat
- Eat treats from a remote trainer like a Manners Minder™ or Pet Tutor™.

For toys, I like dogs to understand how to:

- Tug on cue
- Wait while watching the toy and tug on cue

- Open their mouth to drop the toy on cue (tug or retrieve)
- Follow a rolled or tossed toy and return it to me
- Chase a toy without having to return it to me.

You will see a variety of reinforcement procedures in the example videos for this chapter. When you watch the videos, pay attention to what skills the animal needed in order to access reinforcement. How to get your treat is more than just knowing which behavior to perform: it's also understanding how the reward sequence works.

7.5.2 Stillness as a Foundation Skill

For examinations and any kind of care, we will want pets to be stationary. Teaching stillness with relaxed body language is worthwhile. When we work with pets on stillness, we need to remember that some pets become still or freeze when their FAS score increasing, so monitor all body language rather than just the absence of movement when working on stillness. Stillness exercises may take a single session per exercise for some pets, while others may need days, weeks, or months to learn the stillness exercises. Work at the pet's individual pace, it is worthwhile to be able to build value and a strong reinforcement history for having a still body.

A few exercises to teach that holding still is good:

7.5.2.1 Calm Cookies

Work in a place the pet is comfortable and they are likely to relax like their bed, mat, or even on the sofa. Have a small collection of low or medium value treats available and place one treat in one hand, with several treats closed in your opposite hand. Go near the bed or mat and sit quietly. When the animal comes to investigate, calmly deliver the single treat directly to the pet's mouth in the body position of the animal's choice (sit, stand, down). As they are eating, refill your hand that's next to the animal's nose by moving your opposite hand closer. Try to keep the hand next to the animal's nose stationary without moving it as a target. Gradually increase the pause between treat refills a second (or a fraction of a second!) at a time until the animal can stand, sit, or lie still for 15 treats in a row spread out over 30 seconds (or more).

7.5.2.2 Breakfast in Bed

If the pet already knows how to lie down, use the cue for lying down. The goal is for pets to easily be able to eat the treat while they are lying down without needing to move. Some pets need to learn how to eat while lying down! They will naturally stand up when the treat is delivered. If the pet stands each time to chew, start by delivering the treat to their nose instead of placing it on the floor. Then with each repetition, move your treat hand 1″ closer to the floor before each refill until you can place treats on the floor and the pet can eat them in the down position.

Once the pet can eat while lying down, use the same strategy as calm cookies. When the pet is lying down, place one treat between the pet's front paws *or* next to the outside of one elbow. You may need to experiment to find which position the pet prefers. When the first treat is eaten, calmly and with a smooth movement, deliver a refill treat to the exact same location. Gradually increase the pause between treats by 1 second (or a fraction of a second) until the pet can lie down and eat 15 consecutive treats over a period of at least 30 seconds.

7.5.2.3 Chin Cookies

Chin cookies can be a good precursor to the Chin Rest behavior discussed later in the skills section of this chapter. To practice Chin Cookies, sit on a chair or on the floor at a height where you can comfortably offer your palm at the pet's chin level when they are standing. Keep one hand empty, hold several treats in your opposite hand with closed. Show the pet the closed treat hand, then open your opposite hand flat with the palm facing the ceiling at the pet's chin level, between the pet's current position and your treat hand. When the pet leans forward toward the treat hand, their chin will be resting on your outstretched palm. Move the treat hand to the pet's nose and shift one treat out of your fist into pinched fingers to feed it. Using the same strategy as Calm Cookies, feed successive treats calmly while the pet's chin is touching your palm. Gradually increase the pause between treats until the pet can stand with their chin in your hand for 15 consecutive treats over a period of at least 30 seconds.

7.5.2.4 Pattern Games

Leslie McDevitt has published a number of pattern games in her Control Unleashed program. Specifically, the games Up-Down, 1-2-3, and Chair Game are useful for stillness and can easily be adapted to a cooperative care setting.

There are many more ways to teach stillness, these are simply a few of the author's favorites.

7.5.3 Approaches

Every final veterinary behavior begins with the patient approaching a team member and allowing some form of touch. Begin by shaping approaches. Once you're settled in the training area (likely an exam room), choose where you'd like the animal to work, such as a mat, rug, or low table. Sit or stand near the station. Watch the patient closely. At first, watch the patient's nose. The nose moving toward you will mean the animal is going to look at you, but the nose is often easier for you to watch than the eyes at first. Click when the patient moves his nose toward you, then toss a treat behind the dog so he turns away. Next, click for the dog looking at you, then approaching one step. Again, toss the treat behind the dog so he turns away. By tossing the treat behind, you're setting up the dog for a new repetition. By now, some patients will be running right up to you, while others will need you to reinforce each step toward you incrementally until they are ready to come all the way to you. Avoid reaching toward the patient while training approaches. First, we will teach the patient to come to you, then we will let him initiate touch through targeting.

Some patients will require an entire session or even multiple sessions just to train approaches, while others will approach within a few seconds. Be sure to note in the medical record what you did during the session, where the animal's skill Type began, where it was when you concluded the session, and what your plan is for the next visit.

Video 7.1 shows a short shaping and targeting session with Fifi, a nine-year-old poodle with no history of training and moderate to severe stress in the veterinary clinic. This is her first time hearing a clicker, and her first training session. Each time she glances at or approaches Monique, she earns a click and a treat. In a few repetitions, she is too nervous to take the food, but she eventually approaches and even offers the target behavior.

7.5.4 Targeting

Once the patient will approach, we will invite them to a designated area using the foundation skill of targeting. When we say "targeting" in this section, we will refer to touching your hand, or a target stick or other object of your choice. For simplicity, each of these items will be interchangeably called a target.

Many of these patients have a learning history where the veterinary team member reaching for or touching them predicts something scary happening. Instead of reaching for the patient, let him come to you. For the first few repetitions, roll the treat behind the patient to send him away from you. Sending the patient away uses both food and increased personal space to reinforce the target behavior. If you need to move your hand or body, use the same treat-rolling process to move the patient away from you, then make your movement(s) while the patient is further away at first.

Using a similar procedure to shaping approaches, sit or stand near the station and hold your target (hand, stick, spoon, etc.) slightly away from your body. Watch for the dog to look at the target. Click, take the target away, and toss a treat. Remember: the click should happen during the desired behavior (the glance at the target), and the treat will come after. When the dog turns around, present the target again and click for movement toward the target. Each time, roll the treat past the dog to move him away and set him up for a new repetition. When he turns back toward you, present the target. Eventually, he will be ready to sniff or touch the target. When he sniffs or touches the target, click, remove the target, and drop a treat. The click should occur the *instant* his nose is touching the target. Once the dog has eaten the treat, present the target again, click for a nose touch, remove the target, and treat. By removing the target after each click, you are establishing that the target *appearing* is the cue for the behavior. You may also want to use a verbal cue in addition to the visual cue of the target appearing. A common choice is the word "touch" or "target." If you'd like to use a verbal cue, introduce it when the animal is starting to offer the target behavior frequently, and give the verbal cue at the same time you present the target. The shaping approach makes interaction with the target a contingency for receiving a treat. This is different from luring, where the animal simply follows a treat or treats to move along a specific path.

After the animal has become comfortable touching the target, it is time to teach him to follow. If you're sitting, you may need to stand so you can move and he can follow. If you change body positions, reward a few simple targets in your new body position before trying to teach the animal to follow. Even something as simple as the trainer moving from a sit to a stand can change the pet's comfort level and emotional state. Present the target, and as the pet approaches, move the target 1″ further away from him to encourage him to move toward the target to touch it. The instant he touches the target, click, remove the target, and treat. Step by step, begin moving the target 2″, then 3″, then 4″, reinforcing the behavior of moving to follow and touch the target several times at each increment. When the dog will follow the target for 5–10 steps, you're ready to use it to introduce the station.

7.5.5 Stationing

When deciding on what kind of station to use, such as a rug, mat, low platform, or table, consider what the end goal behavior will be. For a small-dog procedure, a cat procedure, or a medium-sized dog for cephalic venipuncture, an elevated platform may be helpful. For larger dogs, or procedures done from above such as eye and ear medicine or subcutaneous fluids and injections, the floor may be a better place to work. Choose a spot that will be comfortable for both the trainer/handler and the patient. Some patients may need to learn more than one station. For example, the table might be used for a physical exam, but the floor for a nail trim. Each time you change the station, you will need to retrain that behavior, so try to plan ahead and know in advance what you will want and need from the learner (refer to Figure 3.23 for station examples). It can be helpful to use a non-slip mat such as a chunk of yoga mat, a bath mat, or a pet mat which is portable and easy to place on the floor, onto a platform, or onto the table. Then the go to mat behavior can be used to facilitate patient comfort on new surfaces by building on what the pet already knows.

One approach to teaching stationing is to use the foundation target behavior to show the dog how to go to the station. To use a target to build stationing, first sit or stand near the station. Reward the dog several times for following the target, then move the target toward the station. When the dog places a paw on the station, click and treat. In this situation, treat the dog while he is in position on the station rather than tossing or dropping the treat behind the dog. Then have the dog follow the target to move off of the station, click, and treat in position. Move the target over the station, so the dog follows and places both front paws on the station. Click, and treat with the dog in position on the station. Move the target off of the station, click, and treat. Progress moving the target further and further, until the dog has all 4 ft on the station. Reward in position, and then reward again right away for remaining on the station. Repeat the process until you can reward every three to five seconds for remaining on the station to help build duration. Table 7.4 shows one example of a possible training plan worksheet for a session teaching stationing.

Training Tip: Homework for Station Training

Clients, colleagues, and anyone else you're teaching will need a short reminder list about the function and form of any exercise you assign. Here's an example homework debrief provided to a client as a reminder guide for the station exercise:

Introduce the mat as a way to say "Ready for Touching" vs. "Not Ready for Touching"

Mats and platforms are helpful because they have a tactile (feeling) and visual boundary for both animal and person.

To build the mat behavior, start by inviting your pet onto the mat by dropping a treat on the mat.

When your pet comes to the mat and eats, toss or roll a treat behind them so they leave the mat to seek the treat.

Once they have eaten that treat, wait for them to turn back toward you, and drop a treat on the mat again.

Repeat × 3–5 repetitions.

Next: When your pet turns back toward you, tap the mat with a finger or point, then wait for them to move toward the mat before dropping a treat.

Gradually wait longer before dropping the treat, until at the end the treat is dropped once the pet has all 4 paws on the mat.

Training loop:

Pet on mat > Treat drops on mat > Pet eats treat > Toss treat behind pet to reset > Pet returns to mat
Once this loop is created, introduce orienting on the mat.
Practice having your pet:

  - Face to face with you
  - Perpendicular to you facing to the right
  - Perpendicular to you facing to the left

Training loop:

Pet approaches mat > Person provides a hand or finger target or an inviting gesture to show the pet how to orient > Pet comes onto mat and orients > Treat given > Treat tossed behind pet off mat to reset > Pet follows treat and eats it > Pet approaches mat > Person provides information about orienting.

Table 7.4 Sample of a possible Type Three training plan to introduce stationing.

Training plan: Type Three training	
Completed behavior: Go to station and remain there until end of behavior is signaled	Component behaviors: Look at station Move toward station Lean over station with any body part Any one paw Both front paws Any 3 paws All 4 paws All 4 paws, short duration All 4 paws, lengthening duration
Consent point: All 4 paws on station	Consent point: N/A
Preferred reinforcers 1. Cheese 2. Bacon 3. Kibble	
Medications: none	Working area: exam room 2
Foundation behaviors required: Clicker charged Hand target Approaches	Known cues needed: Sit, hand target Additional DS/CC/CCC: Yes XX No
Starting criteria	Look at station
Progression	Patient progressed through all component behaviors as expected until duration was introduced.
Ending criteria	4 paws on station for 3 seconds
Observations	Patient relaxed and comfortable throughout the process, but showed mild loss of interest when duration increased beyond 3 seconds. Attempted to extend interest/working period using cued behavior of "sit" and "touch" when on station, but duration still not available.
Homework	Work on sit, touch, down, and building the repertoire of known cues so we have more alternatives for ping-pong and maintaining behavioral momentum.
Plan for next visit	Increase duration on station, introduce body touching on station if patient is comfortable.

Video 7.2 shows introducing a platform to a Type three dog for the first time. Mushu is a dog who loves to work and understood the clicker and working for food before his first visit. He also has a history of delivering bites during veterinary care and body handling to both strangers and the owner. Using a shaping procedure, Mushu receives clicks and treats for successive approximations. Once he is approaching frequently, a finger target is shown to help invite him onto the platform. Rewards are given both for approaching the platform and returning to the floor as a foundation

for teaching an opt-in/opt-out behavior as well as resetting for the next repetition. *(Author's Note: In Mushu's first visit videos, he is wearing a prong collar. This collar was placed by a trainer elsewhere, and neither I nor the owner could safely remove it without sustaining a bite. Once safely removed, the collar was no longer used by the client.)*

To use shaping, break down the behavior of "go to the station" into many building blocks, such as "look at the station," "move one step toward the station," "move several steps toward the station," "place one paw, then multiple paws, then all four paws on the station," and finally "remain on the station for longer and longer periods." When shaping, watch for the dog to constantly be trying to improve on the prior performances, and attempt to solve the puzzle. The dog should seem interested, engaged, and happy. If the dog checks out, seems uninterested, or begins offering the incorrect behavior, assess yourself and the process. The rate of reinforcement may be too low, which means you're expecting big steps instead of baby steps. The solution in this case is to split those steps into smaller approximations. The dog may not be offering improvements because he doesn't understand the shaping process, or that you're working toward a larger goal behavior. The dog may also be mentally fatigued, or stressed by the process. In that case, take a break, work on another behavior, check for environmental stressors, or stop the session.

Short term luring can also be helpful in speeding the station training process. Roll or toss a treat away. When the animal has followed and eaten the treat, then turns to check in, place a treat on the station. The animal will eat that treat, and you can toss another off the station. Once the pet is easily moving on and off the station, begin feeding intermittently for longer duration on the station, and sending the animal away less frequently.

Training Tip: Two Strikes and You're Out

Maintaining a high rate of reinforcement and a low level of confusion is critical for training success, especially for new learners and new trainers. If an animal makes two errors in a row, pause, assess the situation, and split the criteria down into smaller pieces that are easier for the animal to understand. Multiple errors in a row will decrease behavioral momentum and slow the learning process.

7.6 Teaching Consent, Touch, and Restraint

7.6.1 Consent at the Station

Once the pet will go to the station, it is time to teach her she is in control of the interaction, and her way of controlling the interaction is by using the station behavior. The station becomes the on and off switch for interaction and rewards, and the animal will learn they are in charge of this switch fairly quickly.

When the patient goes to the station, click and treat for stationing, and then give a cue the animal knows well such as sit, down, or target. Click and treat, repeating several times. Then use a target or tossed treat to move the dog off the station, and pause all clicking and treating. Move nearer the station yourself, and when the pet comes to the station, repeat the process of asking for several simple behaviors the pet knows well, and click/treat for each repetition. Generally during this process, the pet will choose to move off the station at some point. Perhaps she will be distracted by an odor, curious about something happening outside the room, or just looking for something else to do. When the pet moves away, carefully observe her. If she is just investigating, wait for her to orient to you and gaze at the station. If she comes back to the station, resume training. If the pet looks concerned, hesitant, or shows any body language associated with escalating FAS, decrease the criteria for coming to the station and switch to the approaches exercise temporarily. If the pet is reluctant to participate in the approaches exercise, end the session and make a new plan for the next session.

Video 7.3 shows Mushu's very first introduction to the idea of interacting on the station and moving off the station to take a break from interacting. He is introduced to small reaches toward him shuffled in with performing some known behaviors such as a hand target. When the reach approaches his threshold of comfort, he moves off the station which is the perfect learning opportunity to teach Mushu he can control the interaction by coming to and leaving the station.

If the patient chooses to leave the station in the middle of training, pause and reflect on what just happened. Did you reach for the animal? Was there a noise outside the room like a barking dog? Did the owner move around or rattle the treat pouch? Have you been working for several minutes and the animal is mentally fatigued? Did the pet's paw slip or any other unsettling movement happen while she was on the station? Use what you learn to increase future success. If it was a reach toward the pet, that pet is not yet ready for that kind of reach. If a dog barking outside was upsetting, remember to feed every time the patient hears that sound until she is no longer bothered by barking. Remember to make notes in the medical record for future sessions about what is successful, but also about anything that causes a pause or setback in training.

When the learner realizes he or she is in control of the training process by choosing to station, or choosing not to station, the need for distance-increasing signals and aggression falls away. We have established a new way to communicate, and the animal will learn we are listening to them. The animals can be excellent teachers for us, just as we can be for them, with mutual communication.

Stationing is only one kind of consent behavior, but it is the simplest one to teach, so we use it the most for examples in this book. Other consent behaviors include chin rest, holding on target, or changes in body position. We will introduce those concepts later in this chapter.

7.6.1.1 Predictably Unpredictable: Variety in Training

When training for other behaviors, such as obedience skills, sport training, or skills training like entering a carrier, it is helpful for the trainer to be extremely consistent in presenting the cue. Same voice, same gesture or signal, same sound, same body position and posture, and same environmental setup. For Cooperative Veterinary Care training, we will introduce predictable unpredictability throughout the training process.

What is predictable unpredictability? Every team member will have a unique way of touching animals, and there is no way to train for every single procedure or handling event an animal may encounter in their lifetime. By intentionally varying where we touch animals, which hand we use, which order we touch which body part, and how intense the touching is at the end of a repetition, we better prepare animals for actual care. The animal knows when they opt-in they will be safe, but they may not know the exact touching or procedure which will occur. By working in a variety of different locations, times of day, environments, and groups of people, clients can normalize husbandry and medical type handling as a routine part of being a pet rather than a special occasion which prompts fear or distress. This homework can really speed the training process for veterinary care.

Keep a bit of variety in your interactions rather than being extremely consistent with every individual touch. For example, switch hands often. If touching the shoulder, touch right and then left. If petting, sometimes pet head-to-tail and sometimes downward along the side or gently against the grain of the fur. Change the duration of the touch rather than constantly increasing difficulty, or always touching for the exact same amount of time with every repetition. It's natural when training to get into a rhythm – but this rhythm can sometimes cause stagnation in the training process. Taking and analyzing video of your training sessions is an excellent way to catch if you're developing a rigid protocol rather than creating a fluid experience. Always be predictable in providing a safe environment, responding by allowing the animal to opt-out or encouraging them to opt-out if they need help, and listening to and responding to the animal's side of the conversation. Be predictably trustworthy!

7.6.2 Teaching Touch

Once the patient will come to the station, and understands the interaction ends if they leave the station, we are ready to begin training to allow touching. For dogs, touching the shoulder or ribs is generally a good place to start, while cats usually prefer cheek or chin touching. But every pet is unique! Owners can be very helpful in developing a Body Map for the pet. Ask clients to make a map of Green, Yellow, and Red areas on their pet. This can be a mental exercise or you can even provide a pet silhouette and ask them to color in the areas on a diagram. Green areas are the ones clients feel the pet enjoys being touched by friends and by strangers. Yellow areas are those the client feels the pet will allow them to touch but probably does not prefer it. Red areas are those the client knows the pet dislikes having touched. The Body Map will help create a training plan for the Touching Game or other touch related exercises.

Training Tip: Body Map Homework

Here is an example homework reminder list for the Body Map assignment:

Pets have general and individual differences in sensation and perception for touch on different parts of their bodies. Personal preference, sensory differences, and learning history will all influence the body map.

Make a body map of your pet:

- GREEN: Areas you can predictably reach toward and touch, and your pet enjoys it.
- YELLOW: Areas you're not sure if the pet will enjoy or not.
- RED: Areas you know your pet shows reluctance and prefers not to be touched.

Early in training, all touching will be in green areas.

As training progresses, touch will always START in a green area, then glide to yellow or red areas.

Through the course of training, the hope would be to change the body map to be more green, with less yellow and red present.

Touching exercises are introduced once the animal shows they are willing and interested in coming to the station by repeating the behavior and remaining on the station for some duration – at least 10 seconds. To begin teaching touch, invite the animal to the station. Watch the patient closely, and reach toward an area marked green on the body map. If the patient stays at the station and looks relaxed, touch in a nonthreatening way. Click *while* you are touching the patient, then treat. The click should mark the instant the touch is occurring, not the time after the touch has already stopped. In some cases, early in the process, the animal may move slightly when you reach to touch them. Click during every touch, and treat after every touch, even if the animal moves. As the patient becomes more familiar with the process, you will be able to increase criteria and click/treat only when the patient stands still for touch in the future.

If you reach out to touch the patient and they look nervous and lean away or start to move away, stop reaching toward them. Toss or roll a treat away to promote movement away from you when they are uncomfortable. This patient needs desensitization and classical counterconditioning to hand movements prior to touching. Move gradually through an exposure ladder for reaching and touching, with each step predicting a click and treat. Start by raising your hand an inch or two from your side, then click/treat. Continue moving your hand toward the patient a few inches at a time, until you can touch the patient. Remember: desensitization should look boring while it is happening. The patient should not show any signs of avoidance when you raise and move your hand. If the patient is showing avoidance or stress, make your hand movements smaller. If any hand movement at all causes stress, go back to asking for simple behaviors at the station, then end the session. Consider slowing the training plan and spending more time targeting where the patient touches you, modifying the environment to be less stressful, modifying the medical management portion of the treatment plan, or some combination of these suggestions.

Once the animal is comfortable with reaching movements, begin nonthreatening touches. Gradually lengthen the duration of the touch, click and treat at the end of the touch. The click should occur immediately before you remove your hand, and the treat be given after your hand is removed. Begin touching in a green area and then gliding to other green areas without paying attention to any special concerns. This is where the Body Map is extremely helpful! Initially, all touching on the station will be in green body areas.

When the pet is comfortable being touched with one hand in each green area for several seconds of duration, switch hands. When the pet is comfortable with either hand, add a second hand to the touching process. Change between hands, and then touch with both hands. For some animals, touching with both hands is considerably different than touching with one hand. One hand means petting; two hands mean an exam or restraint. Train for this eventuality. When you're touching the patient with two hands, you may need to place the clicker under your foot, or change to a verbal marker such as a tongue cluck or the word "yes."

Pets who are comfortable being touched in green body areas for 10 seconds with two hands are ready to have more invasive kinds of touching introduced. To touch yellow areas, always start in a green area and glide to the yellow area. Click at the end of the touch and treat afterward. Repeat the steps with each hand, then both hands. Provide variety during the touching rather than doing it in precisely the same order every time.

Some pets through training will show they are ready to have even red areas touched when on the station. Use the gliding motion and carefully observe the pet's body language during every repetition. Over time, you will find it's time to re-draw the Body Map because the green areas are expending!

Video 7.3b shows Barley. He has learned to hop onto the bench to opt into touching, and hop off the bench to opt out. Barley is a dog who strongly responds to restraint but has learned to play the touching game. We use the bench to opt in and principles he learned about gradual touching to begin introducing some restraint training for him. Notice the touching is broken down into numerous approximations, and the marker happens at the most intense part of the touching repetition.

7.6.2.1 Adding Equipment

Being touched with hands and being touched with equipment are two different things. One addition to the touching game is to introduce touching the pet with assorted objects, both medical and non-medical, during repetitions of gliding hands over their bodies. Ideally, choose a variety of objects, some of which are already well-tolerated such as a hairbrush.

Set up the training mat, and lay the assortment of objects out close enough to easily pick them up and put them down. An example assortment might be a hair brush, a syringe, a stethoscope, a TV remote, a cell phone, and a spoon. *If the pet has a known fear of a specific piece of equipment, do not use it during the early stages of this exercise.* When the pet comes to the mat, alternate repetitions: touching with hands and introducing objects.

To introduce the object, devise an exposure or shaping plan starting at a non-stressful starting point and carefully controlling the intensity of the exposure while watching the animal for signs of discomfort. Every repetition is followed by a treat. Frequently reset the loop by tossing a treat to send the pet away and assess if they are ready to begin again.

Example exposure hierarchy for introducing an object:

- Reach toward the object
- Reach toward and touch the object
- Touch the object and lift it 1″
- Lift it in 1″ increments per repetition until it is head height for the pet
- Lift it to head height and 1″ toward the pet
- Move toward the pet in 1″ increments per repetition until touching the pet in a green area.

Adding two hands – more closely simulating actual care. It would be uncommon to touch a pet only with an object. Usually we touch them with two hands, one holding the object in question. Example of adding a second hand:

- Begin again, but first touch the pet with an empty hand
- Keep your hand on the pet and reach toward the object with your opposite hand
- Keep your hand on the pet and touch the object
- Keep your hand on the pet and lift the object
- Continue as above, until both a hand and the object are touching the pet
- Gradually increase duration, firmness, and intensity of touch
- Intentionally incorporate variety during the training process
- Rotate between objects rather than staying on a single object for many repetitions.

Training Tip: Touching Game Homework Help

One example of a possible homework reminder for clients for the Touching Game:

Once you have a BODY MAP and have introduced MAT/STATION, teach TOUCHING GAME

Touching game means introducing touching into the training loop, so the pet begins to understand that coming to the mat means "Ready for Touching" and moving off the mat means "Not Ready" or is the Pause Button.

(1) Set up your workspace with mat, treats, clicker (if used), and few distractions
(2) Introduce touching into the Mat Loop.
Pet comes to mat > Reach toward green area > TREAT > Toss treat to reset
Pet comes to mat > Reach toward and lightly touch GREEN > TREAT > Toss reset
Pet comes to mat > Lightly then more firmly touch GREEN > TREAT > Toss reset
Pet comes to mat > Variety of duration and nature of touch in GREEN > TREAT > Toss reset

---

(Continued)

(Continued)

---

(3) Watch for any body language of discomfort or approaching threshold:
   Wide eyes
   Look away, lean away, move away
   Tense muscles
   Tense lips
   Slow to respond to cue
   Takes treats too rough or with reluctance
   Yawn or shake off
(4) If you see signs of this body language, PAUSE reaching or touching and toss a reset treat. This will act as a lure to teach the animal to move AWAY when they are feeling worried rather than stay close and become defensive or engage in uncomfortable conflict.
(5) Over time, only at the pet's comfortable pace, begin adding glides from green to yellow areas.
(6) SHUFFLE behaviors. As you and your pet become more proficient, SHUFFLE behaviors. This means using known cues as a way to access rewards in between handling repetitions.

Example:

Mat > Green touch > Treat > Toss reset > Sit > Treat > Target > Treat > Mat > Green/Yellow touch > Treat > Wave > Reset treat

Handling, grooming, and restraint should hopefully become "normal" behaviors for a pet just like sit, target, or any other trick they learn on cue. Shuffling handling in among known cues is a good step toward normalization.

7.6.2.1.1 Adding "Intent"

Some clients may say their pets accept touching with objects, but only when it feels like training for the animal or in a casual moment, but the animal will opt out if the client tries to "do something" to them. I refer to this as handling with "intent." It's very common for animals to avoid handling with intent while allowing other handling, particularly when first starting out in Cooperative Care training with an animal who has an established fear of procedures.

Introducing "intent" into the training process will be important for success with these animals. To introduce intent to the handling practice, I recommend to clients to incorporate it into Touching Game by shuffling. One easy way to introduce intent is to try to take a picture of a body part using a cell phone. The act of focusing on a body part, holding the phone close, and trying to focus will feel very much like examination with equipment to the pet. Use the cell phone as one of the objects during equipment familiarization. When rotating between objects while touching with the opposite hand as described above, introduce the photo procedure into the rotation. *The photo procedure will need to be broken down into multiple approximations for success.*

It's easy to become so focused on training for handling that we forget to provide breaks, fun, and variety for the animal. Sessions will be more interesting, fun, and relaxing if you play a little "ping-pong" when training touching behaviors. To play ping-pong, practice with touches, but between practicing touches, ask for other simple behaviors and tricks the patient knows. This builds **behavioral momentum**. Behavioral momentum is helpful because one success leads to another, and it encourages the patient to stay interested and engaged. By giving the learner some variety, we also reduce the pressure of learning to tolerate something scary (touches), and diffuse some stress before it builds. *This process also normalizes touching into "just another trick," rather than having it seem suspicious or always predicting an exam or other potentially unpleasant experience.*

Training Tip: Shuffling and Ping Pong!
Shuffling handling training into the normal set of behaviors and tricks the pet knows helps normalize the handling behaviors.

7.6.3 Training for Restraint and Sedation

Stabilization and Gentle Control is worth conditioning. So many pets are fearful of being held, even gently. When we introduce any stabilization technique, it is helpful to take a desensitization-minded and shaping approach. Stabilization techniques vary on the position the pet needs to assume and the procedure being performed, but there are some similarities across all stabilization techniques. Here is an example of some of the aspects of stabilization which can be broken down into controlled exposures for enhanced success:

- Handler is at a non-stressful distance to the pet
- The distance is gradually decreased until close together (either animal or handler can move)
- If two people will be working with the animal, both people are present and at a non-stressful distance
- The distance is gradually decreased until both people are close to the pet
- Once the pet is comfortable with proximity of less than half your arm's reach, one person reaches out toward the pet while the other person remains at a distance
- One person touches the pet (See Body Mapping exercise to choose touch locations)
- One person glides their hand over the pet in a number of repetitions until their first arm is around the pet in the desired position
- One person touches with their opposite hand only and the process is repeated with each hand
- One person touches the pet with both hands and simulates stabilization for one second
- Duration is gradually added
- The second person approaches and is closer
- The touching exercise is repeated with the second person closer
- The second person begins exposures for the specific procedure while the first person stabilizes the pet (see specific procedures later in this chapter)
- If examination gloves, loupes, or other equipment will be worn, put it on and then diminish the intensity of handling, returning to a series of less intense exposures to evaluate the patient's response.
- Some patients may need to see or check equipment before the handler puts on the equipment.

Many pets perceive "one hand is petting and two hands is vetting." Also, "one friend, two foes." Changing from touching with one hand to two hands and adding a second person are common points where pets will suddenly show a higher stress level. Putting on examination gloves is another exceptionally common trigger for pets to experience escalating FAS. Watch for these, and plan in advance to introduce them gradually to set pets up for success.

7.6.3.1 Foundation Exercises for Comfort with Stabilization
7.6.3.1.1 Tunnel Game
Video 7.8a

The purpose of the Tunnel Game is to teach animals that being in a confined space is a behavior that will lead to rewards, and can even feel fun and good. Many pets are wary of tight spaces and feelings of being trapped. Using Tunnel Game creates reinforcement opportunities in tight spaces without causing any distress for the pet. For each of these games, make sure the pet is positioned on a non-slip mat or surface when they are in the goal position.

Start by rolling treats alternating directions.

- Roll a treat to your right several feet away
- When the pet picks up the treat, roll a treat to your left several feet away so the pet passes by you
- Repeat several times to make sure the pet can follow rolled treats and change direction.

Next, find a space to work where there is a wall, bench, sofa, coffee table, fence, or other stationary object. Stand or sit facing the stationary object (we will use a wall in this example), far enough away that there is a nice wide gap between your body and the wall. The gap should be wide enough the pet will freely move through it without pausing or noticing a change in social pressure.

Repeat the alternating treat rolling exercise.

- Roll a treat to your right several feet away
- When the pet picks up the treat, roll a treat between you and the wall so it lands several feet away to your left
- If the pet goes between you and the wall, switch and roll to the right again
- Continue alternating until the pet is walking between you and the wall both directions
- If the pet goes around you to avoid the space between you and the wall, move further away from the wall so it is very easy for the pet to travel the desired route.

As the pet becomes proficient at moving back and forth through the gap, add an additional treat to the sequence:

- Roll a treat to the right
- When the pet picks up the treat, drop a treat between you and the wall to encourage a pause in that spot
- When the pet picks up that treat, roll another treat to your left
- When the pet picks up the treat, drop a treat between you and the wall to encourage a pause in that spot, then roll another to the right, and so on.

As the pet becomes comfortable pausing for the treat between you and the wall, slowly close the gap between your body and the wall while also adding duration to the pause in the tightest spot. Only change either the distance or the duration on each repetition. For example:

- Roll a treat to the right
- Move 2″ closer to the wall
- Drop one treat in the gap, then roll to the left
- Drop one treat, then two treats in the gap, then roll to the right (two treats = more duration in the tight gap)
- While the pet is to your right, move 2″ closer to the wall
- Drop two treats in the gap, then roll to the left
- Drop three treats in the gap, then roll to the right
- Move 2″ closer to the wall
- Drop three treats in the gap, then roll to the left.

Continue alternating increasing duration while closing the gap until you can sit or stand so close to the wall that the pet brushes against your legs or feet while they are eating their treats paused in the gap.

When the animal can stand and pause in the gap for at least 10 seconds, substitute a second person for the wall, so the gap is now between two people rather than between a person and an object. Return to the original starting distance. If you were 5′ from the wall to begin, the people will need to be at least 5′ apart to start. Repeat the steps as above, but with the goal of the animal pausing between two people rather than pausing between one person and an inanimate object.

For bonus difficulty, introduce the Tunnel Game in corners rather than just along a flat or straight surface so the animal is pausing while confined in a corner.

7.6.3.1.2 Arm Hoops
Video 7.8a

Arm Hoops is essentially the Tunnel Game but the gap is created between the trainer's arm and their body rather than between their body and another object or another person. From the animal's perspective, the feeling of spatial pressure may be similar, but we are adding in the experience of something present above them rather than just on their left and right sides.

Sit, squat, or kneel in a comfortable position. Extend one arm out to the side parallel with the floor. Begin as with Tunnel Game, by rolling treats in alternating directions: forward and backward to encourage the pet to pass back and forth under your arm. As the pet becomes more comfortable gradually lower the arm to the pet's head height, then add in a bent elbow so the arm creates an arch or hoop for the pet to pass through.

Continue through the progression as with Tunnel Game adding the dropped treat directly in the gap to encourage a pause in the arm hoop, then adding duration remaining under the arm.

The next step is to add a second person, as with Tunnel Game. Begin far apart, then move closer together. The second person can even incorporate aspects of Touching Game once the pet is comfortable in the smallest gap for a duration of at least 30 seconds.

7.6.3.1.3 Center or Middle
Video 7.8b

Center or middle are positions where the animal is between your feet or hands. Medium and large dogs will be positioned between your legs or feet while you sit or stand. Small dogs and cats would be positioned between your hands or arms on a table or platform. The exercise is easier with two people if you're practicing Center between hands instead of feet. This exercise is exceptionally helpful to prepare for jugular blood collection, eye examination, ear treatments, and anything where the animal will be stabilized and their head or front legs would be handled.

The fundamentals of this exercise are similar to Tunnel Game and Arm Hoops, only the position is different.

- Stand with feet shoulder width
- Roll a treat forward to begin
- When the pet picks up the treat, roll a treat backward through the gap between your feet to encourage movement through the gap
- Alternate delivery positions until the pet is freely passing through the gap
- Encourage a pause in the gap by dropping a treat directly between your feet
- Gradually introduce duration or narrowing the gap on each repetition
- Drop one treat, then two treats in the gap, then roll one forward (two treats = more duration in the tight gap)
- While the pet is in front of you, close the gap 2″
- Drop two treats in the gap, then roll a treat behind
- Drop three treats in the gap, then roll a treat forward
- Close the gap 2″
- Drop three treats in the gap, then roll behind, etc. alternating closing the gap and increasing duration.

For working on an exam table or with a smaller pet:

- Two people are needed for safety
- Sit at the end of the table with your forearms shoulder width apart and the forearms resting on the table
- A second person rolls a treat forward
- When the pet picks up the treat, helper rolls a treat backward through the gap between your hands to encourage movement into the space between your forearms
- Alternate delivery positions until the pet is freely passing into and out of the space between your arms
- Encourage a pause in the gap by dropping a treat directly in front of the pet's nose while they are between your forearms
- Gradually introduce duration or narrowing the gap between your arms on each repetition
- Drop one treat, then two treats in the gap, then roll one forward (two treats = more duration in the tight gap)
- While the pet is in front of you, close the gap 2″
- Drop two treats in the gap, then roll a treat away
- Drop three treats in the gap, then roll a treat away
- Close the gap 2″
- Drop three treats in the gap, then roll behind, etc. alternating closing the gap and increasing duration until the pet is pushing through your hands to get into the space between your elbows on the table.

7.6.3.1.4 Squeeze Please

Squeeze Please adds the sensation of pressure being applied to the pet's body.

When the pet is comfortable pausing in the tightest gap, gradually introduce touching and then applying gentle pressure to the pet's sides, back, and belly simulating typical stabilization positions such as around the thorax or flank and under the neck. Remember to isolate each segment of the handling and introduce one segment at a time. For example, one arm, then pressure, the opposite arm, then pressure, two arms without pressure, then two arms with pressure. The same is true with Center or Middle position, but pressure is applied with shins, knees, and then introducing hands over time to stabilize the pet's head and neck.

Practicing these exercises prepares animals to be conditioned for common restraint positions. When the pet is proficient at coming into the positions of Arm Hoops and Center, and can do the Big Squeeze, all we need to do is practice gliding our hands and arms to new places on the body using principles from the Touching Game to create trained restraint.

7.6.3.2 Sedation Training

Sometimes when patients have high levels of FAS, and especially when they have a history of stressful veterinary visits, sedation training is a successful endpoint in the training plan. In other cases, the patient may be able to learn voluntary treatments over a lengthy series of visits, but the owner may not be ready to pursue a long-term training relationship. For these patients, the most practical course is to teach cooperative sedation protocols.

For sedation, some dogs may first need to learn to wear a muzzle. See Section 7.7 for information on muzzle training.

The purpose of sedation training is to create a safe, low-stress experience for the patient, the veterinary team, and the client. Some animals can be trained to accept unrestrained sedation or walking sedation, while others are best trained for light restraint and then injection. When training restraint for injection, determine where the animal will be when sedated, what position the animal will be in, and how the handlers intend to touch the animal to sedate him. How many hands will you use to touch him? Where will your hands be? How many people will be present? How many people will touch him? Where will the injection be given? How long will the injection take? The answers to these questions will guide your plan for each specific patient's sedation training.

The least stressful position for restraint for intramuscular sedation is generally standing or sitting for dogs, and sternal recumbency for cats. These positions are comfortable for the patient and give good access to the epaxial and gluteal muscles. Some sources recommend epaxial muscles as the preferred site for intramuscular injection, while others suggest gluteal muscles. Most medications used for sedation are labeled for intramuscular or intravenous use. In the author's experience, sedating medications labeled for intramuscular use are often effective when delivered subcutaneously, and training for subcutaneous injections is easier for most animals. In any case, it is important to make sure the patient is comfortable with the injection process to reduce patient movement and decrease the risk of potentially serious side effects from intramuscular injections. As with any protocol, pay attention to the animal's signals and be prepared to try something different during the training process. A few dogs may prefer to sit or lie down rather than stand.

Training Tip: Medication Makeovers

Training patients to accept sedation will result in patients who are less stressed and less fearful. Because these patients are more relaxed, they often require lower doses of sedation than they did when they were more fearful. Make sure to calculate drug dosages for the more relaxed patient in front of you rather than simply repeating what was done in the past when the patient's anxiety level may have been much higher.

For this example, we will discuss standing light restraint for a medium-sized dog for intramuscular injection.

Here are some example building blocks for this behavior:

- Come to station with syringe visible in training area
- Allow touching
    - Full body with one hand
    - Full body with two hands
- Allow touching under the neck and over the shoulder with one hand
- Allow touching under the abdomen or over the planned injection area with one hand
- Allow simultaneous touching of the neck and the abdomen
- Allow touching of the neck and abdomen with a light squeeze
- Allow squeezing of the neck and abdomen with gentle pressure
- Allow gentle-pressure squeezing for progressively longer durations
- Allow long-duration gentle pressure while a second person is in the room
- Allow duration pressure while a second person holds a syringe
- Allow duration pressure while a second person approaches with a syringe
- Allow duration pressure while a second person touches
    - Touches of injection area progress in firmness up to a pinch
- Allow duration pressure while a second person simulates injection with a capped needle
- Allow duration pressure with a training needle
- Allow duration pressure during an injection.

Each of these steps is introduced gradually, and every small approximation is followed by a click during handling, and a treat afterward. If at any time the dog tries to move away or leave the station, he is allowed to do so. The temptation to keep going once we have our hands on the animal can be very strong. Remember how much effort we have invested to gain the trust of this animal. Trust comes with routine, predictability, and consistent mutual respect, and the desired behavior gets stronger through reinforcement of good approximations. Table 7.5 shows a sample worksheet for a training session to prepare a dog to allow sedation.

Some animals or teams will never be ready for this training exercise, their fear is simply too great. For those animals, veterinarians should consider prescribing oral and oral-transmucosal medications to decrease the animal's fear sufficiently to allow a rapid IM injection for sedation.

Table 7.5 Sample of a possible Type Three training plan for session 2 of 3 for IM sedation.

Training plan: Type Three training	
Completed behavior: Allow IM sedation Session 2	Component behaviors (approximations): Station – train in advance Light body hug – train in advance Touch injection area Pinch injection area Second person approaches with syringe Second person pinches injection area Faux injection with capped syringe Actual injection
Consent point: At station	Consent point: Stands still without moving away
Preferred reinforcers 1. Peanut butter spoon 2. Squeeze cheese 3. Chicken baby food	
Medications: Trazodone, Gabapentin night before and 2 hours prior	Working area: Exam room 1
Foundation behaviors required: Station Arm Hoop Squeeze Please	Known cues needed: Sit, Hand target, Down, Spin Additional DS/CC/CCC: XX Yes – 2nd person and all touching break down DS/CCC simultaneous with operating cooperatively (OC).
Starting criteria	Station and light hug, second person holding syringe
Progression	Patient progressed through approximations as expected, including faux injection
Ending criteria	Faux injection with capped syringe
Observations	Patient relaxed and comfortable. Second person approaching needed to be broken down so that we reinforced after each step she took toward the dog. Faux injection was well tolerated.
Homework	None required
Plan for next visit	IM sedation for exam, blood draw, radiographs

Generally these protocols begin with oral tablets or liquids administered starting 24–48 hours before the visit followed by oral-transmucosal administration of medications, or even licking some medications from a plate with sticky food. Muzzle training should be undertaken for safety for dogs, and cats should be sedated in their carrier or a light towel cover using the emergency sedation technique.

Video 7.4 demonstrates oral-transmucosal administration training with Border collie Quill. This dog already has the foundation behaviors of coming to a station, body touching and handling, and comfort with syringes.

7.7 Muzzle Training and Protected Contact

Consider this: a fearful, defensively aggressive dog is presented to the hospital. To stay safe, the team member grabs a muzzle and applies it with some difficulty. The dog is then held down by two people, while a third cleans his painful infected ear. The muzzle has now been linked with the stress and pain of the visit, and predicts an unpleasant encounter. When the dog sees a muzzle in the future, it may trigger a strong response. Muzzle training can prevent these experiences.

Muzzle training, or training a pet to wear an Elizabethan collar is a form of protected contact. Protected contact means there is a physical barrier in place for safety. Other forms of protected contact include working with a baby gate or fence between the animal and the trainer, tethering the animal on a leash, or having the pet remain in a crate or kennel and working through the bars. Muzzle training is an excellent idea for all dogs, not just anxious dogs. Elizabethan collar training is helpful for all dogs, in the event they may need to wear one for an injury or surgery recovery. Teach owners to keep a properly sized basket muzzle in the pet first aid kit. If a pet sustains a painful injury, a muzzle can keep the owner safe during transportation and the veterinary team safe during assessment and pain management. However, the dog must allow placement of the muzzle for it to work.

Before undertaking muzzle training or Elizabethan collar training, check with the client to see if they are aware of an existing negative response to either piece of equipment. If the animal already shows high FAS at the sight of the equipment, take care to select equipment which looks very different from what the animal fears before starting the training process.

Muzzle training is a variation on target training. Instead of targeting a hand, target stick, or spoon, the dog is taught to target the inside of the basket with his nose. Many dogs learn to love this game, and happily "get dressed" on cue. Creating this positive emotional response is far preferable to classically conditioning the negative emotional response that is so common.

To wear a muzzle, the dog needs to feel comfortable with:

- Tactile stimulation circumferentially around the snout
- Tactile from the straps on the cheeks and head
- Allowing manipulation of the straps and muzzle
- The sound and sensation of the straps being buckled or clicked closed
- Remaining still for the straps to be unfastened
- Eating treats through the basket (there's a learning curve for both pet and person here)
- Duration of wearing the basket
- Ability to move while wearing the basket
- Ability to respond to known cues while wearing the basket.

In rare instances, some dogs may show intense frustration or resource guarding triggered by food being presented outside the basket. It's quite uncommon, but always closely monitor a dog's body language the first time food is offered through the basket.

Practicing with an object other than the muzzle first is a good way to develop handler and dog mechanical skills and coordination. Some dogs will be reluctant to place their nose into anything narrow, while others are unconcerned. Building this skill into the training plan allows for the most sensitive dogs to be successful.

7.7.1 Exercise: Taking Food from a Narrow Space

A coffee cup, teacup or small takeout container can be used. The exercise is simple. Hold a coffee cup, teacup, pint glass, takeout container, or other object similar in circumference to the planned basket muzzle. Hold the cup with the opening facing the ceiling. Show the dog a treat and with an obvious motion, place the treat into the cup. Turn the cup 90° so the opening is facing the dog and sit still, allowing the dog to investigate and reach into the cup for the treat. Once the treat is gone, turn the cup upward again so the opening is facing the ceiling.

Orienting the cup in a predictable way is really useful because this will later become the visual cue for placing the muzzle. Reinforcement will be available when the muzzle opening is facing the pet, and reinforcement will not be available when the muzzle opening is facing the ceiling.

If the dog is reluctant to place its nose inside the cup, consider ways to get to a starting point of success. Use a more shallow container, or a ring shaped object rather than a cup such as a roll of masking tape. Place the object on the floor without holding it, and feed around an inside the object. Once the dog can eat around and from the object, progressing to deeper objects and holding the object is usually possible.

7.7.2 Exercise: Eating with Snout in a Narrow Space

My favorite training prop for this exercise is a clear plastic cup or takeout container with the bottom cut out to make a clear plastic tube the approximate circumference of the planned muzzle.

Hold the tube with the opening facing the ceiling and hold a treat in the opposite hand. Rotate the cup so the opening is toward the dog, and when they reach forward with their nose toward the opening based on their learning history with the prior exercise, immediately show the treat through the tube. When the dog inserts their nose, they will be able to eat the treat while their nose is in the tube. Repeat several times until the dog is diving their nose quickly into the tube, then begin introducing duration by feeding several treats in succession. When feeding the final treat, remove the tube from the dog's nose rather than the dog moving backward out of the tube.

Once the dog can eat five treats over the period of 5–10 seconds, starting introducing the tube in a variety of orientations so the dog reaches left, right, up, and down to get their nose into the tube. Remember, the opening should face the ceiling when reinforcement is not available, and the opening should face the dog when reinforcement is available.

After the dog can orient left, right, up, and down, it's time to introduce the basket. At first, secure the straps around the top, bottom, or front of the basket so the straps can't move or flop and startle the dog. Present the basket using the same steps as presenting the tube. Use the same body language and positioning, but feed the treat through the front of the basket. It may be necessary to use a cupped hand or push the treat through the basket with a finger. Using a squeeze tube, spray cheese can, or syringe to deliver food may be easier for some people and pets. At the end of each repetition, remove the muzzle before the dog pulls his nose back.

Once the pet is readily placing their nose into the basket and remaining there for five consecutive treats, introduce different orientations up, down, left, right – and a new one – forward. When the dog places his nose into the basket, move the basket 1″ away from the dog in a forward direction so they need to reach further and push harder to place their nose into the basket. Gradually increase criteria of nose-in-basket while leaning forward, walking, and even walking and turning as they work to keep their nose in the basket.

Next, teach the straps. There are a variety of ways to teach the strap portion of the behavior. One is to place the muzzle like a pendant on a necklace. If the dog is already comfortable with wearing a collar or harness, this step may be easy and only take a couple of repetitions. Another is to close the straps at a size that is big enough the dog can slide their head through the closed straps to get their nose into the basket.

Close the strap, fold it forward, and hold the clipped strap on the bridge of the nose of the muzzle (see Video 7.6). Offer the muzzle and when the dog places his nose into the basket, raise the strap 1″, then lower it, reward, and remove the basket. Incrementally increase the raise until you can touch the dog's forehead with the straps while the dog keeps his nose in the basket. Next, begin presenting the basket with the strap held open in front of the basket, so the dog can thread his nose through the loop and into the basket for reinforcement. Gradually change the position of the straps over a series of repetitions until the dog can push his head through the straps into the basket and end up wearing the muzzle loosely while accepting treats. Unclip the strap to remove and reward stillness after removal. When the dog is comfortable wearing the loose muzzle for short periods of time, the step of tightening the straps to fit is added.

An alternate method for teaching straps is for the dog to keep his nose in the basket while the trainer raises first one strap, then the other to touch the dog's face, and works through a series of approximation to get closer and closer to closing the straps behind the dog's head until eventually being able to close them. For muzzles with fixed-length straps rather than adjustable straps, this method will be the only one possible. Choose the method which seems easiest for each individual dog to accept.

Some dogs need protected contact but can't wear a muzzle, for example brachycephalic dogs. Using a large Elizabethan collar may be an option for some dogs. The steps to teaching the Elizabethan collar are quite similar to teaching the muzzle.

Video 7.5 shows a dog voluntarily putting on his own cone for the first time with the client during a consultation. Notice his emotional state, eager participation, and how pleased the client is with the process. The end of the video shows a visit later in Elvis' training process where we use the Elizabethan collar for its intended purpose during a subcutaneous injection.

Video 7.6 Muzzle Introduction. In this video, you will see the use of training props and a basket muzzle to begin muzzle training. Quill the Border collie has never worn a muzzle before, but he has the foundation skills of going to a mat, stillness, interacting with novel objects, and placing his head through a collar and a harness.

Video 7.7 shows several different dogs engaging in muzzle training over the course of several different visits. Observe each dog interacts with the muzzle slightly differently, but each dog willingly either puts the muzzle on themselves, or allows the muzzle to be applied without stress. The dogs can eat through the muzzle, and perform known cues while wearing the muzzle. The muzzle allows these dogs to engage in safer Cooperative Veterinary Care because the likelihood of a bite is greatly reduced and the feeling of needing to restrain the dogs as a primary means of preventing bites is also eliminated.

Working in protected contact behind a baby gate, fence, or through a kennel door or crate may be necessary for safety for a small number of animals. Examples of behaviors that can be performed in

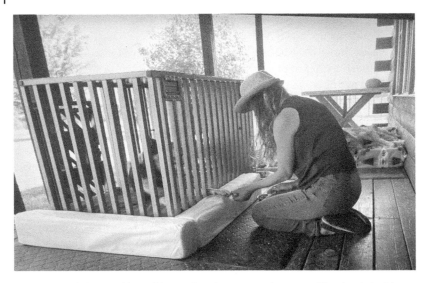

Figure 7.4 A dog working with a trainer in protected contact. The dog is inside a crate, and the bolster outside the crate gives the dog a comfortable place to rest a leg for paw inspection, nail care, or blood collection. Source: Courtesy of Ellen Withrow and Laura Monaco Torelli.

this way would include a trained cephalic or jugular blood collection, nail care of the front paws, or intramuscular sedation. When working in protected contact, remember to always keep your hands on your side of the barrier and the animal must come to you. The purpose of the barrier is to prevent any accidental injury to the trainer. Reaching through the barrier to the animal's side can create a dangerous situation.

Figure 7.4 shows an example of using a physical barrier to work in protected contact with a dog.

7.8 Physical Examination Training

There are many right answers when it comes to how to train a physical examination.

Some exams can be trained using the touching method described in Section 7.6, simply expanding the touches to include all aspects of the physical examination. Other patients might do best with individual cues for each portion of the exam, asking for presentation of specific body parts. Yet another set of patients may be most successful if taught a behavior like the chin rest or extended target for examination (see Section 7.11).

7.8.1 Touch Training for Exam

Physical examination is a series of touches. Using the principles of desensitization and counterconditioning introduced in Chapter 6 for Type Two exams combined with the Type Three touch-training protocol will often result in successful examination training. As always, the key is to progress at a pace that feels comfortable for the patient, maintaining a non-stressful experience, and where the goal behavior is broken down into its many building blocks, with each block representing an opportunity for reinforcement.

For physical examination using touch training, the consent point is staying at the station (or chin rest, target hold, etc.) *and* showing body language consistent with low FAS. Invite the animal to the station, and ask for a few well-known easy behaviors. When the dog is working well, begin practicing touch training as described in Section 7.6 to assess the patient's comfort with contact. Before each touch, show the animal your hand or hands so they know you plan to use your hands to touch them. When the pet seems comfortable based on food acceptance, body language, and staying at the station, initiate touches that are part of a physical examination. Use the guidelines presented in the Touching Game for moving through examination of different body parts, paying attention to the individual pet's Body Map information.

As with the Type One and Type Two physical examinations, begin with less sensitive areas, progressing to more sensitive areas. Save any individual sensitivities, oral exam, paws, rectum, and painful areas for last.

During training sessions, the technician will both train the patient and observe responses, assessing for changes in the patient's stress level. Increases in the stress level are a sign to break down the touching into smaller increments, before the animal withdraws consent by leaving the station.

Begin touching in a less sensitive area, and then glide to the desired exam area. Gradually increase criteria for both pressure and duration as the patient becomes more comfortable. Timing is important: the click should occur at the end of the touch but while your hand is still in contact with the animal. Ping-pong between exam skills and other known behaviors such as "sit," "down," and tricks; this will help keep the session less stressful and more interesting. Also, giving the animal frequent breaks away from the station is important early in the training process, until their mental and emotional stamina is sufficient to work through an entire exam.

Training Tip: Maintain Your Momentum

Remember: known cues are secondary reinforcers. A patient who has learned to sit, touch, lie down, and go to mat has been given a primary reinforcer such as a treat for these behaviors many times. Often, being able to do simple behaviors in response to cues improves the animal's emotional state, and builds behavioral momentum. Keep your learner's momentum high by giving known cues intermittently during training sessions for new skills.

Once the animal is showing comfort with coming to the station and allowing touching, begin using presenting your hands as the signal that reinforcement is available rather than inviting the pet to the station. Toss a treat away from the station. When the animal orients to you, show your hands as you have been prior to touching the animal. Wait to see if they elect to come to the station. If so, begin touching. If they choose not to come to the station, do not touch them or coerce them using cues or food lures to come to the station. The pet is now showing understanding that they have control over whether you will touch them or not! This is a beautiful moment of understanding during the training process. Changing the cue allows the pet to truly decide if they would like to be touched, rather than choosing if they want to come to the station. This is a key of cooperative care training: for the animal to truly opt in, they need to first know what they are signing up for.

Here is a sample progression of criteria for the touch method exam training. Notice many of the steps have sub-steps built in. "Auscultation" as a step is too big. Split touches like auscultation into smaller approximations, then build up to the full diagnostic touch. If the animal appears to have an increase in stress, break down the behavior into even smaller approximations so the animal has a chance to learn the exam will be nonthreatening.

For patients with a strong fear of the stethoscope, *the use of a Bluetooth enabled stethoscope can make it possible for clients to place the bell on the pet without the team member coming so close* until the pet has received adequate training.

- Touch shoulder, glide to prescapular lymph nodes (LN)
- Glide to prescapular LN, palpate gently
  - Gradually increase pressure until diagnostic palpation is achieved
    - Do not increase continually; click and treat for every small pressure (criterion change)
- Move to submandibular LN, repeat process
- Touch hip, glide to popliteal LN
  - Gradually increase pressure until diagnostic palpation is achieved
    - Do not increase continually; click and treat for every small pressure (criterion change)
- Touch shoulder, glide along spine
  - Gradually increase pressure until diagnostic muscle and comfort assessment achieved
- Touch shoulder, glide to lateral chest where auscultation would occur
- Wear a stethoscope in your ears and repeat
- Hold stethoscope in your other hand, repeat
  - Approach with stethoscope
  - Place stethoscope next to the touching hand in a green body area
  - Glide toward the auscultation location, may require multiple approximations
  - Gradually increase pressure and duration until auscultation is diagnostic
  - Glide stethoscope to new locations for continued diagnostic auscultation
- Touch shoulder, glide down spine to flank, glide down flank to abdomen
  - Gradually increase pressure with one hand until diagnostic pressure achieved
  - Add a second hand at lower pressure
  - Gradually increase pressure of both hands until diagnostic pressure achieved
  - Do not increase continually; click and treat for every small pressure (criterion change).

Continue with each component of the examination, until every component has been trained. Some patients will be able to work through a full physical examination in one training visit. For others, the training process may require several visits before the technician can complete a full examination. Once the technician can perform the examination, it is time to involve the veterinarian and begin transferring these skills to a second person. Some patients will readily transfer these skills, while others will take more time to feel comfortable with a new person. Remember: we are making a long-term investment in the patient's welfare, allowing for a lifetime of faster and better veterinary care. For patients with individual sensitivities, for example those who are more anxious about the oral examination, it may be best for the technician trainer to display the oral cavity to the veterinarian, rather than having the veterinarian touch inside the patient's mouth.

Training Tip: Technology for Auscultation

For patients with a strong fear of the stethoscope, *the use of a Bluetooth enabled stethoscope can make it possible for clients to place the bell on the pet without the team member coming so close.* This tool allows auscultation from a distance, reducing social pressure and reducing the size and appearance of the equipment placed on the animal.

Video 7.9 shows Bija, a small mixed-breed dog with a history of defensive aggression and fearful behavior at the veterinary office. This video shows his progression through five visits, culminating with the veterinarian performing most of a physical exam. Monique is the technician trainer in this video.

During the early visits, a combination of desensitization and counterconditioning and operant conditioning are used. The technician breaks the examination process into its component parts, and introduces Bija to the desired responses during examination. At first, Monique works with Bija by performing the approximations as well as clicking and treating. Soon, the owner is brought into the picture. Monique and the owner communicate, so that the technician can do the exam, and the owner can click and treat.

During the final clip, Monique demonstrates to the doctor how Bija has progressed, and how he expects his examination to feel. As Monique demonstrates a portion of the exam, the owner clicks and treats, and the veterinarian replicates Monique's movements. Near the end of the examination, Bija becomes more nervous because the veterinarian moved a bit too quickly for his comfort. Even with this handling error, Bija was able to return to baseline and finish his visit. While the behavior shown in this video may not be "perfect" or FAS 0, it is a functional behavior which has held up long-term and facilitated years of care for Bija.

7.8.2 Naming the Examination

An alternative, or extension, of the touching method is the *named examination*. For the named exam, each portion of the exam is put on cue. These cues are different though: rather than the cue being a signal to the animal that reinforcement is available for a specific behavior, predictor cues tell the animal what the trainer or handler is planning to do next. The patient learns each cue predicts a certain part of the exam, and can be better prepared to participate (Figure 7.5). Predictor cues should not be introduced until the trainer is confident the animal is generally comfortable with touch in that body area.

To use this method, make sure you initiate touch in the same fashion each time you work with the animal. Say the name of the body part you're going to examine ("ear," "eye," "belly," "teeth," "heart," etc.) using the same sound and tone of voice each time you say it. Glide your hand to that body part, then reward after each touch. This is establishing both a verbal and a visual cue for the animal about what is happening next. The process will look like:

- Say "ear."
- Touch shoulder, glide to the ear.
- Click while ear is touched.
- Stop touching the ear, and give a treat.

After a few repetitions, the animal will often begin pressing the cued body part toward the trainer, for example leaning the ear into your hand, leaning his chest against the stethoscope, or turning his rump closer to you for abdominal palpation. If you notice the animal leaning away, shifting their weight, or showing signs of escalating FAS after hearing a predictor cue, this is helpful data. The animal may be uncomfortable with that body part being touched for emotional or stress reasons, or due to physical discomfort.

Another version of named exams involves teaching the animal to prevent a specific body part on cue. Each portion of the exam can even be shaped into a separate behavior, or trick, of presenting the cued body part. For example, cue "teeth," and the dog would present his nose to offer an oral exam, rather than just allowing examination of his teeth. Cue "heart" while holding out a stethoscope, and the dog would move closer and orient sideways to press his chest to the stethoscope. Dogs can

Hand over head: I'm going to touch your nose.

L-shaped finger: I'm going to lift your leg at elbow.

Flat vertical hand: I'm going to lift your ear.

Pinching motion with fingers: I'm going to tent your skin.

Single finger over: I'm going to touch injection site.

Flat hand moving in circular motion: I'm going to rake your hair backward to look at your skin.

Presentation of stethoscope: I'm going to touch you with this.

Flat hand presented low: Give me your paw to touch.

Flat hand presented close to body: I'm going to palpate your belly.

Figure 7.5 Named examination example cues.

even be trained to open their mouths, and hold them open for a detailed oral examination (see links in the Appendix). The limit to what can be trained is only the physical ability of the pet and trainer's motivation and skill set. The process of presenting every body part is an extensive and exciting training project, and would warrant a whole separate guide of its own!

7.9 Treatments, Sample Collection, and Imaging

The recommendations for some treatments will sound familiar to you from Chapter 6, because desensitization and classical counterconditioning will automatically occur when we are using operant conditioning as well. Once the pet learns how to participate in his care and receives plenty of rewards for meeting criteria, he will be developing learned skills through operant conditioning, but also a positive conditioned emotional response, a sign of classical conditioning.

7.9.1 Subcutaneous Injections

Type Three subcutaneous injections build on the training we have done so far of stationing and touch training, combined with desensitizing the injection equipment and sensation.

Invite the animal to the station, and begin the familiar touching routine. Determine where on the body the injection will be given, and focus touching in that area, then begin expanding touches to tenting the skin. Remember: every approximation or building block earns a click and treat. When the skin tent is going well, introduce the syringe approaching, an injection with the capped needle, simulating injection with a training needle, and finally the injection itself. Naming the injection procedure helps to establish a cue, so the animal knows what to expect during future sessions.

Once the injection procedure is trained, only a few clicks and treats will be required to perform the unrestrained injection.

The more savvy a patient becomes to training, the more quickly training will progress.

Video 7.10a shows an example homework session for subcutaneous injection training. The dogs know how to station on a mat, how to move away when uncomfortable. They are introduced to a series of approximations associated with subcutaneous injection. The use of a clicker is optional, but it does serve to mark both the strongest intensity moment of each approximation and also the dog's stillness which is desirable in this context.

Video 7.10b shows Quill's completed real-time injection behavior. Notice his enthusiasm for the mat, and how this affects his feelings about the entire injection process.

Video 7.10c shows several dogs working on injection training at different levels of readiness. Notice the touching plan, timing plan for food delivery, injection mechanics, and whether predictor cues are added varies by dog. These variations are selected based on feedback each individual dog gives during the training process.

7.9.2 Cephalic Venipuncture

For cephalic venipuncture, the patient will need to be at a comfortable height for the technician to perform venipuncture. This may mean the floor or a table depending upon the size of the patient and the height of the technician (Figure 7.6). Foundation behaviors for cephalic venipuncture include stationing, paw target, and the touching exercise. Care should be taken, because we will be working face-to-face with unrestrained patients. Pay attention to food acceptance, body language, and proximity preference. If the patient looks uncomfortable or delays in participation, pause and

Figure 7.6   One example of a position for cooperative cephalic venipuncture training.

assess the situation. Make sure to work safely while training. Protected contact in the form of a muzzle or gate may be indicated.

The key to success will be breaking down the behavior into a series of building-block approximations, and then walking the patient through the approximations in a predictable way, clicking and treating for cooperation with each step. The final training plan will take into account the phlebotomist's preference for patient positioning. Some people may want to hold the limb from the elbow, others may prefer an additional helper to hold the limb, while still others may prefer for the animal to keep their limb on the ground while sitting or lying down.

Here is a sample of *possible* building blocks for the cephalic venipuncture behavior if the plan is for the pet to sit, and the phlebotomist to hold the limb during venipuncture:

- Come to station
- Sit
- Present limb (if this is the planned position)
  - First the paw, then the wrist, then the entire forelimb
- Rest limb on technician's arm (or keep paw on the ground, depending on phlebotomist preference)
- Verbal cue and visual cue are introduced
- Allow technician to touch elbow
- Allow occluding vein while touching elbow
- Rest limb while vein occluded and palpated
- Rest limb while liquid applied
- Rest limb during pinching of the skin and touching with capped syringe
- Rest limb during simulated blood collection with training needle, duration achieved through multiple exposures
- Rest limb during blood collection
- Rest limb during pressure application following blood collection.

Video 7.11a shows practice for cephalic injection positioning and a cephalic blood draw with Kenji. Both of these examples use modeling. Modeling means I have raised the dog's leg to place it in the correct position for blood collection. At first, the modeling movement is the cue. With practice, these dogs learn that a tap to the elbow is the cue to raise their leg and allow me to position it where I need to place it for optimal blood collection positioning.

Video 7.11b shows training cephalic venipuncture for Rye. He is a clicker-savvy dog and learned the behavior from start to finish in two short sessions. This dog is generally cooperative for veterinary care and comfortable in the clinic, but is sensitive to needle sticks. As Monique walks him through the steps, she uses his understanding of paw targeting, adding duration and building a complex behavior to show him how to cooperate for this procedure.

In the first clip, he is working on the table, and in the second clip he is working on the floor. The consent point for this dog is if he chooses to move to any position other than the sit. If he wishes for the process to stop, he can simply stand – he does not even need to leave the station for the procedure to stop.

Watch his body language. Notice he is mildly concerned about the procedure. He licks his lips, tightens his tail tip, and looks away. He chooses to remain engaged in training and chooses to participate without any restraint. The second clip includes him giving his first unrestrained blood sample. He notices the needle stick and does not like the sensation, but remains stationary and cooperates, happy to accept his food reinforcement at the end of the behavior. Cooperative care may not make every patient love needles, but allowing them to have control over the process is what cooperative care is all about. Through repeated experience, Rye showed progressively less and less response to the needle sensation when he was familiar with the procedure and knew what to expect. He now shows no response to the needle sensation at all when his blood is collected.

7.9.3 Lateral Saphenous Venipuncture

For lateral saphenous venipuncture, at least two people will generally be needed: one to provide a target and observe the patient, and another to collect the blood. It is difficult to observe the patient's expression while working alone with a rear limb, but in calmer dogs it may be possible. Many dogs who are nervous will be reluctant to have us working around their hind limbs, and will prefer cephalic sampling. For a standing voluntary lateral saphenous, utilizing a hand target or chin rest can be very helpful. See Section 7.11 and the Appendix for more information.

7.9.3.1 Patient Case History: Leon

Video 7.12 shows Monique working with Leon, a Labrador retriever. After multiple extremely stressful visits as a puppy at a different hospital, Leon developed severe fear of veterinary care including barking, lunging, and snapping when approached with equipment or for examination. He is friendly and happy to interact with loose body language and excellent food acceptance within the hospital from a variety of team members if they are not holding equipment and are not trying to actually examine him. Leon is highly trained and is a Federal Emergency Management Agency (FEMA) Certified disaster search and rescue dog, but has extreme fear of husbandry and veterinary care. As a result, Leon was trained to allow sedation, and his wellness care was conducted under sedation until age seven years when he developed cancer.

Leon's cancer treatment meant he would need to give blood samples every 7–14 days for a period of months and possibly even more than a year. It would be impractical and not ideal for Leon's health to sedate him so frequently, so a program for training venipuncture was undertaken. Leon was too fearful to allow training for jugular blood collection, so lateral saphenous blood collection was trained in order to preserve his cephalic veins for possible intravenous catheters if needed.

Leon came to the clinic twice weekly for blood draw training with Monique for two weeks. In the first session, the mat and touching game were introduced while determining Leon's preference for timing of treats. It was most practical based on Leon's behavior for him to receive his treat after touching was completed. If he was fed during touch, he would eagerly gobble the food and move all around, which is incompatible with the stillness needed for blood draw. Monique assumed this could be attributed to increased FAS as well, so used touch-then-treat timing for his early training. In the second session, rolling onto a hip to present his hind leg, and touch gradient to establish occluding the vessel were introduced as well as the addition of alcohol to the skin. In the third session, the above was repeated while adding in simulated venipuncture with a training needle. In the fourth session, Leon was able to give the blood sample shown in the first part of the video.

Leon's blood draw behavior held up for weekly blood collection for 2 months, and every 2 weeks for 13 months! Leon also relaxed enough over the course of many sessions to eat both during and after touching, rather than only after touching. After the 15 months, Leon's lateral saphenous veins gradually became more compromised from frequent venipuncture. During one visit, neither saphenous vein gave a sufficient quality blood sample, so Monique elected to try to generalize Leon's blood draw training to a cephalic vein.

In a single session of about five minutes, using a combination of desensitization and operant counter conditioning to build on the Leon's existing blood draw behavior, he was able to give a voluntary cephalic sample. Because Leon's lateral saphenous position was the down, Monique chose to perform his cephalic sampling in the down position also. During the later part of this video, you see Leon's first cephalic venipuncture. Notice he is on his mat, in the down position. The handling steps are similar, but the body location is different. Touch-then-treat is used during the approximations, and touch-with-treat is used for the actual blood collection.

7.9.3.2 Jugular Venipuncture

For jugular venipuncture, it is generally helpful to have two people: one to position the pet and to train while the other collects a blood sample. The approximations discussed for cephalic venipuncture are applicable for jugular access just modifying positioning and the body parts being touched, but also requires the animal to raise their head and remain still.

A variety of methods can be used to teach the animal to raise their head and remain still. Chin rest, discussed later in this chapter is one. A prolonged nose target is another, and my preferred method. For larger dogs, this procedure can be performed in the Center or Middle position, or with the dog on a platform or station depending upon the trainer's level of comfort.

Video 7.13 shows examples of jugular venipuncture training. Mushu is a dog shown earlier in this book with a history of FAS 5 defensive aggression for medical procedures. In the video, Monique uses Mushu's foundation behaviors of stationing, duration chin target, syringe conditioning, desensitization to handling, and needle acceptance to rehearse a new behavior for the first time. Mushu has not been asked to train a jugular blood collection before, but his understanding of all the component behaviors allowed Monique to combine them into a functional positioning behavior rapidly. Mushu gave his first jugular blood sample about two weeks later.

The second dog in the video, Mikey, has been taught a ring target. The ring target is a hand positioned so the dog can place their nose into the trainer's hand as a signal they are ready to be handled. If the dog moves his nose out of the trainer's hand, he is asking for a break.

Video 7.14 shows Ada giving her first trained jugular blood sample. Ada has historically shown FAS 4–5 for blood collection. Her owner has conditioned her to wear a muzzle and accept restraint for blood collection at other hospitals, but Ada's fear gradually worsened so her owner requested training appointments to learn a blood draw behavior. Ada learned the ring target, as with Mikey, and series of five conditioning visits were used to teach: comfort with two people, comfort with someone other than the owner touching Ada, coming between Monique's arms, targeting between

Monique's arms, performing other cued behaviors in the location of the planned blood draw, performing the ring target in close proximity, ring target for simulated blood collection adding intensity of touch and duration, and finally blood collection using the trained behavior. The video shows Ada's first trained blood draw.

Video 7.7 in the muzzle example section showed Kenji, a Belgian Malinois X German Shepherd Dog engaging in a practice session using the Center position to establish jugular access. Kenji also has a trained cephalic injection, physical examination including open mouth, and subcutaneous injection behavior.

7.9.4   Ear or Eye Medications

Ear and eye medications are similar to injections and venipuncture, an extension of the stationing and touch training. First, the patient will come to the station, then become accustomed to remaining at the station and holding still during eye or ear medications. Training this skill is especially useful for patients who will be receiving chronic medications, such as those being treated for dry eye and KCS (keratoconjunctivitis sicca), requiring lifelong daily eye drops.

Here is an example list of possible building blocks for the eye drop behavior:

- Come to station
- Touching of the head
- Gliding touch to the upper eyelid
- Raising the upper eyelid
- Touching the head while holding drops in the opposite hand
- Gliding touch to the upper eyelid and raising it while holding drops
- Applying a drop to a less sensitive area
- Applying a drop to the eye.

This list should look familiar; it is similar to the desensitization and counterconditioning list for this same treatment. The difference here is that if the animal moves away, no click and treat will occur. The patient is being given the opportunity to cooperate by coming to the station, giving consent, and holding still, rather than being taught to simply have a pleasant conditioned emotional response to receiving eye drops.

Video 7.15a shows a cat learning to accept ear medications. In the before video, you can see the staff is chasing Mama Kitty around the hospital to try to capture her and apply her ear medication. Mama Kitty is a clinic pet and very comfortable in the hospital, but still fearful of ear medications.

Alicea Howell RVT, VTS (Behavior) trains Mama Kitty using operant conditioning to follow her target, jump onto the table to station, and gradually allow the placement of medicated drops in the ear. While Mama Kitty moves away slightly during a few early repetitions, notice she is unrestrained and free to leave, and she can jump off the table to withdraw her consent to participate at any time. She chooses to stay engaged and an active participant in her own care.

Video 7.15b shows Rye; this time, he is learning to present for eye medications without restraint. Rye is savvy to veterinary training and to the clicker, but he has never received eye drops of any kind before this video. The video shows the power of good foundation behaviors, including the station and the understanding of veterinary training. Notice Monique tries to keep her cues consistent for the eye drop behavior, and the saline is dropped on less sensitive areas first before it is dropped into the eye. You will also notice the use of a verbal marker intermittently, when both of Monique's hands are needed for the procedure.

7.9.5 Imaging

Positioning for radiographs requiring lateral and dorsal recumbency can be stressful for any patient. Cooperative care training allows us to prepare animals in advance, so that in the event they require imaging such as this, they understand the environment and skills required. Remember: cooperative veterinary care can be prevention as well as intervention.

Video 7.16 shows an 18-week-old puppy learning cooperative positioning for radiographs. Before trying this on the x-ray table, Monique taught this puppy how to move onto her side when she said "night," as a trick around the house and then on the floor of the veterinary hospital. This is her first session on the x-ray table. Kestrel gives consent to participate by placing her front feet on the table edge and allowing herself to be boosted onto the table. She is comfortable offering known behaviors like sit and down, so cooperative lateral recumbency is cued and reinforced. The V-tray is also introduced, but it is awkward for Kestrel to roll herself onto her back because of the shape of the tray. Monique gently helps her onto her back, and then using a combination of luring, targeting, and modeling, Kestrel is able to understand how to remain stationary on her back without restraint. As Kestrel becomes comfortable, duration is increased and the sound of the x-ray rotor is introduced.

Small variations in the environment can influence a learner's ability to understand cues and participate in training. In the second half of the x-ray positioning video, personal protective equipment such as a lead apron, thyroid shield, and lead gloves are introduced. Kestrel learns to understand the "night" cue even when given with a gloved hand, and remains stationary while Monique puts on and takes off her gloves, simulating what will happen during a real x-ray. Finally, Kestrel earns clicks and treats for remaining in position while the trainer is in full PPE and the rotor is activated.

7.9.6 Emergency Sedation

In some situations, Type Three dogs may have medical needs that demand immediate treatment. These dogs will generally need sedation prior to treatment, and it is important to have an emergency sedation strategy for these rare events. Figure 7.7 shows positioning techniques for emergency sedation. Notice the dog is muzzled, he is wearing slip leashes, and he is being walked in a very distracting environment. A second team member is approaching him from the side, and will inject

(a)   (b)

Figure 7.7   (a–b) Emergency sedation technique for dogs.

the sedation. In situations like this, taking the time to palpate the muscle prior to injection will often provoke an unwanted response from the patient. Simply inject as quickly as possible. Based on extensive experience, the authors have yet to see an adverse reaction with this technique.

Author's note: Still images are provided rather than video for this procedure, because walking injections are uncommon in the author's hospital. When we are presented with a Type Three dog who needs emergency sedation, the priority is always the welfare of the animal rather than capturing video, and adding a videographer to the situation may unnecessarily increase the dog's anxiety level.

7.10 Grooming

While we are not groomers by trade, veterinary professionals are equipped to provide these services for patients with special needs, such as Type Three dogs and cats. These patients need treatments like nail trims and anal gland expression, but are not good candidates for the untrained owner, or groomers not familiar with desensitization, counterconditioning, and operant conditioning techniques. Poor grooming experiences can cause considerable lasting emotional harm to patients, compromise the relationship between clients and pets, and damage the trust between veterinary professionals and patients. Teaching voluntary grooming behaviors improves the quality of care, and quality of life, for these patients.

Nail care is a prime topic to focus on for voluntary grooming. To trim nails, we will follow the same process used for other treatments. The behavior of nail trimming should be broken down into its small component building blocks, or approximations, and then the patient should be trained to participate in these approximations. If the patient chooses to opt out by moving away from the station, nail trimming should stop, even if the procedure has not been completed. Involving the owner in the training process will often create a functional situation where the owner can take over this routine care procedure at home, reducing the need for the patient to visit the veterinary hospital for nail care.

The example approximations for nail trimming are similar to the exposure ladder for desensitization, but the patient will need to agree to participate in each step to earn a click and a treat, rather than the steps simply predicting the appearance of food (Figure 7.8). Remember to give the patient frequent breaks, only progress at the pace the patient is comfortable, and alternate or ping-pong

Figure 7.8 Example of cooperative nail care training.

Table 7.6 Sample of a possible Type Three training plan for session 1 of nail trimming.

Training plan: Type Three training	
Completed behavior: Nail trim all 4 paws unrestrained Session 1	Component behaviors (approximations): Station Offer or allow paw pickup DS/CCC may be needed Isolate toe, toenail DS/CCC may be needed Clippers to toe Clippers around toenail Sound of clippers near toenail Tactile of clippers tapping nail Clip one nail Clip multiple nails Repeat process for each limb
Consent point: At station	Consent point: Offers or allows paw handling
Preferred reinforcers 1. String cheese tiny bits 2. Chicken breast cubes 3. Cheerios	
Medications: Zylkene daily, Trazodone 2 hours prior	Working area: Exam room 3
Foundation behaviors required: Station Limb handling	Known cues needed: Sit, Paw target, Hand target Additional DS/CC/CCC: XX Yes – Paw, toe, toenail may all be needed
Starting criteria	Station
Progression	Station, shoulder, elbow, carpus, paw, toe, toenail, clipper approach
Ending criteria	Clipper tap on toenail
Observations	Pet was comfortable all the way until isolating a toenail. Toenail isolation was mixed with other skills – sit, hand target, paw target, and spin to decrease possible anxiety and preserve behavioral momentum. Mild stress (lip licks) at sight of nail clippers, but willingly targeted nail clippers with her nose. Ended by tapping toenail with clippers. No nail clipping performed today.
Homework	Owner OK to simulate training seen today, but do NOT clip any nails.
Plan for next visit	Clip one or two nails

with other behaviors during the training process to reduce stress and keep the training process fun. Table 7.6 shows a sample worksheet for a Type Three training session on nail trimming.

Example building blocks for nail trimming:

- Patient comes to the station
- Touching begins in a less sensitive area, shoulder for forelimbs, hip for hind limbs
- Glide touch to the elbow or stifle
- Glide touch to the carpus or hock

- Glide touch to the paw
- Pick up nail trimmers in your other hand, and begin touching process again at the shoulder or hip
- Gradually progress to touching the paw
- Increase duration of paw holding
- Isolate a toe
- Isolate a toenail
- Increase duration of toenail hold
- Approach toenail with clippers
- Tap toenail with clippers
- Encircle toenail with clippers
- Trim one nail
- Trim multiple nails

Video 7.17 shows desensitization and operant counterconditioning for a canine nail trim. Douglas, the dog in the video, has bitten his owners when they try to restrain him for nail trims. He was calmer as a puppy, but as he grew and heavier restraint was used, he became more and more fearful for this procedure. You will see the technician provides a mat, which is the station area for Douglas. If he chooses to walk away and leave the mat, training stops, and when he returns, training resumes. The owners are present and observing as the technician works through an exposure ladder for trimming the nails.

Notice the dog's body language. A few mild stress signals, but he is overall nice and loose with a swishy wagging tail and eager for treats. After the technician demonstrates the technique, she then trains the owners to be able to simulate this technique at home. There is a considerable change to Douglas' body language when the owner attempts the training process. This is likely because the technician has never tried to trim his nails before, so there is no existing negative emotion associated with Monique touching his nails. There is significant unpleasant learning history from when the owner has tried in the past. Douglas still chooses to remain engaged and participate in training, staying on his station and cooperating. With the technician coaching, the owners work together, one handling and the other treating, accomplishing the goal of a nail trim. Pay attention to how nervous the female owner gets when she is told she can trim a nail, and then how happy she is when she successfully does so. Experiences like this improve the quality of life for patient and client, and help bond clients to the practice.

Video 7.18 shows Mikey demonstrating his completed trained nail trim behavior. Mikey has a history of FAS 4 escape behaviors for nail trimming, so his owner signed up for a series of training visits to establish a less stressful grooming routine. To opt in, Mikey comes onto the platform. Before he comes to the platform, Monique shows him the nail trimmers so he knows what he will be opting in for. To opt out, Mikey can either leave the platform, or communicate he is not ready by choosing not to come onto the platform. Notice he receives rewards both for opting in, *and* for opting out. He still finds the actual sensation of the clip mildly unpleasant, but giving him more control over when it happens provides a better quality of life for both Mikey and his owner. Mikey's owner can now clip his nails at home.

7.10.1 Nail Boards

An alternative to conventional nail trimming is to teach dogs to file their own nails using a nail board. Dogs can be shaped to scratch on the rough board, filing their own nails using a scraping or digging motion. Figure 7.9 shows construction steps for making a nail board.

For strength use a 12 inch square of 1/4 inch plywood for the backer

150 grit sandpaper for filing surface

Tape sandpaper to plywood using duct tape

Rubber feet can be added to the back for traction

Sand paper can be changed as needed

Figure 7.9 Steps for constructing your own nail board. Many designs are commercially available as well. Some have a hidden treat compartment, designed to build on the dog's natural behavior of trying to dig to reach hidden foods. Others have bumps or curves to provide a variety of shapes to the scratching surface in an effort to give a more complete nail care to both the central and outer toenails.

As with any shaping process, the completed behavior of scratching on the nail board is broken down into many component parts. These parts include approaching the nail board, touching it with any body part, touching with a paw, touching with multiple paws, moving the paw while touching the board, moving both paws while touching the board, and finally scratching at the board.

Video 7.19 shows Monique demonstrating nail board behaviors with several different dogs. When training the nail board behavior, isolating the scratch is key. Many dogs will place their paw on the board initially without flexing their toes so the toenail is what touches. Watch the dog's paw and toes, and work to time the marker when the dog's toes are in flexion and the nail rather than the paw pad is in contact with the board.

7.11 Additional Consent Options

Stationing is a simple and easy way to establish consent, but it is only one of several commonly trained methods. One popular consent behavior is chin rest. The chin rest is a behavior where the dog is in a standing or lying-down position, and is taught to target a towel, the trainer's hand, a pillow, the trainer's lap, or any other convenient surface with his chin (Figure 7.10). When the dog is keeping his chin on the chin rest, he is showing he is comfortable with the procedure and giving

(a)

(b)

Figure 7.10 (a and b) Two examples of a chin rest behavior, one where the dog is standing and another where the dog is lying down.

his consent. When he raises his chin from the chin rest position, he is communicating that he is withdrawing consent for that moment, and either the repetition was too challenging, more smaller steps are needed, his stress level has increased, or he is mentally fatigued.

Chin rest, presenting a body part, coming to a station, etc. are considered consent behaviors or "Start Buttons" because they allow the animal to communicate if they are ready or not ready **for a certain procedure or event**. This author prefers to use these behaviors for specific contexts, such as injections, nail care, or brushing. The reason is: I can show the animal in advance using a cue such as my hands, the syringe, a toothbrush, or the nail clippers what they are signing up for.

The sequence would look like:

- Animal is attending the person and looks ready to train
- **Trainer shows brush**
- Animal notices brush and puts chin down
- Trainer starts brushing
- Trainer pauses brushing anytime animal raises chin.

If I want to do general handling, I use a more general behavior like coming to a mat or station, which has been associated with foundations like Touching Game where intentional variety is introduced from the very beginning of the process.

Teaching the chin rest takes a little extra time compared to teaching a station, but it is an incredibly useful behavior because in the chin rest position, most procedures can be performed, including physical examination, eye medications, ear treatment and medication, vaccination, venipuncture, urinary catheters for male dogs, sedation, nail care, basic grooming, and other body-handling procedures such as fine needle aspirate, suture removal, hot spot treatment, and more. Any procedure that can be completed in the standing position and does not require access to the chin or ventral neck can be performed using the chin rest behavior with proper training.

The steps for shaping the chin rest include:

- Move toward the rest point
- Touch nose to the rest point
- Lean over the rest point
- Stretch neck over the rest point
- Touch chin to the rest point
- Maintain chin rest position for short durations
- Raise chin when uncomfortable or needing a break (remember to reward this!)
- Maintain chin rest point for extended durations
- Keep chin on the rest point while other procedures are introduced.

The chin rest can also be taught using a combination of luring, capturing, and shaping to speed up the process for some animals. This consists of presenting a small lure, moving it over the chin rest object so the animal's chin brushes the object, then marking and feeding for the contact. After a few repetitions of luring, pause and see if the animal will begin to offer movement toward the chin rest, then approach teaching the rest of the behavior with a shaping plan.

One thing to be aware of with cues like a chin rest or sustained target, is that the animal may stay in the target position in an effort to earn a reward even if they are feeling uncomfortable. Handling exercises in the chin rest may feel more like "proofing" a stay, where the animal is asked "can you still hang onto this behavior even if X is happening?" To avoid motivational conflict, take frequent breaks and watch the animal's body language. As with the station training, monitor the animal for signs of discomfort and encourage them to break the chin rest by sending them away for a reset treat rather than making them so uncomfortable they can no longer hold the target.

Procedures should be broken down into their component approximations, as discussed earlier in this chapter. The chin rest exercise can be combined with stillness training, Touching Game, and touching with intent to create a deep tool box full of useful behaviors.

Video 7.20 shows Debbie Martin RVT, VTS (Behavior) working with Border terrier Chip on grooming. Chip has learned that when he puts his chin down, Debbie will start combing and when he raises his head, she will pause the combing until he is ready to continue again. Taking a teamwork approach with the dog and establishing a language of ready vs. not ready enhances predictability, trust, and autonomy for the animal. (Video courtesy of Debbie Martin and TEAM Animal Behavior and Training.)

Video 7.21 shows Monique and a client working with Sky, who has a trained chin rest behavior. Sky shows her understanding of the chin rest as consent because when she is presented with hands or an object and the opportunity to do the chin rest behavior, she will place her chin when she is ready to proceed. If Sky lifts her chin, the handling is stopped. By empowering Sky to start and stop the handling, she has progressed from allowing very little handling to allowing physical examination, vaccination, and grooming.

Video 7.22 shows Monique introducing the chin rest behavior to puppy Kestrel for the first time via a shaping session. The puppy is using a rolled towel as the chin rest for one session, and Monique's leg for a chin rest in the other session. Monique uses placement of reward after each repetition to further encourage the chin rest behavior. This puppy is demonstrating the chin rest in the down position, an alternative to the standing chin rest. Choose a comfortable position for the patient that will allow the anticipated procedures in the future.

The Appendix contains links to additional videos by other trainers showing training with ready signals.

7.11.1 Target Hold

Similar to the chin rest, the target hold is a consent behavior where the patient is asked to place his nose on a target such as the trainer's hand or a target stick, and remain in that position during treatment. If the patient removes his nose from the target, the procedure stops. If the patient keeps his nose on the target, the procedure continues. Refer to the Appendix for a link showing the target hold as a consent point for unrestrained anal gland expression.

7.12 Type Three Cats

As discussed earlier in this chapter, the veterinary environment presents unique training challenges due to the different social life of cats. It can be almost impossible to make the clinic environment comfortable enough for Type Three cats to engage in operant conditioning training. However, Type One kittens make excellent candidates to start with voluntary unrestrained care from the start.

Type Three cats who are exceptionally stressed are best treated with immediate and preemptive medication for FAS. As with Type Three dogs, the client's goals will dictate the point of success. The successful endpoint of training may be carrier acceptance and sedation training: and that's completely acceptable! Other clients may wish to undertake cooperative care training. House call veterinarians are a great option for cats with trained cooperative care behaviors without the stress of a car ride or visiting the veterinary clinic.

7.12.1 Type Three Cats with Medical Needs

In some cases, Type Three cats will present with true medical needs that cannot be postponed to allow training. In these instances, it is important to have strategies for how to handle the cats without worsening their anxiety whenever possible. Use all the principles introduced in earlier chapters to set up the environment to be as low-stress as possible, assure all your equipment is set up prior to handling the cat, and make a handling plan that allows minimal restraint and short procedures. Figure 7.11 shows one positioning technique for cephalic venipuncture in Type Three cats who prefer to hide.

Video 7.23 shows a cephalic blood draw on a severely stressed cat. This procedure was a need and not a want, as the cat is ill. Notice the cat is allowed to rest in the bottom half of his carrier and the blanket provides a pseudo hiding spot. The first technician uses her hand and the towel to gently rub the chin and be ready to provide restraint if needed while extending the front leg from the towel. Although the cat vocalizes some, he is cooperative, and the blood draw is performed with minimal additional stress.

Figure 7.11 Positioning a cat under a towel for cephalic venipuncture. The towel protects the handler and the cat, and only the limb is exposed for blood collection.

7.12.2 Emergency Sedation Planning

Once a Type Three cat has been provided with pre-visit medications and taught to enter the carrier, she can be brought to the hospital and sedated as necessary for treatment. Refer to Chapter 3 for owner instructions on low-stress transportation practices.

Sedation should be rapid and quiet, using minimal contact and restraint. All equipment and medications required should be gathered prior to the patient's arrival, and a quiet room reserved in advance. Once the cat has arrived, the method of sedation depends upon the type of carrier used and the personality of the cat.

For soft-sided carriers, the cat can be sedated without leaving the carrier by injecting through the carrier's mesh (Figure 7.12). One team member will apply a thick soft towel or small blanket over the carrier and the cat, stabilizing the cat for the injection. A second team member can approach and rapidly administer an intramuscular sedative. Communication between the team members is crucial for this procedure to go smoothly.

For hard-sided carriers, the carrier can be disassembled, and a thick soft towel or small blanket used to sandwich the cat against the bottom of the carrier, stabilizing the cat to allow intramuscular injection (Figure 7.13). With this method, one team member controls the lid of the carrier, while the second team member rapidly introduces the towel at the same moment the carrier is gradually opened. When the cat is stable, the team member who was controlling the carrier top then gives the injection. The carrier top is then replaced so the cat can fall asleep without further restraint.

Video 7.24 shows two team members rehearsing emergency sedation for a cat, first in a soft-sided carrier, then in a hard-sided carrier. This rehearsal is done using a decoy so the team members can practice their technique without causing undue stress to a live patient. Notice the towel used is large enough to cover the carrier and the cat, and thick enough that even if the cat were to bite, no teeth could penetrate the towel. Once the first team member stabilizes the cat, she tells the second team member she is ready, and the injection can be given.

Part 2 of the video shows two team members practicing the sedation technique using a towel sandwich in the hard carrier. A decoy cat is used in this video for training purposes. Observe the

(a)

(b)

Figure 7.12 (a and b) Placing a towel over a soft-sided cat carrier and then administering emergency sedation.

team members working together to coordinate their timing, working quickly to minimize stress on the patient, and communicating quietly but succinctly throughout the procedure.

7.12.2.1 Type Three Training for Cats: Skills and Stationing
One of the most useful skills to train for cats is voluntary carrier entry. (For cats who still experience high FAS on arrival, plan for low-stress sedation strategies once the cat has arrived at the hospital.)

Shaping a cat to move into a carrier is simple, and can be done by almost any pet owner. Often, the best way to teach pet owners this process is by demonstrating with a comfortable cat, or providing video instructions. Video conferencing is a great way to coach owners through training cats while allowing the cat to stay at home, where the stress level is low and the cat is comfortable.

(a)

(b)

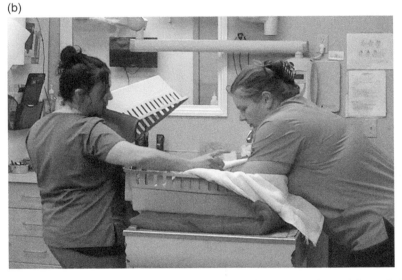

Figure 7.13 (a and b) Sliding a towel into a hard-sided cat carrier and then administering emergency sedation.

Once the cat is shown to have no negative emotional response to the carrier (refer to desensitization and counterconditioning in Chapter 6), shaping to enter the carrier on cue may begin. For successful training, break the carrier entry behavior into many approximations.

Here is an example approximation list for carrier training (this also works great for crate training puppies and dogs):

- Cat looks at carrier
- Cat moves one step toward carrier
    - Cat progresses in one-step increments closer and closer to carrier
- Cat breaks the plane of the carrier entrance with his nose

- Cat places head in carrier
- Cat places head and one paw in carrier
- Cat places head and both front paws in carrier
- Cat steps with all 4 ft into carrier
- Cat moves far enough into carrier for the body, all four paws, and tail to be inside carrier
- Cat remains in carrier while door is closed.

In Chapter 6, Video 6.3 showed Alicea Howell demonstrating the training process for voluntary carrier entry with Mama Kitty. Notice this behavior is shaped from start to finish without the cat being picked up or physically manipulated in any way. She is free to participate or not, and can walk away at any time if her stress level increases. By training the cat to enter the carrier voluntarily, she can be transported to the clinic much more easily.

Cats can learn to participate in nail care, grooming, vaccination, examination, and blood collection just like dogs or any other animal. All of the techniques and concepts discussed so far can be applied to both dogs and cats (and many other animals!) Training cats is different from training dogs in a few ways. Cats generally benefit from shorter sessions, many cats satiate hunger sooner (fewer repetitions because they will stop accepting food when satiated), and most cats are more sensitive to changes in environment than dogs. We discussed earlier in the chapter that most dogs are familiar with car rides, walking on a leash, and visiting different places at least sometimes, while many cats are only in their carrier or the car when they are going someplace unpleasant. Cats are just as smart as dogs, and just as trainable!

Video 7.25 shows a senior cat, Malt. Malt receives Adequan® injections. Through a series of sessions, Tabitha Kucera RVT, VTS (Behavior), CCBC, KPA-CTP has conditioned a Medication Station for Malt. Notice how the cat eagerly comes to the station. Tabitha provides a preferred food treat, then uses Touch Gradient to prepare Malt for the injection, monitoring her responses throughout. After the injection, Malt finishes her food reward. Teaching a station is a great way to prepare cats for medications of any kind.

Video 7.26 shows Chip, another cat trained by Tabitha. Chip also has a trained station behavior, but the timing of food delivery is different. Notice when Tabitha cues "Meds," Chip comes running with his tail up and tipped, vocalizing, and rubbing. He receives his oral medication (which clearly does not taste wonderful) and then a favorite food treat. The elevated feeding platform makes a nice visual target, predictor of treats, and an easy way for Chip to eat his food while standing.

7.13 Conclusion

Type Three training isn't just for Type Three patients: *every patient is a great candidate for voluntary care* (Figure 7.14). However, Type Three patients *require* this type of interventional training because Type One and Type Two training efforts will fail due to the pet's individual preferences, learning history, or both. Using operant conditioning combined with the principles of desensitization and counterconditioning is a powerful technique that empowers pets, facilitates cooperative low-stress and stress-free care, improves the quality of patient care, and helps clients feel more comfortable bringing pets to the clinic. Veterinary technicians, veterinarians, trainers, and owners can all learn to apply these cooperative veterinary care techniques to improve the well-being of animals.

Figure 7.14 Voluntary lateral radiograph position training with a puppy as preventive care.

8

Additional Patient Resources

8.1 Introduction

Training is an amazing tool to improve a patient's ability to cooperate for care and tolerate necessary treatments. In a perfect situation, every patient will respond well to training, every client will support the training process, and every treatment can be completed with zero patient stress. Rather than holding out for perfect, we need to be practical. Some patients will require more than training in order to recover from prior stress or trauma. Some patients will have fear responses that are so strong, it is impossible to find a nonstressful starting point for training. Some clients will not have a desire to follow through with training visits beyond training for sedation. Some animals are only semi-domesticated, such as feral cats, and training is not an option.

If you find yourself feeling stuck, as though you're not sure how to help a patient, or how to best proceed, first remember to *stop*. Do no harm. Consider what additional services within the clinic and beyond may help this patient.

8.2 Nutraceuticals and Pharmaceuticals

The most common adjunct to training is medical management of fear, stress, and anxiety. Medications should always be prescribed by a veterinarian, based on their assessment of the patient. There are a wide variety of medications commonly used for animals, but few Food and Drug Administration (FDA)-approved medications for these indications in pets. However, widespread use has shown these medications to be safe and effective in most cases.

There are two basic medical modalities of behavioral medication in veterinary medicine: baseline medications and event-based medications. There are also a variety of supplements available for event-based or baseline use.

8.2.1 Baseline Medications

Baseline medications are prescribed by the veterinarian when patients require daily treatment for anxiety-related behaviors or disorders. Baseline medications fall into several categories, but the most common category used in veterinary practice is selective serotonin reuptake inhibitors (SSRIs). Tricyclic antidepressants (TCAs), monoaminoxidase inhibitors (MAOIs), and combination drugs are also selectively used in pets [1, 2]. Because pets can't talk and tell us precisely how they feel during treatment, we must observe behaviors and infer whether the medications are

Cooperative Veterinary Care, Second Edition. Monique Feyrecilde.
© 2024 John Wiley & Sons, Inc. Published 2024 by John Wiley & Sons, Inc.
Companion website: www.wiley.com/go/feyrecilde/cooperative

helping the pet. The owner's observations are generally the most helpful, and the veterinary team can guide the owner's observation skills by teaching them what to watch for.

At the time of publishing, there are two baseline behavioral medications approved for use in pets: Reconcile® (fluoxetine, PRN Pharmacal) and Clomicalm® (clomipramine, Virbac). Both are approved solely for the treatment of separation anxiety [3]. For this reason, it is important to obtain consent from your clients for extra-label use of behavioral medications. There is one event-based medication approved for use in dogs: Sileo® (dexmedetomidine oromucosal gel, Zoetis). Sileo is approved for the short-term relief of signs associated with noise phobia in dogs [4].

Many animals who are fearful in the veterinary hospital and anxious about treatment have concurrent anxiety in other contexts. Animals with global phobia, social anxiety disorders, separation distress, separation anxiety, social conflict, conflict aggression, fear-related aggression, cognitive dysfunction, noise phobia, and many other diagnoses are often prescribed a baseline medication [1, 2]. A majority of baseline medications require four to six weeks to achieve stable serum levels and allow assessment for effectiveness. Most of these medications are established to have a wide margin of safety in animals and have published doses in most drug references (e.g. Plumb's [3]).

Pets who are prescribed a baseline medication *must* also be prescribed a behavioral therapy plan. The purpose of medication is to mitigate anxiety and fear to the point at which behavioral therapy is useful. Some animals require lifelong treatment, but others can be weaned off medication if behavioral therapy is sufficiently helpful.

8.2.2   Event-based Medications

Event-based medications are short-acting anxiolytics that are used to briefly ameliorate predictable periods of anxiety. One commonly used family of anxiolytics for animals are benzodiazepines. Examples include alprazolam, clonazepam, lorazepam, chlorazepate, and so on [1, 2]. Another event-based medication that is rapidly gaining popularity in veterinary medicine is trazodone, which is a tetracyclic antidepressant and SARI (serotonin antagonist and reuptake inhibitor) [5]. The analgesic and anticonvulsant medications gabapentin and pregabalin are also known to affect gamma-aminobutyric acid (GABA), and can reduce anxiety [6]. Alpha-2 agonists like clonidine, dexmedetomidine, and detomidine are sometimes prescribed. Beta-blockers such as propranolol are also used as event-based medications in special circumstances [7, 8].

Training Tip: There Is No Magic Pill
Behavioral modification is the most important part of every treatment plan. Remember, the purpose of medications is to relieve suffering, improve welfare, and facilitate behavioral modification. There is no medication that will treat and resolve behavioral concerns without the benefit of a behavior modification plan.

Event-based medications can be given to pets who will be experiencing a sudden stressor. Examples include veterinary visits, travel, fireworks or other loud noises, unavoidable separations from dogs with separation distress, and exposure to any fear-provoking stimuli. These medications begin working right away, and do not require administration for days or weeks to see a result. For veterinary phobias, administration the night before the appointment and again 30 minutes to 2 hours prior to leaving home (depending upon the medication) has been documented as a preferred protocol for many commonly prescribed anxiolytics.

Like any medicine, behavior medications will sometimes cause an unwanted reaction, or not be effective at the initial prescribed dose. For this reason, any event-based medication should be given as a test dose during a nonstressful period to assess for any unwanted response and see if the medication is likely to be helpful for the patient.

Often, pets with anxiety disorders are treated using both a baseline medication and an event-based medication for breakthrough stress. This is not usually indicated when anxiety is limited to veterinary phobias, but rather for disorders affecting the quality of the animal's home life. For example, a pet with separation anxiety is likely to take fluoxetine every day, but may require an additional event-based medication or combination of medications for periods of unavoidable separation, especially early in the course of treatment.

8.2.3   Nutraceuticals

Nutraceutical supplements can also be helpful for veterinary phobias and other anxieties. There are many commercially available supplements for anxiety reduction. Some of these products have considerable effects with respect to serotonin and other neurotransmitters. Nutraceuticals should always be selected with the veterinarian's guidance. Many nutraceuticals are classified as dietary supplements, but they do affect neurotransmitters and can have synergistic effects with other medications as well as serious side effects. Always question clients carefully about possible over-the-counter product use prior to prescribing any supplements or medications to avoid drug or drug–supplement interactions. The most frequently discussed serious adverse reaction to behavior medications is called *serotonin syndrome* [1]. This syndrome can cause serious and even life-threatening clinical signs, but it is *extremely* rare. Serotonin syndrome is usually a result of high doses of medication, or combinations of two or more serotonin-affecting medications or supplements (remember: medications such as mirtazapine, metoclopramide, dextromethorphan, and tramadol and more are not behavior medications, but certainly affect serotonin) [1, 3]. It is important for veterinarian prescribers and veterinary technicians to understand the mode of action and what to expect when medications are prescribed. Proper client education is a key to appropriate therapy and avoiding serious side effects.

8.2.4   Acepromazine: Don't ACE Fear!

Acepromazine is a tranquilizer, but it does not treat anxiety [1]. Because acepromazine slows the body down but does not calm the mind, it should not be used as a single agent for the treatment of anxious pets. Imagine you're having a root canal. Because you move around too much, the dentist gives you some gas to make you feel a little groggy and then injects Novocain® to numb the tooth. Unfortunately, the injection doesn't work well, and you're in a lot of pain during the root canal. Because you're sleepy from the gas, you can't move and talk to object to the pain; you're too groggy to move much and show how upset you are. To the dentist, you look just fine, but you're becoming more and more fearful. Now, think about the next time you need to visit the dentist, even for a cleaning. You'll probably be afraid. The same thing happens when we give acepromazine to pets. They become groggy and slow in their movements, but their mental suffering is unchanged or, based on some studies, may even be intensified [9].

8.3   Professionals and Their Roles

Every patient benefits when a full team of support is available. This team may include a veterinarian, a **veterinary technician**, a **veterinary technician specialist in behavior** (VTS Behavior), a trainer, a veterinary behaviorist, and/or an applied animal behaviorist. It is important for veterinary team members to understand the unique role that each of these professionals fulfills in caring for fearful and phobic patients.

The veterinarian's role is to diagnose conditions and prescribe treatment. If an animal has a behavioral disorder, such as separation distress, global anxiety, noise phobia, social phobia, and so on, this diagnosis should be made by a veterinarian. The veterinarian may be a general practitioner, a veterinarian who is also an applied animal behaviorist, or a veterinary behaviorist. Veterinary behaviorists are board-certified specialists in behavior. These highly trained professionals have completed a residency, and passed the rigorous examination to become diplomates of the American College of Veterinary Behaviorists. Veterinary behaviorists can provide additional support for any patients the general practitioner would like to refer.

The technician's role is to support the veterinarian and the client. For behavior patients, the technician will take a history, assist with examination, and educate the owner about the diagnosis, any medications prescribed, and direct implementation of the treatment plan. The technician can design treatment plans for patients requiring preventive care, but a veterinarian's orders are needed for patients requiring intervention. Veterinary technician specialists in behavior have completed extensive additional education in behavior, have a minimum of 4000 hours of clinical experience in behavior, and have passed the national board exam to be certified as members of the Academy of Veterinary Behavior Technicians. These highly qualified professionals may support the veterinarian with even the most challenging behavior patients.

A trainer or applied animal behaviorist can assist the owner with behavior modification and training, but should not diagnose behavioral disorders, nor recommend or prescribe specific medications. If a trainer or behaviorist is working with a client's animal and thinks the owner should explore medications, the client should be referred to his veterinarian for this service and discussion.

To assure every patient receives the highest level of care available, veterinary teams should take time to assure on-staff technicians are trained to educate clients about treatment plans, provide prescribed training, and educate clients about medications. Veterinary teams should be familiar with local positive reinforcement trainers, certified applied animal behaviorists, and veterinary behaviorists, so that an entire team can work together when necessary for patients who need collaborative care.

In some cases, the roles of technician, technician specialist, trainer, and applied animal behaviorist may intersect, just as the roles of veterinarian and applied animal behaviorist may intersect. It is important to remember the technician can provide a huge range of services for clients and patients, but must refrain from diagnosing disorders and prescribing medications. Refer to Table 8.1 for a summary of the qualifications for different behavior and training professionals.

Table 8.1 Breakdown of professionals recommended by the authors and their qualifications.

Behavior professional	Credentials	Degree required	Training school	Exam written/practical	CE	Code of ethics
American College of Veterinary Behaviorists	DACVB	DVM with residency	No	Yes/no	Yes	Yes
Certified Applied Animal Behaviorist	CAAB ACAAB	PhD MS	No	Yes/no Yes/no	Yes Yes	Yes
Academy of Veterinary Behavior Technicians	VTS (Behavior)	Credentialed technician	No	Yes/yes	Yes	Yes
Karen Pryor Academy	KPA CTP	None	Yes	Yes/yes	Yes	Yes
Certification Council for Professional Dog Trainers	CPDT-KA	None	No	Yes/no	Yes	Yes
Certification Council for Professional Dog Trainers	CPDT-KSA	None	No	Yes/yes	Yes	Yes

References

1 Overall, K. (2013). *Manual of Clinical Behavioral Medicine for Dogs and Cats*. St. Louis, MO: Mosby.

2 Shaw, K. and Martin, D. (2015). *Canine and Feline Behavior for Veterinary Technicians and Nurses*. Ames, IA: Wiley.

3 Plumb, D.C. (2015). *Plumbs Veterinary Drug Handbook*. Stockholm, WI: PharmaVet.

4 Korpivaara, M., Laapas, K., Huhtinen, M. et al. (2017). Dexmedetomidine oromucosal gel for noise-associated acute anxiety and fear in dogs: a randomised, double-blind, placebo-controlled clinical study. *Veterinary Record* https://doi.org/10.1136/vr.104045.

5 Gruen, M. (2008). Use of trazodone as an adjunctive agent in the treatment of canine anxiety disorders: 56 cases (1995–2007). *Journal of the American Veterinary Medical Association* 233 (12): 1902–1907. https://doi.org/10.2460/javma.233.12.1902.

6 DePorter, T., Landsberg, G.M., and Horwitz, D. (2016). Tools of the trade: psychopharmacology and nutrition. In: *Feline Behavioral Health and Welfare*, 245–267. St. Louis, MO: Elsevier.

7 Ogata, N. (2011). The use of clonidine in the treatment of fear-based behavior problems in dogs: an open trial. *Journal of Veterinary Behavior: Clinical Applications and Research* 6 (2): 130–137. https://doi.org/10.1016/j.jveb.2010.10.004.

8 Overall, K. (1997). Pharmacologic treatments for behavior problems. *Veterinary Clinics of North America: Small Animal Practice* 27 (3): 637–665. https://doi.org/10.1016/S0195-5616(97)50058-1.

9 Endersby, S. (2014). Noise phobias and fireworks. *Veterinary Nursing Journal* 29 (10): 332–334. https://doi.org/10.1111/vnj.12183.

9

Implementation Strategies

9.1 Change Is Never Easy

Change is never easy. The uncertainty of change brings discomfort, fear, and anxiety for us, just like the veterinary setting can bring anxiety for some of our patients. Changing the entire veterinary industry's view of our daily patient interactions will take time, but the change has already begun. I feel privileged to be on the forefront of this change, providing education for veterinary professionals around the world with great pleasure. I have watched as the veterinary community has started to embrace the approach of treating the patient's mind *and* body. The desire to change for the better becomes stronger with each passing year, but perceived obstacles can slow or stall change if we are unprepared for them.

The single most important factor influencing successful change is clinic culture. The veterinarians and support staff must commit to making every patient experience as pleasant as possible, and to helping clients understand how deeply each of us cares for the total well-being of our patients. As the clinic culture begins to change, the team will start to feel the effects: fewer bites and scratches, fewer distressed patient vocalizations, fewer distressed clients, and improved satisfaction with how we interact with patients.

Next, clients will begin to notice. The client may make remarks like "Wow, he did not even growl at you. He always tries to bite at the vet's office," or "I've never seen him so calm at the doctor's office." These happy clients will have happy pets who take up less time and effort for treatments. Happy clients will tell their friends about the great experience their pets have at your hospital, bringing even more clients who are interested in the very best care to your doorstep.

When the team and the clients all expect cooperative, low-stress care and positive experiences in the veterinary clinic, it is easy to provide this care. Unrealistic and outdated expectations are a primary obstacle to change. When the client comes to expect patient-centered low-and no-restraint care, we are obligated to be able to provide it.

9.2 Proposing Change

Achieving change "from the bottom up" can be a challenge. Most of our readers are probably veterinary support staff. As technicians, the authors understand how challenging it can feel to get managers and veterinarians to embrace change. Do not be afraid to be the voice of change in your hospital. Advocate for your patients! Advocate for your patients in a way managers and veterinarians will embrace rather than resist: with a great plan.

Cooperative Veterinary Care, Second Edition. Monique Feyrecilde.
© 2024 John Wiley & Sons, Inc. Published 2024 by John Wiley & Sons, Inc.
Companion website: www.wiley.com/go/feyrecilde/cooperative

9.2.1 Identify Solutions

The first step to change is identifying solutions rather than seeking out problems. A solution-based approach will promote cooperation and teamwork. A problem-based approach will often encourage defensiveness and resistance. No one likes to be told they are doing things wrong. One example of identifying a solution would be a proposal for nonslip surfaces. A problem-based approach would be to say, "Animals are afraid of slipping but our patients are slipping all the time because we have the wrongs surfaces in our exam rooms." A solution-based approach would be "I have an idea to improve patient comfort in exam rooms, and it is simple: provide non-slip surfaces for them. I would like to be in charge of this project." While this may seem like a matter of semantics, *how* we say something is often more important than *what* we say when it comes to gaining support for change.

9.2.2 Start Small

Once you have moved through your practice and looked for the solutions you'd like to suggest, consider the impact each proposed solution would have on the practice, and rank them from lowest impact to greatest. In general, smaller changes are easier to make than larger ones. Trying to make a huge change will often meet with resistance, and then only be maintained for a short time before the clinic reverts back to the old way of doing things. By selecting small changes, it is easier for the team to adapt.

Breaking down change into small steps takes advantage of what we know about learning and shaping. Throughout this book, we have discussed desensitization and shaping. Both of these methods work because they take a larger stimulus or more complex behavior, and break it down into nonthreatening and achievable building blocks. The same technique works with veterinary teams. Break changes into smaller chunks to build larger change over time. For example, if the change we want to make is "Every patient has a pleasant visit every time," that change is too vague and too large to accomplish all at once. Instead, break it down into smaller ideas, such as improving exam room surfaces, providing a variety of treats in every room, or scheduling frightened cats at the quietest time of the day.

In addition to the change feeling feasible, some managers and veterinarians will appreciate less costly changes first before making what feels like a large financial investment in something new. Veterinarians are well-known for being thrifty! When you are ready to propose a solution, make sure you calculate the anticipated cost of the change and present it with your proposal. When possible, projecting the anticipated revenue (if it can be quantified) will also help managers and veterinarians feel more comfortable.

9.2.3 Choose Measurable Changes

When embarking on the project of spearheading change, choose measurable changes at first. "Every patient, every time," is difficult to measure, because it is subjective and broad. At first, choose changes that will be easy to measure, and devise a system for measuring the effects of the change in advance.

If we continue with our example of nonslip surfaces, we can begin to build our proposal. You may go to your supervisor and propose adding nonslip mats to two exam rooms for one month. You have already calculated how many mats will be needed and how much they will cost. How will you measure the effects of this change? One way would be by having the support staff vote. In the proposal,

Table 9.1 Sample proposal worksheet: A worksheet to guide proposals for changes to promote patient-centered veterinary care at the hospital level.

Patient-centered care proposal		
Proposed change		
Incremental changes (if any)		
Date	Proposed start date	Assessment date
Assessment type	Assessment team	
Enhancements to patient care		
Enhancements to hospital, team satisfaction and safety, etc.		
Financial benefits	Financial costs	
Anticipated challenges	Marketing tools (if any)	

designate a time period, such as two weeks or one month, for the testing period for this change. In addition, designate a method to measure the change. In our example, we would suggest trying the mats for two weeks, and proposing a voting date where each member of the team is allowed to vote yes or no for keeping the change, and offer feedback if they would like to do so.

By making a formal and carefully thought-out proposal to leadership, you show you are serious about advocating for change. Your effort to include the entire team in the decision-making process will improve confidence and support, and will contribute to a positive change in clinic culture. Being organized, thoughtful, and inclusive are all good ways to gain support from management and make effective change over time. Table 9.1 is a worksheet for planning a proposal for change in your own practice.

9.3 Overcoming Obstacles: Common Concerns and Questions

When I speak with members of the veterinary community, the same questions and perceived obstacles present themselves repeatedly. Be prepared to answer these questions for yourself and your team when you propose changes within your hospital. Recognizing these obstacles in advance will better prepare you and your practice for the changes ahead.

9.3.1 Perception: It's Too Costly

The costs of not providing patient-centered care will far outstrip the costs of doing so. Fees for equipment, treats, and team training are a small price to pay for increased client base, increased client satisfaction, improved safety, and improved job satisfaction.

To start, there is the cost of lost clients. How many clients do not return to the clinic after a negative experience? According to the Bayer/AAFP study, 58 percent of cat owners are reluctant to visit the veterinary office due to patient stress [1]. So reluctant in fact that almost 40% of them feel avoidance and stressful feelings about even calling the veterinary hospital on the telephone. Losing clients due to perceived patient stress is a reality. Changing client perceptions of stress will encourage those clients to return to the hospital.

Providing compassionate and cooperative care requires fewer team members for a procedure. The ear cleaning and treatment that may have required three or four team members now requires only one or two. Working within the patient's comfort means low or no restraint. Manpower requirements are reduced by at least *half*. Reducing the number of team members required per procedure saves time and money.

Paying close attention to animal communication and working to keep animals comfortable and cooperative will reduce team injuries. Defensive aggression toward team members is a primary cause of injuries within the clinic. Injuries are costly for the hospital due to medical costs, labor and industry claims, and lost revenue due to employee absences.

Client loyalty and satisfaction are also increased when we work with the owner present. Clients understand more clearly the treatments provided, adding to their perceived value of services. When clients better understand and appreciate the treatments provided, we answer fewer financial concerns and complaints, saving the team time, money, and frustration.

While there is always some monetary investment with change, the money saved and improvement to the practice will make this one worthwhile investment.

9.3.2 Perception: It Takes Too Long

Using compassionate, cooperative, and low-stress methods really does not take more time. In the cost example, we discussed how fewer team members are required per pet when the pet is cooperative and calm. Returning to the example of a large dog with otitis, say three people are involved in restraint and one person is treating the ears, with the procedure taking 15 minutes. Multiplying four people × 15 minutes each = 60 minutes of team time. Consider also the time invested to figure out that four people would be required. Starting and stopping the procedure, relocating the patient to the treatment room, and pulling other team members away from other patients all cost time. If only two team members are involved, even if the procedure requires 20 minutes to allow for training, two people × 20 minutes each = 40 total minutes invested. Table 9.2 shows an example of the possible time investment and financial cost comparison associated with manual restraint and chemical restraint for a large dog's ear flush.

Using these methods also improves patient cooperation over time, decreasing the number of team members and time required for future visits. Investing some time and patience during our early relationship with patients sets us up for a future of efficient care, because animals are willing participants rather than defending themselves against us.

Video 9.1 gives an example of time comparison between the use of force and the use of cooperative methods for weighing a large dog. The first clip shows a team member lifting the large dog onto the scale. The second clip shows the second team member using her body in the correct position and a treat trail to lure the dog onto the scale in less than half the time.

Video 9.2 shows a completed trained scale behavior in an 18-week-old puppy. This puppy happily rushes in the door of the veterinary hospital to be weighed. Her training program incorporated classical conditioning and operant conditioning. Notice her positive emotional response in addition

Table 9.2 Risks, benefits, and associated costs with sedation for otitis treatment.

Procedure	Staff time required	Risks	Financial profile
Otitis treatment: conscious, active patient	20 minutes × 3 team members = 60 total minutes	Patient injury Team member injury iatrogenic behavioral injury Incomplete treatment Client perceives patient stress Decreased client trust	Team time cost = $40 Fee to client = $100 Profit = $60
Otitis treatment: sedated patient	15 minutes × 1.5 team members = 22.5 total minutes	Adverse drug reaction (rare)	Team time cost = $15 Cost of medication = $1–15 Fees to client: Sedation = $75–150 Ear flush = $75 Profit = $120–200

This table uses an assumed hourly wage of $25 plus benefits for cost calculations.

to her cooperative skill of moving onto the scale mat and lying down. Imagine a world where each of your canine patients makes weighing this easy!

Video 9.3 uses the example of removing a fearful cat from the carrier for an examination. In the first clip, the technician tries to remove the cat through the door. First she coaxes, then she reaches, then she tries to dump the cat out through the door. Eventually she gives up, and the cat is still in the carrier. The second clip shows the same technician, same cat, and same carrier. In this version, she disassembles the carrier around the cat. This version requires less than half the time, and results in the technician being able to work with the cat.

9.3.3 Perception: But This Is How We've Always Done It

Veterinary professionals love animals. Our mission is to relieve animal suffering and improve animal well-being. Agreeing to change how we practice forces us to admit we have room for improvement. The emotions associated with this change, especially for established practitioners, can be complex. We may feel guilt for things we have done in the past. The screaming cats we have stretched, the struggling dogs we have forced into lateral recumbency while two people lay on them for grooming, the defensively aggressive dogs we have caught on a rabies pole or squeezed in a cage door while they urinated and defecated in terror, the cats we caught in an induction chamber and watched struggle and crash against the sides while they are induced – we each did those things because we had been taught it was for the best. We were told receiving veterinary care was in the animal's best interest in that time, no matter what was required to accomplish the goal. We may even have felt pride in being able to handle the most dangerous patients without being injured. It takes time to process these feelings of guilt and fear of change, and to embrace the idea of treating patients with a different mindset and aiming for a different result.

Criticism of people and their techniques will only worsen the guilt and fear into defensiveness and resistance. Successful change is built on recognizing strengths and positive actions, and building them up. Look for positive remarks to make. Some examples of positive remarks might include:

"I noticed you recorded in the chart Oscar did well standing while eating peanut butter for his blood draw. Thank you so much; we read it before we drew his blood today, and it made his visit go much more smoothly."

"Fluffy was showing really anxious body language when I walked by. It was great how you stopped trying to get the blood sample and Dr. Smith prescribed anxiety relievers."

"You have such a nice way of calming cats. Can you help me by feeding Precious while I try to give her vaccinations?"

If you know a certain team member is nervous around defensive dogs, or anxious around frightened cats, discuss these fears in a positive way. Acknowledge your appreciation for how sensitive the team member is to the patient's signals and body language, and reassure them they will not be required to participate in that patient's care until they feel relaxed and ready. Forcing team members to interact with patients they fear can predispose the team member to mistakes, and worsen anxiety for both pets and people over time.

Some team members may express concern about giving so many treats and so much food during visits. They may worry about gastrointestinal (GI) upset or nutritional imbalances. There are a variety of ways to approach this concern. First, your hospital can implement follow-up calls. Simply call and check on the patient the following day, and see if any GI upset or other side effects were noted. Lastly, you can cite the experience of experts. The authors have both conducted next-day calls to check for any trouble related to treats in patients, and have found rare instances of GI upset. Subjectively, these occurrences seem less frequent than stress-induced colitis or motion sickness was in the past.

9.3.4 Perception: I'm Not Sure What to Do

It is difficult to embrace change when we feel uncertain, and anything new always comes with some uncertainty. Providing standard operating procedures and a written standard of care, including a behavioral standard, will help clear up expectations. New team members should be provided with good training sessions, such as shadowing an experienced team member, and with excellent reference materials (such as this text!). Continuing education can be provided in-clinic, or by visiting conferences and symposia to help keep the team motivated and all on the same page.

Knowledge is power, and developing a united set of protocols for when to progress, when to stop, why to stop, and how to talk with clients will help decrease uncertainty and increase confidence and progress.

Lastly, you do not always have to know exactly what to do. You just need to know what is normal, what is abnormal, what is within your scope to treat, and where to refer cases when necessary. The team should be familiar with the nearest veterinary behaviorist who is a Diplomate of the American College of Veterinary Behaviorists. Furthermore, the team should be familiar with local applied animal behaviorists and local trainers.

If you do not have a trainer in-clinic for classes and skills, it is important to know how to choose a trainer for referrals. Trainers should embrace low-stress and positive reinforcement methods. They should be familiar with the principles of desensitization, classical counterconditioning, operant conditioning, and basic problem solving for pets. The trainer should have an open-door policy for observers, always welcoming clinic staff to come and watch, or potential clients to watch a class before signing up. The American Veterinary Society of Animal Behavior (AVSAB) has an excellent free handout for download with tips on how to evaluate and choose trainers.

9.3.5 Perception: We Might Make Clients Angry

Veterinary medicine is a customer service industry. We have long been taught that the veterinarian knows best when it comes to diagnostics, surgery, and prescriptions, but in all other ways the client is always right. Furthermore, there is a long-standing dogma in the profession that we should be able to "do anything" to animals, because we "have a way with them." We must keep our eye on the most important aspect of the care we provide: being the best possible advocate for the animal.

Increasing client understanding about emotional welfare for patients takes a multi-faceted approach. Expectation management is really helpful. Some suggestions for increasing client visibility of your hospital's desire to provide safer and happier veterinary care:

- Send a pre-visit questionnaire by email before appointments to ask how clients perceive their pet's care experience. Automate this into reminders so it does not require extra staff work. The questionnaire can ask if the pet shows signs of motion sickness, pain, fear of specific kinds of handling or experiences, and what their favorite rewards are. An example is available for viewing on the Fear Free Happy Homes website. This gets clients thinking about alleviating fear at the veterinary hospital before they ever leave home.
- Build an emotional reporting system into your medical record. Using the Fear Free FAS Score or another system of your choosing, note the animal's experience through the visit and any success strategies. Assure the client receives a copy of their record via email or patient portal access after each visit.
- Post passive education in exam rooms such as posters or videos highlighting the aspects of body language associated with stress and your team's commitment to provide the least stressful visit possible.
- Share videos and photos on your social media of pets having low stress visits.
- Include information about what to expect during the visit in your appointment confirmation. "We are committed to providing a low stress visit for Fido. Please bring his favorite treats to your appointment. If we notice Fido's stress level increasing, we may pause his appointment to make a lower-stress handling plan."

Communication is everything when we are talking with clients about quality of care. The client may arrive with a goal-oriented mindset with a dog we have not seen in two years. The client would like to have an exam, vaccinations, a heartworm test, fecal sample, vaccinations, a nail trim, and anal gland expression, and have the infected ears diagnosed and treated. A visit like this is unlikely to be completed all in one try, even for the most comfortable and patient dog.

The technician is the first line of communication in setting a good client expectation for this visit. Use a script such as "Dr. Jones is going to start with Fido's checkup. Based on what she sees, she will explain to you which treatments she thinks we should perform today when we start treatment for his ears, and which treatments would be better to do when we see him for his ear follow-up in 10 days." This script begins to introduce the client to the ideas of: wants versus needs, prioritizing care based on the animal's medical needs, and dividing care into more manageable segments.

During the examination, the veterinarian can continue this important message. "Mrs. Smith, I am so glad you brought Fido to see me. His ears are quite painful, and you are right, they are infected. Because his ears are painful, I'd like your permission to give him a pain reliever that will also make him feel sleepy. We can clean and medicate his ears, and collect his heartworm test and perform his grooming if he is staying nice and relaxed. When you return in 10–14 days, I'd like to give Fido's vaccinations after the infection has healed."

Additionally, the whole team can have a good script for if we need to stop. Be honest with clients. Express your empathy for the patient, pointing out signs of stress and fear to the client. Explain your desire to provide the very best care, which includes awareness of emotional harm we could be causing. Describe the importance of maintaining a good trusting relationship between the patient and the medical care team, so you can continue to provide a whole lifetime of excellent care for your patient. Showing clients that we care about patients, and we want to care about them for an entire lifetime, demonstrates how much we value both physical and emotional wellness in the hospital.

Finally, the team needs to be prepared to provide relief from stress and fear in the clinic, using short-term aids such as anxiolytic medications and long-term aids like training visits and happy visits, to achieve the goal of long-term stress-free patient care.

9.3.6 Perception: It's Hard to Know When to Hit Pause

Knowing when to hit the "Pause Button" during an appointment or a treatment relies on every team member understanding the hospital's behavioral standard of care, and feeling empowered to prevent iatrogenic behavioral injuries (IBIs). Every veterinarian and every team member needs to be on the same page, and provide a united message with good continuity for clients. If one technician forcibly restrains a vocalizing puppy for vaccination, but the next technician refuses, both the client and the patient will trust us less. The client may say things like "He was fine last time," or "Just hold him down and do it quickly." These remarks are signs of a lack of continuity of message within the team rather than signs of a problem with low-stress techniques.

If this situation happens, always have a supportive message about your teammates. It can be easy to criticize a teammate without thinking about it. Even saying something as simple as "Jennifer is still learning" or "Maybe I can figure out a different way to do this" can damage the client's confidence in the team and sound judgmental. Focus on the animal in front of you, and remark only on what you can observe today as well as the proposed plan for today's visit.

Using the resources provided, propose adopting a behavioral standard of care for your clinic, focused on improving the patient experience, increasing team safety, and preventing IBIs. Figure 5.1 suggested a scoring system for the emotional state of pets, based on the types of training we have introduced. This scoring system dovetails with the detailed flowchart provided by Dr. Colleen Koch we introduced in Chapter 4 (Figure 4.2). Use these to guide your decisions when filling in Table 9.3, a guide to making your own standard of care.

Table 9.3 Developing a behavioral standard of care.

Designing a behavioral standard of care
(1) Review the hospital's mission statement; assure emotional wellness is included.
(2) Select an assessment tool for measuring patient stress.
(3) Determine "pausing scores" within your assessment tool (e.g. "Moderate" = pause).
(4) Define exactly who can stop a procedure (everyone who handles patients).
(5) Educate the team about the behavioral standard of care.
(6) Educate clients about the behavioral standard of care.
(7) Designate a person(s) to monitor patient care, and assure it meets the standard of care.

Use these steps to begin your hospital's journey toward adopting a behavioral standard of care for every patient, every visit.

9.3.7   Perception: I Am Afraid …

Of being injured while working with an unrestrained animal.

Of being called a follower or part of a new "fad."

Of clients thinking I am afraid of patients.

Clients will not understand.

Fear inhibits behavior in pets and people alike. Fear of working with animals comes largely from being expected to get everything done during a single visit all the time, and without sedation or medications of any kind. Restraint beyond light stabilization is only necessary when animals are fearful and trying to escape or defend themselves. By carefully observing our patients, and training them, medicating them, and choosing not to push them over their threshold, we can remain safe while working using light stabilization or trained behaviors for patients. When consulting with clinics, the majority of bites and scratches I have heard about and observed have occurred during failed attempts to restrain a patient who was showing defensive aggression.

Some clients may be judgmental if you change your style of care. The client may say that you are just trying to take part in a new fad, or you are afraid of their patient and cannot handle him. In the 1890s, Ivan Pavlov began characterizing classical conditioning. *The Behavior of Organisms* by B.F. Skinner was released in 1938. Learning theory is nothing new. Taking the time to learn it is a new widespread feature of veterinary medicine.

Our commitment to keep animal stress levels low and minimize defensive aggression may read as fear or reluctance to owners because they are accustomed to a different kind of care. Reiterate to yourself and to the client the purpose of stopping and making a new plan: to provide the very best care while causing the least possible amount of stress, improving patient wellness, and preserving the trusting relationship between veterinary professionals and patients.

Use direct education and passive education to teach owners what to expect at the veterinary hospital. Hang posters of relaxed and fearful animal body language cues. Provide handouts describing the special approach and services you provide. Create Purr Packs and Wag Bags that include: pheromone wipes, a nutraceutical stress reliever, a dose of anxiolytic medication, and instructions for easy administration and a stress-free ride to the clinic. Post displays with flyers advertising your Purr Packs and Wag Bags in each exam room to start the discussion about comfortable care. If you need to reschedule a visit, communicate in advance with the client about any financial changes associated with additional visits so there are no surprises.

9.4   Making Change for the Right Reasons

Clients and team members will embrace the change to cooperative and low-stress care, and making prevention of IBIs a priority, when we approach it from a position of empathy and positivity. Every client who brings a patient to the hospital loves that pet enough to go to the trouble of coming in. If the animal is acting fearful or defensive, the owner may be anxious, embarrassed, or angry. Education is the key.

Demonstrate and teach empathy for these animals and their owners. Avoid labels like "bad," "mean," "tough," "spoiled," or "dominant." Simply describe what you see: an animal who stops taking treats, moves away, looks away, or becomes tense as a form of communication (Table 9.4). Translate for the animal, and communicate the meaning of these subtle signals to the owner. You're an expert! Show the owner each sign and signal, and explain that the patient is simply worried about what will happen next.

Table 9.4 Flipping the script.

Label	Example replacement
Bad	None (not an appropriate term for pets)
Dominant	None (not an appropriate term for pets)
Mean	Fearful, anxious, stressed
Fractious, aggressive	Fearful, anxious, stressed
Stupid	None (not an appropriate term)
Spoiled	Fearful, anxious, stressed
Stubborn	None (not an appropriate term for pets)

Avoid the use of labels for animals in the veterinary hospital. Instead, describe emotions or behaviors. Some terms have no replacement, because they are inappropriate for pets and especially for the veterinary setting.

Reassure the owner that you and your team are perfectly equipped with the tools and knowledge needed to help this patient, and you'll guide them through every step of the process together, even if it means more than one visit.

9.4.1 Family Presence for Veterinary Care

Family presence has been studied extensively in human medicine in recent years, and the amount of research in this area appears to be growing. Historically, family presence in hospitals has been discouraged. Very limited visiting hours even for family, disallowing family members to be present during emergency treatment, and especially excluding family during end-of-life or life-threatening emergencies and codes.

The reasons for this have been myriad, but the most common threads were worry that the family member would be unable to "handle" seeing the procedure, and worry that they would interfere/get in the way and decrease the quality of medical care provided. Here are some findings from research on the human side:

- 94% of parents would choose to repeat the experience of attending their child's invasive procedure [2].
- Parental anxiety was statistically significantly reduced related to the procedure, but not to the diagnosis/prognosis [2].
- While 93% of professionals questioned *before* the procedure thought family presence would be a hindrance, *after* the procedure 94 percent of nurses felt the parental presence was helpful to the child [2].
- Residents are less likely to feel positive about family presence compared to attending and more experienced professionals [3].
- There is a low prevalence of negative outcomes or effects of family presence in trauma and ER [4].
- When a structured program is present, providers initially opposed to family presence show a striking reversal of opinion after observing the effects of family presence during procedures and treatment [5].
- Family presence does not negatively affect the time efficiency of the pediatric trauma resuscitation nor time from admission to CT result [6].

Veterinary clinics may have policies in place to protect client safety by instituting hands-off or staff-only-contact edits. Even in staff-only-contact clinics, family presence can be valuable. Concerns about client safety in the presence of animals who are receiving treatment can be reduced by having clients stand within view but out of reach while a veterinary team member stabilizes the pet. It can be safe to have clients give treats during a variety of treatments, at the discretion and instruction of the veterinary team.

Regardless of a hospital's individual policy, setting clear boundaries and expectations in an honest and caring way is the key for success. Statements such as, "I know you and Milo have a special bond. I would like to keep you together while we are working with him. To do that safely, I need you to please follow these instructions…" are acceptable and appropriate.

9.4.1.1 Calming the Patient

- Modulate client behavior by giving good, detailed instructions about what TO DO.
- Keep clients SAFE. Make sure clients are not going to receive bites or scratches when they are present.
- Allow the pet to see and hear the client, but touching may or may not be appropriate.
- If using treats (do it!), make sure to figure out a safe administration method and give the client clear instructions about what is expected.
- Check with the client to assure they are comfortable with needles, blood, and medical procedures before proceeding. Some clients will need to step out of the room for their own welfare and this is best determined in advance.

Family presence is calming for many pets. Hearing the owner's voice, seeing the owner, receiving treats and attention from the owner, and being able to seek comfort will all help patients relax in many situations. In human medicine, healing times are hastened, overall hospital stays are decreased in length, and patient perception of time spent in the hospital is more favorable if the family is encouraged to be present.

If the pet is separated from the client and becomes noticeably more fearful, reuniting the pet with the client and making a new plan about client presence and probably the use of medicines to reduce anxiety is often a helpful strategy. Some patients may benefit from tailored admission and discharge protocols for inpatient procedures, where the client stays with the patient during initial sedation and is present during recovery once the pet is sternal. For practitioners worried about the impact of emergence delirium on the client – we should be even more worried about its impact on the pet! Prevention of stress and appropriate well-rounded anesthesia protocols should reduce emergence delirium to almost zero, and rapid administration of medications to relieve emergence delirium can be done when proper IV access is present and the nursing team is directly supervising the patient's recovery.

In rare instances, a veterinary team member may feel that the animal is being made more anxious by a client using a high-pitched voice, rapid stroking, or strong restraint. Many clients are anxious coming to the veterinary clinic, and they need to be able to trust the veterinary team. The veterinary team can and should direct the client how to remain safe but also be most helpful.

9.4.1.2 Example Scripts

"Mrs. Smith, I have a handful of tiny treats here for you. I would like you to drop one into this dish for Fluffy to eat every two seconds. Before you drop each treat, tell Fluffy you'll be dropping it by saying her name and then 'treat'."

"Mr. Jones, I've prepared this long-handled spoon with cheese for Fido to lick while I draw his blood. Please stand to my left and hold the cheese where he can reach it, but please touch only the spoon and not Fido until I let you know we have collected this sample."

"Ms. Johnson, I'd like your help while I trim Missy's nails. When I say 'treat', please give her two licks from this special mat I've prepared with delicious treats."

"Mr. Adams, Dr. Jackson needs to feel Sammy's knee. This might hurt, so I would like you to stand here on my right where Sammy can see you and speak softly to him, but please do not reach out to touch him until we are done."

9.5 Conclusion

My hope is this book has empowered you to look at your patients in a new light, and commit to giving every patient the best possible veterinary experience every time they visit the hospital. By improving awareness of patient sensation, perception, and communication; creating a behavioral standard of care; understanding learning theory; and learning about the training options and methods available, you are already off to an amazing start. I hope you are excited to work with patients who are less stressed, more relaxed, and willing to participate in their own care. I hope you are inspired to consider the more advanced training methods of operant conditioning and fully voluntary patient care for the future. And, lastly, I hope I have reignited your love of animals and reminded you of our true mission as veterinary professionals: to improve *all* aspects of the lives of animals.

References

1 Volk, J., Felsted, K.E., Thomas, J.G. et al. (2011). Executive summary of the Bayer veterinary care usage study. *Journal of the American Veterinary Medical Association* 238 (10): 1275–1282. https://doi.org/10.2460/javma.238.10.1275.

2 Powers, K.S. and Rubenstein, J.S. (1999). Family presence during invasive procedures in the pediatric intensive care unit: a prospective study. *Archives of Pediatrics and Adolescent Medicine* 153 (9): 55–958. http://dx.doi.org/10.1001/archpedi.153.9.955.

3 Fein, J., Ganesh, J., and Alpern, E.R. (2006). Medical staff attitudes toward family presence during pediatric procedures. *Pediatric Emergency Care* 20 (4): 224–227. https://doi.org/10.1097/01.pec.0000121241.99242.3b.

4 O'Connell, K.J., Farah, M., Spandorfer, P., and Zorc, J. (2007). Family presence during pediatric trauma team activation: an assessment of a structured program. *Pediatrics* 120 (3): e565–e574. http://dx.doi.org/10.1542/peds.2006-2914.

5 McGahey, P. (2002). Family presence during pediatric resuscitation: a focus on staff. *Critical Care Nurse* 22 (6): 29–34.

6 Dudley, N., Hansen, K.W., Furnival, R.A. et al. (2009). The effect of family presence on the efficiency of pediatric trauma resuscitations. *Annals of Emergency Medicine* 53 (6): 777–784. https://doi.org/10.1016/j.annemergmed.2008.10.002.

Index